Handbook of Aviation
and Space Medicine

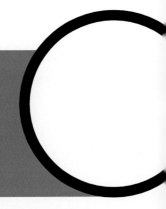

Handbook of Aviation
and Space Medicine

Edited by

Nicholas Green, Whittingham Professor of Aviation Medicine, RAF Centre of Aviation Medicine, RAF Henlow, Bedfordshire, United Kingdom

Steven Gaydos, US Army Senior Aviator and Master Flight Surgeon board certified in Aerospace, Occupational and Emergency Medicine, Director of Graduate Medical Education, US Army School of Aviation Medicine, Fort Rucker, Alabama

Ewan Hutchison, Consultant in Aviation and Occupational Medicine and Head of Medical Assessment, Civil Aviation Authority, Gatwick Airport, West Sussex, United Kingdom

Edward Nicol, Consultant Cardiologist, Chair of the NATO Aviation Cardiology Working Group and the RAF Consultant Advisor in Medicine, Aviation Medicine Clinical Service, RAF Centre of Aviation Medicine, RAF Henlow, Bedfordshire, United Kingdom

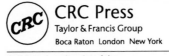

CRC Press
Taylor & Francis Group
Boca Raton London New York

CRC Press is an imprint of the
Taylor & Francis Group, an **informa** business

CRC Press
Taylor & Francis Group
6000 Broken Sound Parkway NW, Suite 300
Boca Raton, FL 33487-2742

© 2019 by Taylor & Francis Group, LLC
CRC Press is an imprint of Taylor & Francis Group, an Informa business

Contributions from Squadron Leader Matthew Adam, Wing Commander Sentiru Baladurai, Flight Lieutenant Joseph Britton, Lieutenant Colonel Alaistair Bushby, Wing Commander Agustin Cabre, Colonel Ian Curry, Victoria Cutler, Wing Commander Joanna d'Arcy, Wing Commander Gary Davies, Lieutenant Colonel Claire Goldie, Wing Commander Nicholas Green, Group Captain Gwynne Harper, Dr Michael Harrigan, Wing Commander Peter Hodkinson, Squadron Leader Jonathan Hynes, Major Damian Jenkins, Group Captain Jon Kendrew, Wing Commander Ian Mollan, Wing Commanded Edward Nicol, Wing Commander Ivor T. Owen, Squadron Leader Bonnie Posselt, Wing Commander Joanne Rimmer, Group Captain Andrew Timperley, Surgeon Commander Malcolm Woodcock © Crown Copyright 2019

No claim to original U.S. Government works. This applies to contributions from Captain Nathan Almond, L. Renee Boyd, Colonel (Ret) William P. Butler, Dr J. Lynn Caldwell, Colonel Kristen Casto, Steven Chervak, Dr James Clifford, Colonel Steven Gaydos, Major John Houk, Colonel (Ret) Russ S. Kotwal, Captain Joseph T. LaVan, Dr Ben Lawson, Colonel Mark McPherson, Major (Dr) Joseph J. Pavelites, Colonel Richard A. Scheuring, Captain Alfred F. Shwayhat, Dr Anthony Tvaryanas

Printed on acid-free paper

International Standard Book Number-13: 978-1-138-61786-5 (Paperback)
International Standard Book Number-13: 978-1-138-61787-2 (Hardback)

This book contains information obtained from authentic and highly regarded sources. While all reasonable efforts have been made to publish reliable data and information, neither the author[s] nor the publisher can accept any legal responsibility or liability for any errors or omissions that may be made. The publishers wish to make clear that any views or opinions expressed in this book by individual editors, authors or contributors are personal to them and do not necessarily reflect the views/opinions of the publishers. The information or guidance contained in this book is intended for use by medical, scientific or health-care professionals and is provided strictly as a supplement to the medical or other professional's own judgement, their knowledge of the patient's medical history, relevant manufacturer's instructions and the appropriate best practice guidelines. Because of the rapid advances in medical science, any information or advice on dosages, procedures or diagnoses should be independently verified. The reader is strongly urged to consult the relevant national drug formulary and the drug companies' and device or material manufacturers' printed instructions, and their websites, before administering or utilizing any of the drugs, devices or materials mentioned in this book. This book does not indicate whether a particular treatment is appropriate or suitable for a particular individual. Ultimately it is the sole responsibility of the medical professional to make his or her own professional judgements so as to advise and treat patients appropriately. The authors and publishers have also attempted to trace the copyright holders of all material reproduced in this publication and apologize to copyright holders if permission to publish in this form has not been obtained. If any copyright material has not been acknowledged, please write and let us know so we may rectify this in any future reprint.

The views, opinions, or positions expressed by Ministry of Defence (MoD) or Department of Defense (DoD) employees represent those of the individual contributors and are not to be considered necessarily representative of position, policy, or decision of the MoD or DoD or their respective components.

Visit the Taylor & Francis Web site at
http://www.taylorandfrancis.com

and the CRC Press Web site at
http://www.crcpress.com

Contents

Foreword

Human flight and medicine have been linked for centuries. When man first ascended into the skies, one of the pioneer balloonists was an apothecary. As such flights became ever more daring, it was apparent that exposure to the environment at altitude could have significant, even fatal, consequences. However, scientific study made strides to understand the physiological challenges flight posed and tried to develop means of reducing that risk.

During World War I, the need for aeromedical specialists to select and advise aircrew became clear. Throughout World War II, as aircraft and their life support systems became more capable but more complex, greater medical and scientific knowledge were essential to enhance flight safety and operational capability. After the war, the continued need to give medical officers comprehensive aeromedical knowledge led to the creation of bespoke courses at the former Royal Air Force Institute of Aviation Medicine at Farnborough in the UK. That such training was equally necessary for civilian doctors in airlines and aviation regulators resulted in their early inclusion after the Diploma in Aviation Medicine was established more than 50 years ago.

Although there had been at least one large tome of aviation physiology produced previously, it was in 1978 that a comprehensive UK textbook of aviation medicine was first published. Initially in two volumes, this covered the full range of the topic, including clinical medicine and aviation psychology. Over time, the textbook has become so much more than a book for a specific course, forming an essential reference used by practitioners in their clinics, surgeries or laboratories. Now named "Ernsting's", after Air Vice-Marshal John Ernsting, who had been so active in the field throughout his long career and was known to generations of military and civilian doctors working in aviation medicine, the book can now be found in aeromedical units across the world and in the offices of engineers engaged in the design and development of aircraft life support and escape systems. The Institute's original course book, currently in its fifth edition, has become the specialty's default reference, and a new generation of trainees in aviation and space medicine have come to the text to be taught the art and science of the discipline, reflecting the spread of the specialty into commercial passenger health, space medicine and even uninhabited air vehicles.

"Ernsting's" is a textbook that is written to address the requirements of a large and varied audience, with differing needs and expectations. However, for one group in particular, that of the postgraduate student studying frantically for an essential profession examination, what is also required is a pithy, concise primer that delivers sufficient information to refresh the memory and distil the core of a subject into easily digestible bites. That is exactly what this new handbook does. Written by authors who have a direct association with the application of aerospace medicine across its many aspects and the requirements for success in its postgraduate examinations, their insight into the essentials is unquestionable. Using a consistent bullet-point format, this handbook will be of huge value to all those facing board certification or specialist qualifications in aerospace medicine, or simply seeking a convenient précis of the issue in question. Largely echoing the topic structure of "Ernsting's", readers will easily access the subjects of interest, finding very concise, listed text augmented by familiar diagrams and figures. The editors are well-established leaders in their fields and, moreover, they have managed to develop an admirably consistent style throughout the book. The many contributors are drawn from across the world of aviation and space medicine, on both sides of the Atlantic, and from the military and civilian spheres. There is an interesting range of familiar names in the contributor list, augmented by those emerging as the next generation of enthusiasts for the specialty.

I am sure this book will be an invaluable aid to all those studying aerospace/aviation and space medicine as they prepare to demonstrate they have acquired the broad and detailed knowledge of the science and medicine required for its practice in the varied and challenging environment of flight.

David Gradwell BSc PhD MBChB FRCP FRCP(Edin)
FFOM(Hon) DAvMed FRAeS
Professor of Aerospace Medicine, King's College London
President, Association of Aviation Medical Examiners
Past President, Aerospace Medical Association

Foreword

When the editors first asked me to write a foreword for this important new book, I was honored, but I asked if this effort was in competition with the trusted textbooks on aviation and space medicine that line my shelves, especially the cornerstone textbook, *Ernsting's Aviation Medicine*. I have the greatest respect for that tome, its editors and contributors, and the book's namesake, John Ernsting (JE). I was very fortunate to have known JE and am the proud owner of a well-used second edition which he graciously signed for me many years ago, hence my question. The editors assured me this *Handbook of Aviation and Space Medicine* was in fact complementary, similar in structure to *Ernsting's Aviation Medicine* (now in its fifth edition), so the two can be used in parallel, with the Ernsting text as the definitive reference.

So with this understanding, I heartily agreed to write this foreword. But why me? Well, for one, I am board certified in aerospace medicine, now for almost 30 years. I have served as a flight surgeon and a mission-ready fast jet pilot, having flown the F-4 Phantom before medical school, and then the F-15 Eagle, F-16 Falcon, and the RAF Hawk as a dual-rated pilot and flight surgeon. My time in the Hawk was as the US Air Force Exchange Officer assigned to the RAF Institute of Aviation Medicine at Farnborough in the late 1990s, performing the duty of Senior Medical Officer/Pilot. During this time, I was fortunate to work alongside some of the editors of and contributors to this book. And that long-time professional collaboration and friendship has persisted throughout the years, up to and including my appointment as the USAF Surgeon General, my last US Air Force duty before retirement.

In the editors' own words, this *Handbook of Aviation and Space Medicine* is intended to be a soft-cover quick reference and revision guide. Having now reviewed the book, I completely agree this is a different type of reference, in an easy-to-scan format, that gives the reader the essential facts related to topics ranging from atmospheric science, to the basics of fixed wing, rotary wing, and space flight, as well as up-to-date topics such as remotely piloted aircraft. Additionally, this book is truly international, with about a third of the contributors and one of the editors being from the US aerospace medicine professional community.

I think this handbook will serve as a ready reference for the busy practitioner in the increasingly complex duties of our aviation and space medicine roles. And with the rapid evolution of technology and the challenges that humans will face in these systems, this format will lend itself to being more readily updated. I particularly appreciate the readable format, which makes it easy to glean the most salient points in describing the aviation and space environment, countermeasures to environmental and occupational stressors, and the clinical conditions aerospace medicine practitioners will be faced with for disposition decisions. I wish I had possessed this reference when I was actively involved in the practice of aerospace medicine, and I congratulate the editors and contributors on providing such a useful new reference.

Thomas W. Travis MD MPH
Lieutenant General, USAF, Retired

List of Contributors

Squadron Leader Matthew Adam
Registrar in Infectious Diseases and General Internal Medicine
Royal Free Hospital
NHS Foundation Trust
London, UK

Captain Nathan Almond
Program Director of the Navy Residency in Aerospace Medicine
Naval Aerospace Medical Institute
Pensacola, Florida

Wing Commander Sentiru Baladurai
Consultant Nephrologist
Aviation Medicine Consultation Service
RAF Henlow

David Bigmore
Principal Engineer
QinetiQ
Farnborough, Hampshire, UK

L. Renee Boyd
Emergency Medicine Physician
University Hospital in Cleveland
Cleveland, Ohio

Flight Lieutenant Joseph Britton
Aviation and Space Medicine Registrar
RAF Centre of Aviation Medicine
RAF Henlow
Bedfordshire, UK

Lieutenant Colonel Alaistair Bushby
Consultant in Army Aviation Medicine
HQ Army Air Corps
Middle Wallop, Hampshire, UK

Colonel (Ret) William P. Butler
Retired Professor of Aerospace Medicine
USAF School of Aerospace Medicine
Wright-Patterson Air Force Base
Dayton, Ohio

Wing Commander Agustin Cabre
Officer Commanding Aviation Medicine Unit
Royal New Zealand Air Force
Bedfordshire, UK

Dr J. Lynn Caldwell
Senior Research Psychologist
Naval Medical Research Unit Dayton
Wright-Patterson Air Force Base
Dayton, Ohio

John A. Caldwell
Senior Experimental Psychologist
Coastal Performance Consulting, LLC
Yellow Springs, Ohio

Colonel Kristen Casto
Director of the Public Health Directorate
US Army Surgeon General's Office
Falls Church, Virginia

Dr Rae-Wen Chang
Consultant in Aviation and Occupational Medicine
Chief Medical Officer
NATS, Swanwick Centre
Hampshire, UK

Steven Chervak
Human Factors Engineer
US Army Public Health Center
Aberdeen Proving Ground
Aberdeen, Maryland

Professor Anthony Cleare
Professor of Psychopharmacology and Affective Disorders
Institute of Psychiatry, Psychology and Neuroscience
King's College London
London, UK

Dr James Clifford
Head of Endocrinology
Naval Medical Center
San Diego, California

Dr Des Connolly (Wing Commander Retired)
Principal Medical Officer and Fellow
Applied Sciences
QinetiQ
Farnborough, Hampshire, UK

Colonel Ian Curry
Consultant Advisor Aviation Medicine
MOD
Southampton, UK

Victoria Cutler
Human Factors Design Engineer
Lockheed Martin
Bedfordshire, UK

Wing Commander Joanna d'Arcy
Consultant Cardiologist and General Physician
RAF Reader in Aviation Medicine
Aviation Medicine Consultation Service
RAF Henlow
Bedfordshire, UK

Wing Commander Gary Davies
Consultant in Respiratory and Acute Medicine
Clinical Director Acute Services
Chelsea and Westminster Foundation Trust
London, UK

Dr Sally Evans
Chief Medical Officer
UK Civil Aviation Authority
Gatwick Airport
West Sussex, UK

Colonel Steven Gaydos
Director, Graduate Medical Education
US Army School of Aviation Medicine
Fort Rucker, Alabama

Lieutenant Colonel Claire Goldie
Consultant in Aviation
Occupational Medicine and Helicopter Pilot
British Army

Wing Commander Nicholas Green
Whittingham Professor of Aviation Medicine
RAF Centre of Aviation Medicine
RAF Henlow
Bedfordshire, United Kingdom

Tracy L. Grimshaw
Principal Psychologist in the Human Performance Group
QinetiQ
Farnborough, Hampshire, UK

Group Captain Gwynne Harper
Deputy Assistant Chief of Staff Aviation Medicine
Tri-Service Lead for Aviation Medicine
RAF Centre of Aviation Medicine
RAF Henlow
Bedfordshire, UK

Dr Michael Harrigan
Consultant Occupational Physician
British Airways Health Service
Harmondsworth, UK

Dr D. Helen M. Hoar
Captain B747-400
Virgin Atlantic Airways
Crawley, UK
and
Aviation Medical Examiner
Bristol, UK

Wing Commander Peter Hodkinson
Consultant in Aviation and Space Medicine
RAF Centre of Aviation Medicine
RAF Henlow
Bedfordshire, UK

Major John Houk
Assistant Professor of Occupational Medicine
Senior Flight Surgeon and Battalion Surgeon
7th Special Forces Group
US Army
Eglin AFB
Okaloosa County, Florida

Dr Martin Hudson
Senior Aviation Medical Examiner
UK CAA, EASA, FAA, CASA and Transport Canada

Dr Ewan J. Hutchison
Consultant in Aviation and Occupational Medicine
Head of Medical Assessment
Civil Aviation Authority
West Sussex, UK

Squadron Leader Jonathan Hynes
Medical Officer Pilot
RAF Cranwell
Cranwell, Lincolnshire, UK

Dr Tania Jagathesan
Consultant in Occupational and Aviation Medicine
Civil Aviation Authority
West Sussex, UK

Soo James
Principal Scientist in Military Acoustics
QinetiQ
Farnborough, Hampshire, UK

Major Damian Jenkins
Defence Medical Services Senior Registrar in Neurology
Fellow in Medicine at St Hugh's College
Oxford University
Oxford, UK

Group Captain Jon Kendrew
RAF Consultant Advisor in Trauma and Orthopaedic Surgery
Royal Centre for Defence Medicine
Queen Elizabeth Major Trauma Centre
Birmingham, UK

Colonel (Ret) Russ S. Kotwal
Aerospace Medicine and Family Medicine Physician
Director of Strategic Projects
Department of Defense Joint Trauma System
San Antonio, Texas

Captain Joseph T. LaVan
NAMI Officer in Charge
Pensacola, Florida

Dr Ben Lawson
Technical Director
Naval Submarine Medical Research Laboratory
Naval Submarine Base
New London, Connecticut

Dr Vivienne Lee
Team Leader for Flight Physiology
Human Performance
QinetiQ
Hampshire, UK

Wing Commander Matthew E. Lewis
RAF Consultant Advisor in Aviation Medicine
RAF Centre of Aviation Medicine
RAF Henlow
Bedfordshire, UK

Dr E. Jane Marshall
Consultant Psychiatrist and Visiting Senior Lecturer in the Addictions
Psychiatrist Advisor to the Civil Aviation Authority
Addictions Clinical Academic Group
South London and Maudsley NHS Foundation Trust
London, UK

Colonel Mark McPherson
Consultant for Aerospace Medicine
US Army's Office of the Surgeon General
Falls Church, Virginia

Wing Commander Ian Mollan
Consultant Occupational Medicine Physician and Aeromedical Examiner
RAF Centre of Aviation Medicine
RAF Henlow
Bedfordshire, UK

Wing Commander Edward Nicol
Consultant Cardiologist
Chair of the NATO Aviation Cardiology
Group and the RAF Consultant Advisor in Medicine
Aviation Medicine Clinical Service,
RAF Centre of Aviation Medicine
RAF Henlow
Bedfordshire, United Kingdom

Wing Commander Ivor T. Owen
RAF Exchange Flight Surgeon and Chief
Aerospace Medicine (Interoperability)
USAF/SG3P, Defense Health Headquarters
Falls Church, Virginia

Major Joseph J. Pavelites
Director
Occupational Medicine Residency
United States Army School of Aviation Medicine
Fort Rucker, Alabama

Dr Mark Popplestone
Aviation Medicine Specialist
Qatar Airways
Doha, Qatar

Squadron Leader Bonnie Posselt
Speciality Trainee (Year 6) in Aviation and Space Medicine
RAF Centre of Aviation Medicine
RAF Henlow
Bedfordshire, UK

Wing Commander Joanne Rimmer
Consultation Gastroenterologist
Aviation Medicine Clinical Service
Centre of Aviation Medicine
RAF Henlow
Bedfordshire, UK

Dr John Roberts
Consultant in Aviation and Occupational Medicine
Qatar Airways Group Medical Director

Professor David Russell-Jones
Clinical Director of Outpatients Specialties in Endocrinology and Diabetes
Royal Surrey County Hospital
Surrey, UK

Colonel Richard A. Scheuring
Associate Professor
Military and Emergency Medicine
Uniformed Services
University of the Health Sciences
Bethesda, Maryland

Captain Alfred F. Shwayhat
Medical Corps
US Navy
Chairman Emeritus and Staff Endocrinologist
US Navy Medical Center
San Diego, California

Dr Tim Stevenson
Occupational Physician
The Healthy Company Ltd
Brighton, UK

Group Captain Andrew Timperley
Chief Medical Officer
RAF High Wycombe
Buckinghamshire, UK

Professor Mike Tipton MBE
Extreme Environments Laboratory, DSES
University of Portsmouth
Portsmouth, UK

Dr Michael J. A. Trudgill
Consultant in Aviation and Occupational Medicine
Head of Medical Oversight and Training
Civil Aviation Authority
West Sussex, UK

Dr Anthony Tvaryanas
Preventive Medicine Physician
Wright-Patterson Air Force Base
Dayton, Ohio

Dr Andrew Weller
Principal Thermal Physiologist
Human Performance
QinetiQ
Farnborough, UK

Dr Elizabeth Wilkinson
Consultant in Aviation and Occupational Medicine
Chief Medical Officer at British Airways PLC
Waterside, UK

Surgeon Commander Malcolm Woodcock
Consultant Ophthalmic Surgeon
RAF Centre of Aviation Medicine
RAF Henlow
Bedfordshire, UK

The editors and publisher would also like to thank and acknowledge the reference work *Ernsting's Aviation and Space Medicine*, Fifth Edition, its editors David Gradwell and David Rainford, and its many contributors. The *Handbook* draws upon the structure used in *Ernsting's* for ease of reference by readers wishing to use both texts in parallel.

CHAPTER 1

Fixed wing aircraft

Contents

1.1 DEFINITIONS

Aircraft that use lift generated by wings to sustain flight, including:

- Powered aircraft that gain thrust from an engine.
- Gliders that use air currents to climb.
- Microlights and powered hang gliders.

Aircraft controls usually include control column/joystick/yoke, throttle(s) and rudder pedals.

1.2 AIRCRAFT ROLES

Fixed wing aircraft form bulk of aviation due to flexibility, cost effectiveness, speed and range, capacity. Wide variety of roles and types exist:

Fighter, fighter/attack
- High speed, including supersonic, pressurised (low differential), high altitude, very manoeuvrable, high G loading, ejection seat, single pilot operation, usually short-duration missions (maximum around eight hr with in-flight refuelling).

Military transport/parachute drop
- Moderate speed, pressurised (high differential), medium altitude, generally medium to low manoeuvrability, long duration missions, multi-crew operations, may feature deliberate depressurisation (e.g. parachute drop).

Commercial
- Moderate speed, pressurised (high differential), medium (to high-medium) altitude, low manoeuvrability, long duration, two pilot operations (one pilot operation for some business jets).

General aviation
- Usually low speed, unpressurised, low altitude, single pilot operation.

1.3 OPERATING ENVIRONMENT

ATMOSPHERE

- Composition of altitude relatively constant until around 300,000 ft altitude.
- Typical composition shown in Table 1.1 and Figure 1.1.

Table 1.1 Composition of the atmosphere

GAS	PERCENT VOLUME
Nitrogen	78.08%
Oxygen	20.95%
Water	0 to 4%
Argon	0.93%
Carbon Dioxide	0.04%

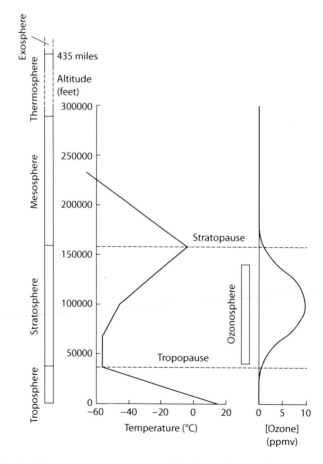

Figure 1.1 Relationship between temperature, altitude and layers of the atmosphere.

- Ozone (O_3):
  - Found highest concentration at 100,000 ft; less than 1 part per million by volume (ppmv) below 40,000 ft.
  - Very strong oxidant; 0.6–0.8 ppmv for two hr reduces vital capacity and forced expiratory volume; 1 ppmv causes lung irritation; 10 ppmv causes pulmonary oedema.
  - At normal engine power settings, air entering cabin has passed through engine compressors at high temperatures, breaking O_3 down to molecular oxygen.
- Layers of atmosphere shown in Table 1.2 International Civil Aviation Organization (ICAO) standard atmosphere (1964) closely represents pressure and temperature characteristics of the real atmosphere at temperate latitude of 45° North:
  - Used as basis for calibration of flight instruments and to allow accurate comparisons between the performance of various aircraft and aircraft systems.
- Absolute pressure = gauge pressure + local atmospheric pressure
  - Cabin absolute pressure = cabin differential pressure + atmospheric absolute pressure.

Table 1.2 Layers of the Earth's atmosphere

LAYER	DETAIL	AVIATION IMPLICATION
Troposphere	• Sea level to 30,000 ft (8 km) at poles or 56,000 ft (16 km) in tropics • Temperature falls with increasing altitude at uniform rate of 2°C/ 1000 ft (Environmental Lapse Rate) • Tropopause above Troposphere (constant temperature of −56.5°C)	• Most commercial and military fixed wing aviation occurs in this layer • All weather in this layer
Stratosphere	• From Tropopause to around 50 km (164,000 ft) • Initially isothermal at −56.5°C, then temperature rises to around 0°C at Mesosphere	• Military aviation sometimes occurs in this layer • −56.5°C is lowest theoretical temperature encountered in fixed wing aviation
Mesosphere	• From Stratopause to around 80 km • Atmospheric composition altered	
Thermosphere	• Up to 600 km • Karman line at 100 km commonly represents boundary between Earth's atmosphere and outer space	

2

Rotary wing operations

Contents

Key Facts

Unique missions include:
- Utility/general transport.
  - Tourism.
  - Law enforcement.*
  - Offshore oil platforms.
- Heavy lift – sling loads, internal cargo.
  - Logging.
  - Construction.
- Medical evacuation.*
- Search and rescue.*
- Reconnaissance.*
- Attack.*

*Frequently involve advanced vision aids such as night vision goggles (NVG), forward looking infrared (FLIR) or millimetric waveband radar (MMWR) presented to the pilot via helmet-mounted device or instrument panel.

2.1 BASIC FLIGHT DESIGN AND AERODYNAMICS

- Main blades turn at set RPM creating relative wind over airfoils; generates total rotor thrust and lift.
- Torque effect of main rotor (fuselage rotation) countered with tail-rotor thrust in the opposite direction (see Figure 2.1), by contra-rotating systems in tandem, or contra-rotating coaxial design.
- Main rotor force vector (total rotor thrust):
  - Magnitude controlled with collective (power) setting.
  - Contributes to lift and thrust components for direction of flight (see Figure 2.2).
- Three related controls (see Figure 2.3).
  - Cyclic: Differentially changes angle of incidence on blades around the main rotor controlling direction and magnitude of horizontal thrust; 'tilting' rotor disk in intended direction of flight (operated with right hand between legs or right-sided 'side stick').

- Collective: Collectively changes angle of incidence on all main rotor blades contributing to total force vector and lift (operated with lever in left hand).
  - Pedals: Control pitch (thrust) of constant RPM tail rotor counteracting main rotor torque and controlling heading/yaw.
- Special circumstances.
  - Effective translational lift: With forward airspeed, aircraft effectively 'outruns' rotor downwash (approximately 16–24 kt); induced drag decreases rapidly and rotor efficiency (lift and thrust) increases significantly at set power.
  - Dissymmetry of lift: Difference in lift between advancing and retreating half of rotor disk caused by differential velocity at forward speed.
  - Retreating blade stall: Retreating rotor blade operates at high angle of attack; retreating blade can no longer compensate for dissymmetry of lift.
  - Autorotation: Controls manoeuvring and arrest rate of descent with engine failure; preserves potential energy and control in rotor system by disengaging from the engine (free-wheeling unit) through lowering collective and reducing angle of attack.

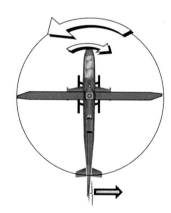

Figure 2.1 Tail rotor counter to torque effect (fuselage rotation).

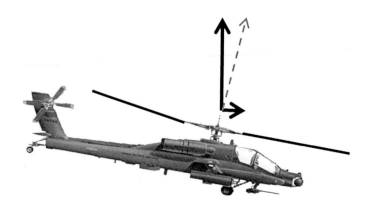

Figure 2.2 Main rotor force vector (total rotor thrust).

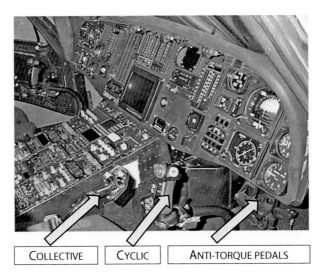

Figure 2.3 Helicopter flight controls.

2.2 AEROMEDICAL ISSUES/STRESSORS OF FLIGHT

- Noise (see Chapters 23 and 24).
  - Can exceed 100 dBA in cockpit/cabin of some airframes; varies across frequency spectrum; noise-induced hearing loss of occupational concern.
  - Passive or active protection usually provided concomitantly with communication headsets or helmet.
- Vibration (see Chapter 23).
  - Multiple sources, including aerodynamic contributions, as well as engine, transmission, gearboxes, blades.
  - May be transmitted or even amplified to aircrew.
  - Issues include fatigue, motion sickness, visual stability, spinal pain, others.
- Hypoxia (see Chapter 9).
  - Unpressurized, but many aircraft can easily attain altitudes in physiologically deficient zone as mission requires.
  - Aircrew-borne or aircraft supplemental oxygen systems of varying types and performance characteristics.
- Thermal extremes (see Chapter 19).
- Motion sickness (see Chapter 28).

2.3 SELECTED AEROMEDICAL ISSUES

- Ergonomics: simultaneous control of three related controls can place pilots in maladaptive posture for extended periods ('helo hunch').
  - Forward flexion of trunk and shoulders; kyphosis and loss of normal lumbar lordosis (right forearm resting on thigh to control cyclic).
  - Leftward rotation and lateral bend (asymmetric collective control with left arm).

- Loss of support base of feet while sitting with pelvic tilt (feet dorsiflexed on pedals).
- Integration of pilot, control geometry, cockpit design, personal protective/survival equipment often challenging.
- Spinal pain.
  - Lumbar: exceedingly common problem in aircrew across platforms; multifactorial aetiology, including posture, vibration, anthropometrics, history of previous injury, protective equipment, others.
  - Cervical: head-supported mass, off-axis CofG due to helmet-mounted devices, posture, increased workload for visual scan with narrow device field-of-view, others.
- Fatigue.
  - Sustained high workload, stress, multiple takeoff/landing missions, challenging ambient conditions.
  - Circadian dysrhythmia, operational tempo/long duty hours, austere living environments (see Chapter 33).
- Aircrew equipment.
  - Needs to be optimized for rotary wing operations (see Chapters 20 and 21).
- Accidents and survivability.
  - Risks include low-altitude/low-airspeed operations, night flying and reliance on night vision devices, degraded ambient conditions (degraded visual environment), ground obstacles (see Chapters 17, 18 and 35).
- Spatial disorientation (see Chapter 27).
  - Cause of significant RW accidents; disproportionate severity with respect to loss of life/aircraft destruction.
  - Brownout/blowing dust; whiteout/snow, fog/smoke, low illumination.

CHAPTER

3

Maritime aviation

Contents

3.1 HISTORICAL NOTES

- Initial aviation operation off ships by UK Royal Navy and US Navy:
  - Other navies with successful shipboard/maritime aviation include Japan, Russia, India, Italy, Thailand and France.
  - China in initial stages of carrier aviation program (first Chinese aircraft carrier was operational in 2012).
- Steam catapult revolutionized shipboard aviation by launching heavier aircraft with higher takeoff speeds and heavier payloads; next-gen catapults utilise mag-lev technology.
- Angled flight deck (landing area angled 10.5 degrees outboard from midline) enabled aircraft that missed arresting wires to avoid impacting other aircraft on flight deck, markedly decreasing shipboard aviation mishaps.
- Rotary wing aircraft allow for operations on smaller platforms and function as a rescue unit during carrier fixed wing operations (plane guard).

3.2 SHIPBOARD ENVIRONMENT

- Noise and vibration transmitted throughout hull of ship; vibration and noise can damage hearing and disrupt crew rest/sleep.
- Rocking of ship at sea:
  - Seasickness risks dehydration and impacts readiness for flight.
  - Increased risks of injuries in passageways and while transitioning between decks (ladderwells).
  - Shifting of unsecured objects (missile hazards).
  - Complicates aircraft movement on constrained flight deck (on CVN, ~60 aircraft taxi, land, takeoff in close proximity on four-acre 'airfield' see Figure 3.1 and 3.2).
- Sustained around-the-clock operations.
- Prolonged separation of military deployment coupled with loss of privacy in close quarters can exacerbate mental health issues and social problems.

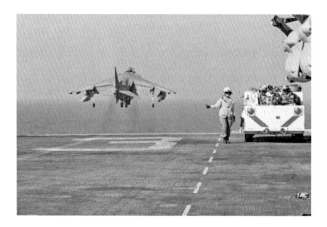

Figure 3.1 Carrier-borne short takeoff operations.

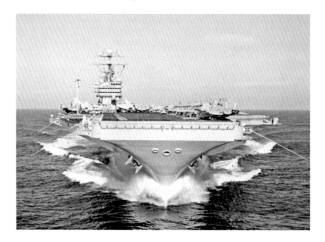

Figure 3.2 Typical large aircraft carrier.

- Infectious disease outbreaks due to close quarters include respiratory illnesses (respiratory viruses, influenza, tuberculosis) and enteric/food-borne illnesses.

3.3 UNIQUE ASPECTS OF AVIATION IN MARITIME ENVIRONMENT

- Launch/recovery.
  - Positive Gx from catapult launch results in somatogravic illusion (perception of nose-up lasting up to 30 sec).
  - Landing at average sink rate of 4–7 m/s.
  - Landing at angle to flight path (10.5 degree angled flight deck).
  - Stopping distance of 100 metres.
- Visual illusions (see Chapter 27).
  - Flying over the water with lack of visual features may result in autokinetic illusion.

- Rotary wing operations over water may lead to visible downwash producing vection illusion affecting ability to hover.
- Approach to ship includes absence of fixed points making approach difficult.
- Lighting issues:
  - Ship may be isolated island of light in otherwise low or no light environment.
  - Decreased visual contrast at night and in haze.
- Lack of fixed features can decrease ability to navigate or maintain altitude.
- Lack of diversion airfield in case of adverse weather or aircraft malfunction – military ships required to be capable of aircraft recovery 100% of the time.
- Temperature extremes affect personnel and aircraft.
- Mishaps over water:
  - Egress issues for helicopters (see Chapter 22).
    - Tendency to invert due to high centre of mass and sink quickly.
    - Disorientation due to turbulence/inversion/lack of visual cues/darkness underwater.
    - Periodic simulator training for underwater egress.
    - Compressed air bottle in survival gear increases time for egress.
  - Prolonged water immersion can cause hypothermia, dehydration (see Chapter 22).
    - Multi-person inflatable rafts with high-visibility materials and radio beacons protect aviators from environment/increase chances of rescue.
  - Double-lift strop to improve survival and rescue of aviators from sea.

3.4 AVIATION MEDICINE IN SHIPBOARD ENVIRONMENT

- Aviation medicine assets are principal providers of health service support to the ship's crew and embarked personnel:
  - Medical response to casualties.
  - Aviation medicine physical exams and qualification.
  - Aeromedevac support.
- Austerity in space and personnel:
  - For example, US Navy CVN Medical Department responsible for approximately 5000 personnel in CVN crew, embarked air wing and staff and other ships in Carrier Strike Group with wide geographic dispersion. Limited resources include:
    - Three to five primary care providers.
    - Physical therapist.
    - Psychologist.
    - Operating room, general surgeon, anaesthesia support.
    - Limited chemistry, limited haematology, limited bacteriology.
    - Basic radiology (plain film and limited ultrasound only).
    - Preventive medicine.
    - Capacity for 52 inpatients and three intensive care patients.
  - Isolated environment requires ability to function for extended periods without additional resources.
  - Resupply is time/distance constrained.

- Medevac issues:
  - Limited resources necessitate urgent/emergent medevac for some injuries/illnesses.
  - Rotary wing medevac limited to littoral operations, but many aviation capable ships operate well outside these regions.
  - Fixed wing operations extend medevac range:
    - Require catapult high acceleration launch (approximately 4 G); stretcher patients not aligned with acceleration in Gx axis, so unstable fractures may not be eligible for fixed wing medevac.
    - Medical attendants required to be strapped-in during critical phases of flight.
    - Long duration evacuation flight may challenge clinical oxygen supply and battery life of monitors.

4

Parachuting

Contents

4.1 BASIC TERMINOLOGY

- Chute: shortened vernacular for 'parachute'.
  - Round: non- (or minimally) manoeuvrable (see Figure 4.1).
  - Square: manoeuvrable, forward travel (see Figure 4.2).
  - Cruciform: non-manoeuvrable, anti-oscillation.
- Jump: shortened vernacular for 'parachute jump'.
- Pilot chutes: deploy larger chutes from storage.
- Drogue chutes: for lateral directional control and stability.
- HALO: High Altitude, Low Opening.
- HAHO: High Altitude, High Opening.
- Harness: fabric webbing fitted to jumper over clothing.

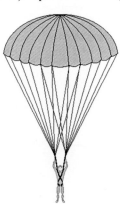

Figure 4.1 Round parachute.

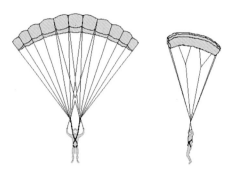

Figure 4.2 Square parachute.

- Risers: fabric straps connecting harness to suspension lines.
- Suspension lines: arrayed cords attached to fabric canopy.
- Canopy: lightweight fabric providing aerodynamic drag (see Figure 4.3).
- Freefall: falling with minimum aerodynamic drag, no chute (see Figure 4.4).
  - Used by most sport parachutists and members of specialized military units.
  - Jumper deploys chute at desired opening altitude.
  - Pilot chute usually deployed via rip cord (see Figure 4.5).
  - Commonly paired with 'square' or ram-air manoeuvrable chute.
- Static line:
  - Used primarily by the military and smoke jumpers.
  - Maximises time under deployed canopy for low altitude jumps.
  - 'Static line' refers to a cord or strap remaining attached to aircraft fuselage anchor.
  - As the jumper leaves aircraft, static line breaks the opening tie and pulls the parachute away from jumper.
  - Once fully elongated, static line breaks from chute.
  - Untethered jumper falls downward under canopy (see Figure 4.6).
  - Often paired with 'round' non-manoeuvrable chute.
  - Some round chutes are manoeuvrable, while some square chutes are not.

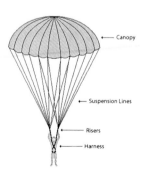

Figure 4.3 Parachute components.

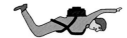

Figure 4.4 Freefall parachuting.

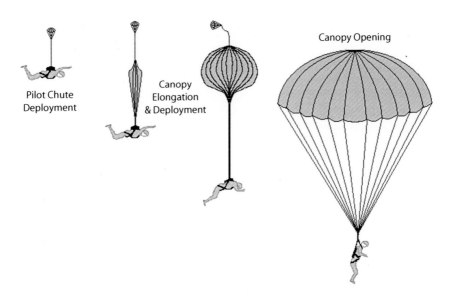

Figure 4.5 Parachute deployment.

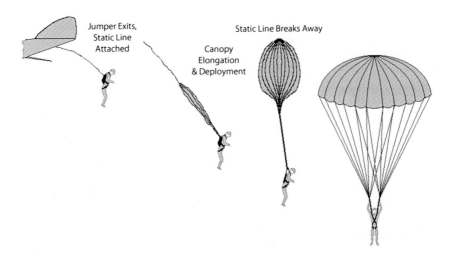

Figure 4.6 Static line jump.

4.2 HISTORICAL BACKGROUND

- First documented parachute design as early as 381 AD.
- First manned jumps in 1200s in China and 1617 in Europe.
- First modern jump in 1783 by Frenchman Louis-Sebastian Lenormand; coined French term *'para'* (to shield) *'chute'* (fall).
- First jump from aeroplane in 1912 by US Army CPT Albert Berry (disputed by some as Grant Morton in 1911).
- First freefall in 1913 by American Georgia Broadwick.
- Early high jump in 1960 by USAF COL(r) Joseph Kittinger at 102,800 ft, fell for 4 min and 36 sec with a stabilizing drogue chute, speeds up to 614 mph, 18,000 ft AGL opening.
- Recent high freefall in 2012 by Australian Felix Baumgartner at 128,100 ft AGL, freefell for 4 min 22 sec, speeds up to 833.9 mph before deploying his first drogue parachute, opened at 5,000 ft AGL.

4.3 PARACHUTE OPERATION

- Purpose:
  - Slow descent/increase atmospheric drag by cupping air:
    - Increase air pressure at leading surface.
    - Decrease air pressure at trailing surface.
  - Orient body for safe descent and landing.
- Carriage:
  - Packed assembly on back in protective covering.
  - Easier transport.
  - Near centre of gravity.
  - Facilitate desired upright landing attitude.
  - Direct opening forces in $+Gz$ and $-Gx$ directions.
- Deployment:
  - Activation by rip cord or static line.
  - Chute drawn out of stowage and away from jumper.
  - Inflates against the rushing air.
- Manoeuvre:
  - Via contorting canopy's shape.
  - Vector cupped air vice direction of travel.
  - Some canopies convert forward momentum into additional lift through wing shaped design.
  - Temporarily diverting the rearward flowing air downward by 'flaring' can slow forward flight, turning a canopy or giving a momentary added lift.
  - Shrinking the vertical canopy surface area or stalling lift-inducing forward momentum increases descent.
- Landing:
  - Minimise sudden bodily stops.
  - Flare and absorb blow with squat extending (see Figure 4.7).

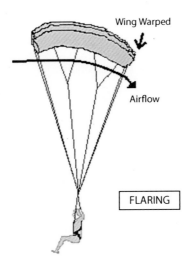

Figure 4.7 Parachute flaring.

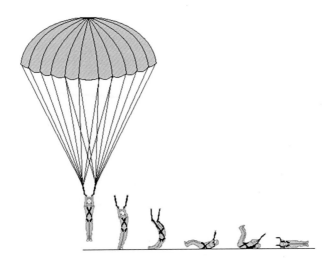

Figure 4.8 Parachute landing fall (PLF).

- Crumple entire body to ground – British developed modern 'parachute landing fall' (PLF) used by most militaries today.
- PLF: land with feet and knees together, executing an oblique roll to the outer side of the leg, thigh, buttocks and muscular upper back (see Figure 4.8).

4.4 NICHE PARACHUTES

- Extremely high altitude: spacecraft or record setting:
  - Use nested layers of automated and command activated parachutes.
  - Controlling spin is critical.

- Velocity:
    - Terminal (jumper in the spread-eagle position) (see Figure 4.4):
        - About 110–125 miles/hour in 12–15 sec.
        - Over a distance of about 1500 ft.
    - Horizontal:
        - Unaided: may approach 25 mph.
        - Wing suits: over 70 mph.
- Ejection seats:
    - Use of strong explosive forces or rockets (7–20 G).
    - Automated sequence deploys the chute as shown (see Figure 4.9).
- Aircraft fuselage parachutes:
    - Designed to land the entire aircraft with all occupants still secured inside fuselage.
    - Uses explosive charges to fire a pilot chute(s) into the airstream (see Figure 4.10).

4.5 STATISTICS

- General parachute characteristics are shown in Table 4.1.
- Differences between civilian and military parachutes shown in Table 4.2.
- Parachute accidental mortality rates shown in Table 4.3.
- Parachute accidental morbidity rates shown in Table 4.4.

4.6 PARACHUTE INJURIES

- Most common acute injury classification: fractures, sprains, strains and contusion/concussions.
- Most common *fracture* locations:
    - 35% ankle or foot (foot strike landing pressure focused on the 1st and 4th/5th metatarsal regions).
    - 25% lower leg.

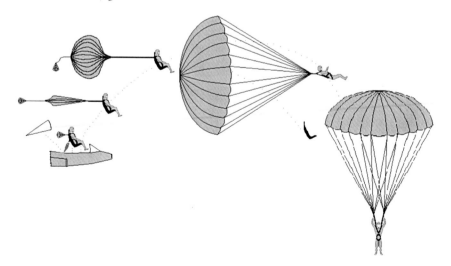

Figure 4.9 Ejection seat parachute.

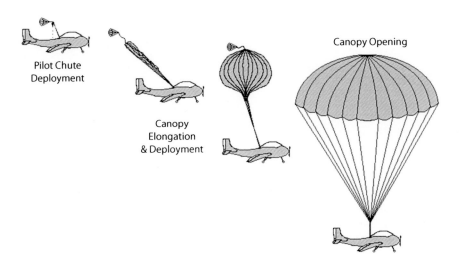

Figure 4.10 Aircraft parachute.

Table 4.1 General parachute characteristics

PARACHUTE TYPE	DEPLOYMENT METHOD	DEPLOYMENT ALTITUDE (ft)	PACKED WEIGHT (lbs)	FORWARD SPEED (mph)	DESCENT RATE (ft/sec)
Military Freefall (MC-4)	Rip Cord	2000–30,000	26–28	15–25	14–18
Military (T-10/11)	Static Line	>500	29–38	0	18–24
Military Reserve (T-11)	Rip Cord	As needed	15	0	18–19
Typical Solo Freefall (ram-air)	Rip Cord	>2000	~15	<10	15–20
Typical Tandem Freefall (ram-air)	Rip Cord	>2000	~30	15–20	15–19
Cirrus Aircraft Parachute System	Emergency Rocket Assist	As needed	Integrated ~200	0	<28
ACES 5 Ejection Seat (GR7000)	Emergency Rocket Assist	As needed	Integrated	0	<24

- 20% pelvis/vertebral column.
- 20% upper limb.
- 12.5% hip/femur.
- Classic injury associated with a military parachute landing fall: supination of ankle and lateral leg/knee strike causing ankle ligament complex damage, fracture upper third of fibula, dislocation of proximal fibular head, isolated knee injuries.
- Associations with increased acute injuries:
  - Increased jumping with equipment.
  - Jumping at night.
  - Conducting military PLF with feet apart.

- Female gender.
- Inexperience.
- Increased ambient temperature or wind speed.
- Increased body weight.
- Decreased physical fitness.
- Increased age.
- Anatomical distribution of parachute injuries identified from published literature shown in Figure 4.11.
- Typical parachute landing injury mechanism shown in Figure 4.12.
- Typical injuries with particular phases of civilian skydiving shown in Table 4.5.
- Parachute opening shock shown in Figure 4.13.

Table 4.2 Comparison of civilian and military parachutes

	MILITARY (ROUND, NON-MANOEUVRABLE)	CIVILIAN (SQUARE, MANOEUVRABLE)
Jump altitudes	Lower (500–1250 ft AGL typical)	Higher (12,000–15,000 typical)
Chute deployment method	Static line predominantly	Rip cord predominantly
Time in freefall	None	~60 sec
Time under canopy	<60 sec	>60 sec
Rate of descent	>18 ft/sec	<20 ft/sec
Planned ground impact rate	18–24 ft/sec	<5–10 ft/sec
Actions on ground contact	Parachute landing fall	Squat/running deceleration

Table 4.3 Parachute accidental mortality rates

POPULATION	TYPE	DATE	RATE (per 1000)
US Army	All, Static Line	1940–1941	.2
US Army	All	1951–1965	.02
Danish Parachute Jumpers Association	All	1979–1983	.05
BASE Jumping	All	1985–2009	~60–90× freefall rates
US Parachute Association	All	2000–2015	.0082
US Parachute Association	Tandem	2006–2015	.002

Table 4.4 Parachute accidental morbidity rates

POPULATION	TYPE	DATE	RATE per 1000 JUMPS
US Army	All	WWII	21–27
US Army Combat Operations	All	1944–1973	10–20
Civilian, Worldwide	All	1944–1998	4.37±2.08
Military, Worldwide	All	1944–1998	5.61±3.78
US Army, 82nd ABN DIV	All, Static Line	1942–2014	11
US Army	All	1951–1965	3.1
US Forest Service Smoke Jumpers	All, Static Line	1992–2010	7
US Army Rangers, Combat Operations	All, Static Line	2001–2003	120
US Army (T-10D/T11)	All, Static Line	2010–2013	8.4
US Parachute Association Members	All	2015	.005

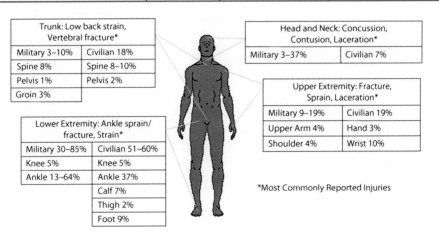

Figure 4.11 Anatomical distribution of parachute injuries from the literature.

4.7 CHRONIC INJURY PATTERNS

- Common complaints of seasoned paratroopers usually focus on the knees and back.
- 2013 Japanese study found that military parachuting was not an independent risk factor for developing degenerative lumbar disc disease.
- Sparse data on chronic knee injury patterns exists.

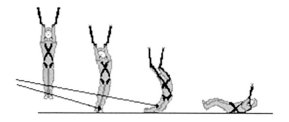

Figure 4.12 Parachute landing fall injury.

Table 4.5 Typical injuries with particular phases of civilian skydiving

PHASE	RATE	INJURY	CAUSE
Exit	2%	Upper extremity strains	Snagged gear or bodily parts, collision with aircraft
Freefall	3%	Contusion, fracture or even death	Collisions with other jumpers
Parachute Opening	9%	Back, face lacerations, neck and posterior auricular injuries	Opening shock, riser tension
Descent under Canopy/Landing	65–85%	Lower extremity and back sprains/fractures, head contusion	Hard or awkward impact with ground

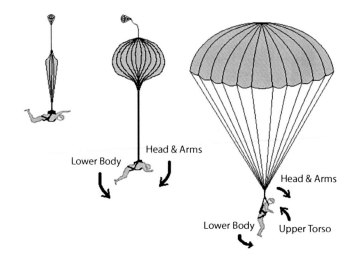

Figure 4.13 Parachute opening shock.

4.8 NICHE INJURIES

- Ejection seat injuries:
  - Associated with low altitude or high speeds, striking the canopy, wind blast to unsecured extremities, and ejection forces (see Chapter 18).
  - Injury rates depend on seat design and whether ejection is within seat performance envelope.
- Jumping while pregnant:
  - Increased nausea in pregnancy is a risk.
  - No evidence to support risk from hypoxia or catecholamine release.
  - 79.3% of injuries happened in the final trimester.
- Aeromedical concerns during high-altitude parachute jumps:
  - Hypoxia.
  - Decompression sickness (ground treatment facilities should be identified).
  - Cold injury.
  - Barotrauma.

CHAPTER 5

Remotely piloted aircraft systems

Contents

> **Key Facts**
> - Although unmanned, there is significant human participation within the system.
> - Wide spectrum of capabilities and complexity within various classes and operations.
> - Medical assessment of remote pilot should include level of cognitive, sensory and physical function, and risk of sudden and subtle incapacitation per national civilian and/or military authority regulations.
> - Occupational and human performance issues should be understood and addressed by aerospace medicine practitioners.

5.1 OVERVIEW OF RPAS

- Unmanned Aircraft System is overarching ICAO class terminology.
- Remotely Piloted Aircraft System (RPAS) is a form of UAS which is not autonomous and is subject to direct pilot control.
- Removing pilot from the aircraft creates novel operational and technical issues.
- ICAO RPAS Manual (2015) provides generalizable framework.
- Although the aircraft is unmanned, there is significant human participation within the whole RPAS, not just control of the aircraft.
- Aeromedical challenges include lack of sensory cues, design of controls, data transmission delays, automation, management of workload/attentional resources, crew handover issues and fatigue.

5.2 ASSESSMENT OF MEDICAL FITNESS

- Remote pilot should have a current medical assessment of level of cognitive, sensory and physical function, and risk of sudden and subtle incapacitation, as per national civilian and/or military authority regulations.
- Medical examiner should consider the specific remote pilot and work environment, platform and mission when assessing medical fitness and determining what is acceptable versus unacceptable with respect to risk to life (RtL) and mission effectiveness.

Table 5.1 Examples of categorization of aggravating and mitigating factors

MITIGATING FACTORS	AGGRAVATING FACTORS
• Operation in visual line-of-sight (VLOS) • Operation in segregated airspace • Overflight of low population density • Flight termination system • Redundancy • Frangibility of RPAS structure	• Extended range operation beyond VLOS • Operation in non-segregated airspace • Overflight of congested areas/high population density • Weaponisation • Failure mode (high kinetic energy) • Complexity

- Stratification of medical certification varies significantly between licencing authorities.
- Medical fitness qualification levels may become increasingly stringent with increasing aircraft weight (surrogate for hazard).
- Beyond weight, there are numerous factors that must be considered in the assessment of RtL:
  - What RPA(s) the remote pilot is to fly.
  - Mitigating and aggravating factors (see Table 5.1).
- The ICAO Class 3 medical assessment (certificate), applicable to air traffic controllers, is recommended as the baseline for remote pilots flying in non-segregated international airspace:
  - Most remote pilots work on the ground, as do air traffic controllers.
  - Represents a professional level of fitness.
  - Class 3 fitness level appropriate for most, but not all, remote pilots.
- Class 3 medical assessment issued for air traffic controllers should not be automatically considered valid for a remote pilot.
- Class 3 medical assessment should reflect that it was issued for a remote pilot versus an air traffic controller.
- Remote pilots may be airborne, in which case certain pilot medical requirements may be appropriate.

5.3 ROLE OF AEROSPACE MEDICINE PRACTITIONERS

- Perform medical assessments for remote pilots:
  - Understand the physical and mental requirements for a particular Remote Pilot Station (RPS) work environment.
  - Assess medical fitness and determine if a remote pilot is acceptable or unacceptable to work safely in the RPS.
- Recommend occupational interventions for human factors related to RPS work environment stressors.
- Give advice and support to operators and line managers on health and well-being matters (such as fatigue and 'deployed-in-country' military operations).
- Provide expertise on human factors during RPAS accident and incident investigations.

6

Space flight

Contents

Key Facts

Hazards of space flight include:

- Space environment:
  - Reduced (partial) or microgravity (μg).
  - Radiation (trapped radiation, Galactic Cosmic Radiation [GCR], Solar Particle Event [SPE]).
  - Extravehicular activity (EVA) (i.e. spacewalks):
    - Vacuum, pressure differential, decompression sickness.
    - Micrometeoroids, orbital debris.
    - Thermal extremes.
  - Interplanetary microbial life (potential).
- Spacecraft environment:
  - Toxic atmosphere.
  - Alterations of atmospheric gas concentrations (O_2, CO_2).
  - Combustion.
  - Thermal control.
  - Isolation and confinement.
  - Noise and vibration.
  - Closed-loop life support environment.

Continued…

Continued…

- Payload and construction activities.
- Nutrition and waste production.
- Fatigue.
- Space mission environment:
  - Remoteness and communication delay.
  - Flight activity (propulsion, G-forces, impacts).
  - Circadian de-synchrony.

6.1 INTRODUCTION

- Space is a unique, isolated and extreme environment with terrestrial analogues used for surrogate training (see Figure 6.1).
- Space medicine combines many medical specialties to mitigate effects of spaceflight on human physiology and prevent and treat problems associated with living in space environment.

6.2 MICROGRAVITY

- Physiologic effects and hazards of reduced or microgravity include:
  - Space motion sickness.
  - Neurovestibular.
  - Cardiovascular.
  - Musculoskeletal.
  - Immune/haematopoietic.
  - Behavioural and psycho-social.
  - Neuro-ophthalmological.

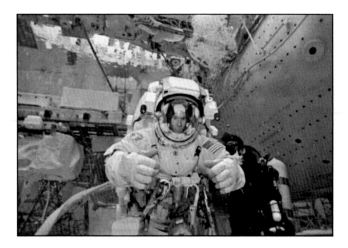

Figure 6.1 NASA flight surgeon in Extravehicular mobility unit (EMU) training in the Neutral Buoyancy Laboratory.

6.3 SPACE MOTION SICKNESS

- Affects 66–95% of crew members; 10% cases severe.
- Symptoms range from loss of appetite to nausea and vomiting.
- Onset from post-orbital insertion to 24 hr; peak at 24–48 hr; resolve at 72–96 hr.
- Aetiology may include:
  - Orientation illusions.
  - Influence of otolith organ asymmetry.
  - Sensory-motor conflict.
  - Cephalad fluid shift of 2 litres from lower extremities.
- Usually treated with IM promethazine or PO meclizine.
- Parabolic microgravity simulation flight motion sickness treated with activity reduction, 1 G orientation and medication.

6.4 NEUROVESTIBULAR EFFECTS

- In-flight changes in neural feedback function produce postural imbalance and loss of coordination post-flight.
- Aetiology includes neurovestibular-otolith and proprioception readaptation.
- All crew members affected to various degrees.
- Post-flight symptoms range from vertigo and gait instability to nausea and vomiting.
- Onset from landing to 48–72 hr.
- Countermeasures include avoidance of rapid head movements, slow progressive activity, medication.
- Visual impairment intracranial pressure (VIIP) syndrome: astronauts experience poor vision after spaceflight, sometimes lasting years; related to neuro-ophthalmological changes including:
  - Hyperopic shifts; globe flattening.
  - Optic disc oedema and increased optic nerve sheath diameter.
  - Choroidal folds.
  - Raised intracranial pressure.

6.5 CARDIOVASCULAR EFFECTS

- Loss of hydrostatic gradient with in-flight fluid redistribution towards upper body and chest.
- 'Puffy head–bird leg syndrome' effects on crew members may include lack of thirst, frequent urination, nasal congestion, dulled sense of taste, facial oedema.
- Baroreceptor-endocrine-diuretic response.
- Body functions with less total fluid volume.
- Deconditioning effects on the heart include:
  - Decreased maximum power outputs during exercise.
  - Less oxygen uptake during exercise.
  - Less circulating blood volume upon terrestrial return.
  - Orthostatic hypotension upon reintroduction to gravity environment.
- Post-flight orthostatic symptoms common in 20–67% crew members with dizziness, light-headedness, 'grey out', syncope.
- Countermeasures include G suits, exercise, medication, pre-landing fluid loading.

6.6 MUSCULOSKELETAL EFFECTS

EFFECTS

- Atrophy of antigravity muscles of trunk, thigh, calf.
- Decrease in leg strength approximate 20–30%; extensor muscles > flexor muscles.
- Bone demineralization 1–2.4% per month in lower extremities and lumbar spine.
- Losses specific to weight-bearing bones; rapid and not necessarily linear.
- Loss of total body calcium; increased faecal and urinary calcium.
- Increased risk of kidney stones, possible fractures, intervertebral disk disease.
- Increased incidence of in-flight back pain (53–68%); fatigue; decreased strength and stamina; muscle stiffness and soreness.

IN-FLIGHT COUNTERMEASURES

- Treadmill.
- Cycle ergometer.
- Resistive exercise device (e.g. Advanced Resistive Exercise Device [ARED] aboard ISS).
- ISS exercise plan includes 2.5 hr/day, 6 days/week.

POTENTIAL OPERATIONAL IMPLICATIONS

- Decreased intra/extravehicular work capacity.
- Decremented landing proficiency.
- Reduced egress capability.

6.7 IMMUNE SYSTEM AND HAEMATOPOIETIC EFFECTS

- Aetiology of spaceflight-induced alterations in immune response may include microgravity, radiation, stress response, and other undetermined causes.
- Depression of lymphocyte function affects approximately 50% of crew members.
- Clinical implications may include latent virus reactivation, delayed wound healing.
- Reduction in circulating red blood cell mass ('spaceflight anaemia').

6.8 BEHAVIOURAL AND PSYCHO-SOCIAL EFFECTS

- Changes in crew mood and morale affect virtually all crew members to some degree.
- Symptoms variable with possible operational effects:
  - Interpersonal conflicts.
  - Anxiety and depression.
  - Sleep disturbances.
  - Performance decrement.
  - Decline in team compatibility.
- Aetiology various and may include:
  - Workload.
  - Sleep habits and facilities; chronobiology.
  - Inter-individual crew personalities and 'crew space'.

- Exogenous factors such as diet, temperature, noise, atmosphere.
  - Lack of family contact.
- Treatment focuses on underlying cause.
- Space analogue environments for evaluation and training:
  - Submarine and undersea facilities; Antarctic; remote/austere environments/locations.

6.9 HABITABILITY AND CREW ENVIRONMENT

- Noise: upper limit of 74 dB (average per 24 hr).
- Temperature: hot cabin >90°F with 90% humidity.
- Water: quality tested for iodine levels, microbes, and pH at L-15 and L-3 days.
- Waste: waste collection system.
- Toxic products and propellants:
  - Generic and payload-specific compounds.
  - Fire/smoke and toxic spills.
  - Quick-don mask.
  - Compound specific analyser-combustion products; monitors O_2, CO, HCl and HCN.
  - Air sample bottles (analysis post-flight only).
  - Containment Clean-up Kit.

6.10 HEALTH RISK AND HAZARDS DURING EXTRAVEHICULAR ACTIVITY (EVA)

- Separation from spacecraft (see Figure 6.2).
- Micrometeoroid/orbital debris.
- Worksite injury (e.g. crush, electrical).
- Foreign body injury (e.g. inhalation, ocular).
- Suit trauma:
  - Onycholysis.
  - Shoulder and other orthopaedic injuries.
  - Bruising, abrasions and paraesthesia.

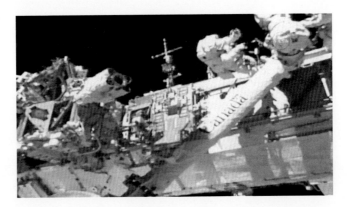

Figure 6.2 Astronauts on EVA work on the latching mechanism on the 58-foot robot arm of the International Space Station, October 2017.

- Toxic substances.
- Life support system failures.
- Thermal injury.
- Radiation.
- Hypobaric suit pressure; suit leak and decompression injury:
  - Type I or Type II ranging from joint discomfort to unconsciousness and death.
  - Prevention includes various protocols of 100% O_2 pre-breathe nitrogen displacement and pressure step-downs.
  - Treatment includes re-pressurisation, aspirin, 100% O_2, fluids.

6.11 SPACE RADIATION ENVIRONMENT

- Exposure based on orbital altitude/inclination, duration and solar activity.
- Crew members are radiation workers with limits for mission and career exposure (see Chapter 14).

6.12 FLIGHT/CREW SURGEON ROLES AND RESPONSIBILITIES

- Critical:
  - Medical certification of astronauts for training and missions.
  - Medical care of astronauts and their families.
  - Support during medical consultations.
  - Perform annual evaluations of retired astronauts.
  - Astronaut selection exams.
  - AOD exams/certification.
- Operational:
  - Provides medical support for space missions.
  - Medical oversight of crew training.
  - Medical support to crew members prior to launch.
  - Monitor EVAs.
  - Participate in contingency/rescue management during launch/landing.
  - Serve as part of the Flight Control Team in Mission Command Center (see Figure 6.3).

6.13 FUTURE SPACE MEDICAL ISSUES

- Long duration deep space or planetary missions:
  - Increased radiation exposure.
  - Isolation from reduced communication from Earth.
  - Lack of resupply.
  - Lack of immediate return or ground-launched interventions for contingencies and emergencies.
- Expected illness and challenges:
  - Orthopaedic and musculoskeletal problems.
  - Infectious, haematological and immune-related disease.
  - Dermatological, ophthalmologic and otolaryngologic problems.

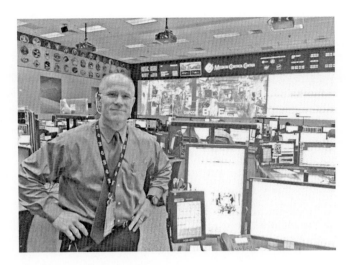

Figure 6.3 Flight surgeon console at Mission Control Center, Houston.

- Acute medical emergencies:
    - Wounds, lacerations and burns.
    - Toxic exposures and acute anaphylaxis.
    - Acute radiation illness.
    - Dental, ophthalmologic and psychiatric illness.
- Chronic diseases:
    - Radiation-induced disease.
    - Dust-related exposure.
    - Presentation or acute manifestation of nascent illness.

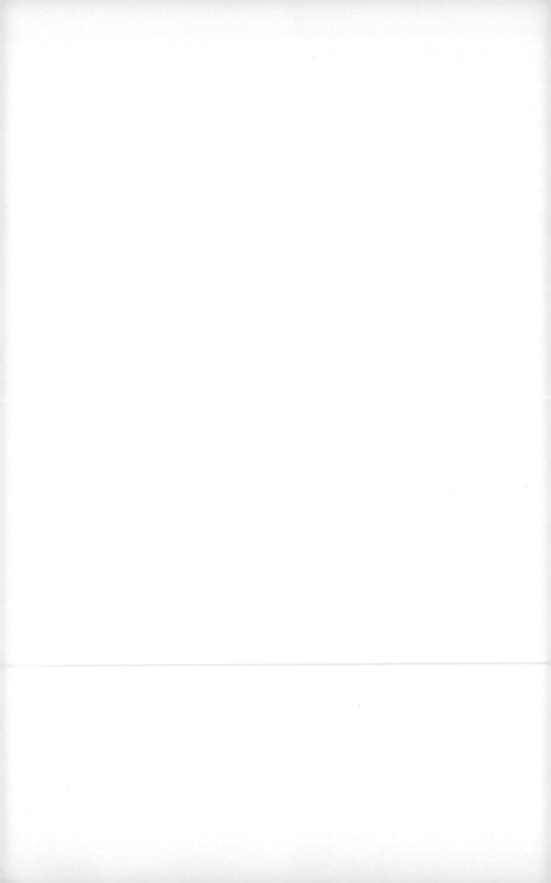

CHAPTER

7

Pressure change

Contents

Key Facts

- Pressure is a measure of force per unit area.
- Atmospheric pressure is the weight of the column of air above the aviator and decreases with altitude.
- The composition of air is 78% nitrogen, 21% oxygen and 1% other gases.
- With an increase in altitude, the composition of air does not change, but the partial pressure of the components decreases.
- Gas expands with increasing altitude (wet gas expands more than dry gas at the same altitude).
- Hypobaric hypoxic hypoxia results from insufficient pO_2 at increasing altitude.
- Rapid decompression may cause nitrogen to come out of solution in the body, forming bubbles.
- Gas dysbarisms and barotrauma occur when trapped gases in body spaces expand on ascent (or atmospheric gas cannot enter lower pressure body spaces on descent).

7.1 WHAT IS PRESSURE?

- Pressure is a force exerted by a substance per unit area on another substance with SI units of pascals ($1\ Pa = 1\ N/m^2$).
- Atmospheric pressure is the pressure of ambient air to which the aviator is exposed:
  - Closely approximated by weight of column of air above the aviator.
  - As altitude increases, there is less overlying atmospheric mass, so atmospheric pressure decreases (as well as air density) with increasing elevation.
- Standard Atmosphere (atm):
  - Defined as 101325 Pa (1.01325 bar); 760 mmHg (torr), 29.9 in Hg, 14.7 psi.

7.2 WHAT IS THE COMPOSITION OF THE ATMOSPHERE?

Partial pressure (pX): pressure that would be exerted by one of the gases in a mixture if it occupied the same volume on its own:

$$pX = (Atmospheric\ Pressure) \times (\%\ of\ gas)$$

- Earth's atmosphere is a mixture of gases composed of approximately 78% nitrogen, 21% oxygen and 1% other gases: argon, carbon dioxide, water vapor, etc. Each exerts its own partial pressure.
- At 5486 m (18,000 ft) the atmospheric pressure is half that at sea level (380 mmHg or 0.5 atm) – see Figure 7.1.
- At 5486 m, the $pO_2 = (380\ mmHg) \times (21\%\ O_2) = 80\ mmHg\ (0.11\ atm)$.

ATMOSPHERIC CHANGES WITH ALTITUDE

- Percentage composition of air generally does not change with altitude.
- Partial pressures for components of air decrease with increasing altitude.
- The atmosphere can be broken into three physiological zones: Efficient, Deficient and Space Equivalent (see Table 7.1).

7.3 GAS LAWS

- **Pascal's Law** states that a pressure change applied to one part of a fluid (i.e. gas or liquid) is transmitted without loss to every portion of the fluid and to the walls of the container:
  - Changes in pressure due to altitude changes are transmitted equally throughout the body.

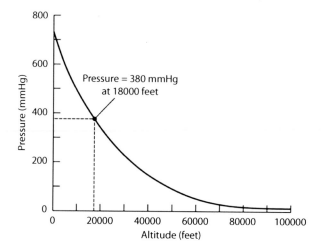

Figure 7.1 Relationship between pressure exerted by the atmosphere and altitude.

Table 7.1 Physiological zones of the atmosphere

ZONE	ALTITUDE	PRESSURE RANGES	CHARACTERISTICS
Physiological Efficient Zone	Sea Level–3810 m Sea Level–12,500 feet	1.00–0.69 atm 1.01–0.70 bar 101–70.0 kPa 14.7–10.1 psi 760–523 mmHg	Body has adapted to operate in the lower regions of this zone. Minor trapped gas problems (ears, sinuses and GI tract) occur in the lower region. Mild hypoxia with dyspnea, dizziness, headaches and fatigue in the upper region with longer exposures or with exertion. Atmospheric pO_2 ranges from 160 to 76 mmHg (21.3–10.1 kPa). Pressurized aircraft generally maintain a cabin pressure equivalent to or less than 2400 m (8000 feet).
Physiological Deficient Zone	3800–15,240 m 12,500–50,000 feet	0.69–0.11 atm 0.70–0.11 bar 70.0–11.0 kPa 10.1–1.62 psi 523–87.0 mmHg	Majority of flying is conducted in this zone. Lack of atmospheric pressure can lead to hypoxia and decompression sickness. At 5486 m (18,000 ft), atmospheric pressure is half that at sea level or 0.5 atm (360 mmHg). Atmospheric pO_2 ranges from 76 to 15 mmHg (10.1–2 kPa).
Space Equivalent Zone	15,240 m–1609 km 50,000 ft–1000 miles	0.11–0.0 atm 0.11–0.0 bar 11.0–0.0 kPa 1.62–0.0 psi 87.0–0.0 mmHg	Very hostile to humans. "Armstrong's line" is at 19,202 m (63,000 ft) and any unprotected exposure above this level causes body fluids to boil (ebullism). Atmospheric pO_2 is negligible.

- **Boyle's Law** states that the volume of a gas is inversely proportional to pressure applied to it (with temperature held constant):
    - Pressure changes allow gas to expand in body cavities (inner ear, sinuses and GI tract) with increasing altitude.
    - Volume flow of a gas is not the same as its mass flow, the difference increasing with altitude:
        - As an example, a mass flow of 4 L (NTP)/min will provide a volume flow of about 8 L (ATPD)/min at an altitude of 18,000 ft due to gas expansion in accordance with Boyle's Law.
- **Charles's Law** states that the volume of a gas is directly proportional to absolute temperature:
    - Can be combined with Boyle's Law to form universal gas law (pressure, volume and temperature of a gas are constant $P_1V_1/T_1 = P_2V_2/T_2$).
- **Graham's Law** states that gas will diffuse from an area of high concentration to an area of low concentration:
    - Transfer of gases between the atmosphere and the lungs, lungs and blood, and blood and the cell.
- **Dalton's Law** states that the total pressure of a mixture of gases is the sum of the partial pressures of each of the mixture's components.
    - Ascent to altitude reduces total atmospheric pressure as well as each of the partial pressures associated with total atmospheric pressure.
- **Amagat's Law** states that the total volume of a gas mixture at constant temperature and pressure is equal to the sum of the individual volumes of constituent gases.
    - Wet gas within the human body expands more than dry gas at the same altitude (evolving water vapor adds extra volume); sea level dry gas volume expands 6 times at 43,000 ft; equivalent wet gas volume expands 9 times.
- **Henry's Law** states that the mass of gas dissolved in a liquid is proportional to the partial pressure in the gas above the liquid:
    - Rapid reduction of environmental pressure causes bubbles of nitrogen to form in the blood and tissues.

7.4 EFFECTS OF PRESSURE CHANGE ON THE HUMAN BODY

- Reduced atmospheric pO_2 causes hypoxia (see Chapter 9).
- Reduced atmospheric pressure may cause decompression sickness (see Chapter 8).
- Change in atmospheric pressure may cause gas dysbarism:
    - Gases that occupy spaces in the body such as inner ear, GI tract and sinuses expand and contract with changes in atmospheric pressures.
    - If these spaces cannot equilibrate with ambient pressures, pain and injury may result (see Table 7.2 and 7.3 and Figure 7.2).

PULMONARY BAROTRAUMA

- If the magnitude of pressure change and rate of decompression are too great, gas expansion may cause over-distension and tearing of lung tissue, with rupture of blood vessels and pleura.

Table 7.2 Typical gas dysbarisms

AILMENT	SYMPTOMS	TREATMENT
Ear block (tympanic membrane barotrauma)	Pain increases with descent. May begin with full feeling in affected ear that may progress to pain. Can also cause vertigo.	• Do not fly with symptoms of upper respiratory infections. • Level off from descent. • Pressure equilibration manoeuvres (see Table 7.3). • Ascend and clear ears again. • Attempt use of spray nasal decongestants. • If no relief, land as soon as practicable. • (See Chapter 61)
Sinus block	Pain may increase with ascent or descent. Pain behind cheekbones and in upper teeth (maxillary block). Pain behind eyebrows and corner of eyes (frontal block).	• Do not fly with symptoms of upper respiratory infections. • Level off from ascent/descent. • Pressure equilibration manoeuvres. • Ascend and try pressure equilibration manoeuvres again. • Attempt use of spray nasal decongestants. • If no relief, land as soon as practicable.
Gastrointestinal tract	Progressively increasing pain in abdominal area with a corresponding increase in altitude.	• Prevent by avoiding gas forming foods, carbonated beverages and chewing gum. • Relieve gas by belching or passing flatus. • Descend to pain-free altitude. • If no relief, land as soon as practicable.
Tooth block	Pain in a single tooth that worsens with a corresponding increase in altitude.	• Prevent by proper dental care. • Level off from ascent. • Descend to pain-free altitude. • If no relief, land as soon as practicable. • Seek dental care.

- Animal and cadaveric studies indicate that pulmonary barotrauma may occur when gas expansion increases the transthoracic pressure differential to more than 80 mmHg; likely to occur with a high initial lung volume and if the airway (glottis) is closed or obstructed.
- Consequences may include:
  - Arterial gas embolism (AGE): Gas entering the blood vessels may pass to the left side of the heart and enter the systemic circulation.
  - Bubbles passing to the cerebral circulation may result in cerebral arterial gas embolism (CAGE). CAGE is a form of decompression illness that may be life-threatening and is likely to warrant early hyperbaric recompression therapy in a specialist centre.
  - Pneumothorax if gas enters the pleural cavity.
  - Surgical emphysema, if gas enters the soft tissues of the neck, face and arms.

Table 7.3 Pressure equilibration manoeuvres

MANOEUVRE	DESCRIPTION
Valsalva	Pinch the nose closed. Close the mouth and inflate nose with breath.
Frenzel	Pinch the nose closed. Move the soft palate to the neutral position. Use tongue as a piston and push air towards the back of the throat.
Toynbee	Pinch the nose closed and swallow.
Edmonds	Tense the soft palate and throat muscles while pushing the jaw forward and down. Perform a Valsalva manoeuvre.
Lowry	Combination of Toynbee and Valsalva. Pinch the nose closed. Inflate nose with breath and swallow at the same time

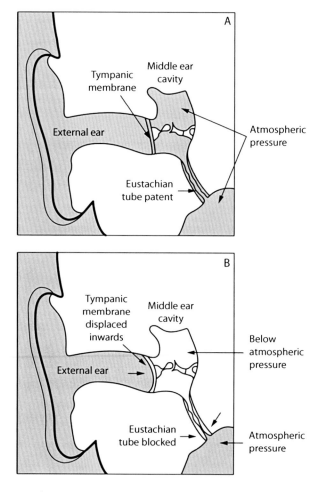

Figure 7.2 Diagram of external and middle ear (A) at a constant altitude with a patent Eustachian tube and (B) during descent with an occluded Eustachian tube.

- Rapid decompression could occur during positive pressure breathing, for example, for protection from +Gz acceleration (PBG). Experimental work provides reassurance that rapid decompression across a 5 psi pressure differential, while breathing under positive pressure up to 60 mmHg, is safe and does not significantly increase transthoracic pressure, providing the glottis remains open and pressure relief valves vent gas from life support system pipework.

Sub-atmospheric decompression illness

Contents

Key Facts
- Decompression illness results from acute exposure to reduced ambient pressure.
- Wide range of clinical presentation including musculoskeletal, cutaneous, pulmonary, neurological.
- Symptoms thought to be caused by bubble formation in circulation and tissues.
- Treatment includes 100% oxygen and re-pressurisation/hyperbaric oxygen therapy.

8.1 DEFINITIONS

Sub-atmospheric decompression illness (DCI) results from hypobaric decompression to ambient pressures less than 1 atm. May occur during ascent to altitude in aircraft, use of extra-vehicular activity spacesuit, or decompression in hypobaric chamber.

Sub-atmospheric DCI includes:

- Decompression sickness (DCS):
  - DCS first recognised in divers/compressed air workers in 1850s as 'caisson disease'.
  - Compressed air and sub-atmospheric DCS have different features.
- Arterial gas embolism (AGE):
  - May arise from pulmonary barotrauma or venous gas emboli through patent foramen ovale or pulmonary shunts.
  - May lead to cerebral arterial gas embolism (CAGE) where occlusion of cerebral vessels may produce ischaemia.
    - CAGE more likely during breath hold in decompression.
    - Symptoms of unilateral paresis, facial weakness, dysphasia or focal neurological symptoms.
    - Requires urgent recompression therapy (short delay to move to centre of excellence acceptable).

8.2 MECHANISM OF DCS

- Body tissues saturated with about 1 L of nitrogen at sea level breathing air.
- On ascent to altitude, nitrogen 'off-gassed' from body (partial pressure in tissues exceeds that in inspired air).
- Rate of off-gassing may be too slow:
  - Leads to supersaturation of nitrogen in some tissues.
  - Nitrogen then forms bubbles.
- Bubbles cause local mechanical effects, block vessels, trigger inflammation.
- Site and size of bubbles determine symptoms.
- Fatty tissues more likely to form bubbles (higher nitrogen content, poor blood supply).
- Venous gas emboli (VGE) can be seen on cardiac ultrasound; usually cleared by the lungs; VGE are poor predictor of DCS symptom severity, but DCS unlikely without VGE present; usually observed in research situations.

8.3 CLINICAL PRESENTATION

MUSCULOSKELETAL – BENDS

- Limb pain comes on over a few minutes.
- Usually near major joint:
  - Most often knees and shoulders.
  - Less often elbow, wrist/hand, ankle or hip (rare).
- Poorly localised, deep seated.
- Mild ache to severe pain (can worsen progressively).
- No better/may be worse on moving limb.

- Local pressure can give relief.
- The most common manifestation of sub-atmospheric DCS (74% of presenting symptoms at 28,000 ft).

CUTANEOUS – CREEPS

- Skin symptoms with itching, tingling and formication.
- Common, usually mild and transient.
- Occasionally blotchy, mottled skin rash (*cutis marmorata*) or urticarial appearance, may persist for days.
- 7% of presenting symptoms at 28,000 ft.

PULMONARY – CHOKES

- Respiratory distress.
- Constriction pain around chest.
- Difficulty taking deep breath, may trigger paroxysmal coughing.
- Almost inevitably progresses to collapse if remain at altitude.
- Less than 5% of presenting symptoms at 28,000 ft.

NEUROLOGICAL – STAGGERS

- No common pattern in aviation.
- Relatively rare.
- May include paralysis (temporary), paraesthesia; loss of proprioception, seizures.
- Unlike diving, do not get spinal bends with lower motor neuron paralysis and sensory losses.

NEUROLOGICAL – SYNCOPE/COLLAPSE

- Loss of consciousness may be sudden.
- Usually late feature.
- 9% of symptoms at 28,000 ft.

NEUROLOGICAL – VISUAL DISTURBANCE

- Patchy scotomata similar to migraine, often with headache.

NEUROLOGICAL – AUDIOVESTIBULAR

- Loss of balance.
- Dizziness, vertigo, nausea, vomiting.
- Hearing loss.

CONSTITUTIONAL

- Non-specific malaise, fatigue, difficulty concentrating or sense of being unwell.
- May progress to cardiovascular collapse without other symptoms.

CLASSIFICATIONS OF DCS

- Type I (musculoskeletal, cutaneous) or Type II (neurological, pulmonary).
- Descriptive: 'early' or 'late' symptoms, 'progressive' or 'plateau', 'relapsing' or 'resolving'.

EVOLUTION OF SYMPTOMS

- 80% persist until descent; 12% clear at altitude; 5% clear but recur; 3% ease partially.
- Progressively worsening symptoms warrant immediate action to avoid progression to collapse.

8.4 PREDISPOSING FACTORS

PHYSICAL

- Final altitude:
  - Decompression to less than half baseline pressure usually required (Haldane's principle).
  - But DCS can occur below 18,000 ft (rare).
  - DCS uncommon below 25,000 ft.
  - Increasing risk with increasing altitude.
  - 'Operational' altitude threshold (prolonged exposure, breathing 100% oxygen) thought to be 20,500 ft, but cases do occur below.
- Base altitude:
  - Equilibration to a different base altitude alters threshold.
  - Diving will lower the base altitude.
  - Delay ascent to altitude for 12 hr after diving to ≤2 atm (10 msw) and for 24 hr after dive to >2 atm (deeper than 10 msw).
- Rate of ascent:
  - Fewer bubbles if decompress slowly.
  - Little practical significance in aviation.
- Duration of exposure:
  - First 5 minutes are relatively safe (e.g. after rapid decompression).
  - Risk increases from 20 to 60 minutes as bubbles form and grow.
- Repeated exposure:
  - Possible increased risk with repeated decompression; details not well understood.
  - Aim for at least 24 hr between exposures.
- Temperature:
  - Increased incidence with cold.
- Breathing gas composition:
  - Higher breathing gas oxygen concentrations are more protective.
  - Hypoxia increases incidence and severity of symptoms (see Figure 8.1).
- Exercise:
  - Significantly increased risk with even minor activity.
  - Symptoms worse and occur at lower altitudes.

PERSONAL

- Age – Increased risk above 25 years, especially above 42 years.
- Individual – Highly variable risk within and between individuals.
- Gender – Ovarian cycle may modulate risk.
- Body habitus – Increased risk if obese.
- Injury – Recent joint/limb injury may predispose to musculoskeletal DCS ('bends').
- Infection – After-effects seem to increase risk.

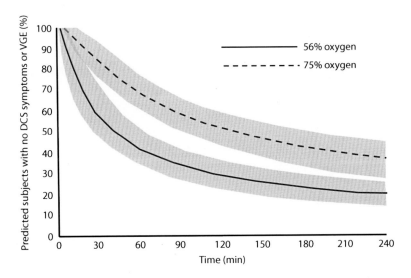

Figure 8.1 Influence of breathing gas oxygen content on risk of decompression sickness (95% confidence intervals shaded).

- Alcohol – Delayed influence to increase risk, possibly related to dehydration.
- Previous DCS – Past susceptibility seems to increase risk of recurrence.

8.5 DIFFERENTIAL DIAGNOSES

- Flight stresses:
  - Hypoxia.
  - Pressure (alternobaric) vertigo.
  - Acceleration atelectasis.
  - Abdominal distension (gas expansion).
  - Motion sickness.
  - Clothing 'pinch points'.
- Psychological stresses:
  - Fear/anxiety.
  - Claustrophobia.
  - Hyperventilation.
- Medical:
  - Myocardial infarction.
  - Pneumothorax.
  - Cramp/limb pain.

8.6 IN-FLIGHT MANAGEMENT

- Descend:
  - Rapid descent to <10,000 ft will usually promote recovery and abolish symptoms.
- Use 100% oxygen:
  - If possible lie flat and rest, keep warm.

- Land:
    - Transfer to medical care as soon as possible.

8.7 POST-FLIGHT MANAGEMENT (ACTIVE TREATMENT)

- Clinical diagnosis:
    - Maintain high index of suspicion.
    - Symptoms are DCS until proven otherwise.
- Continue 100% oxygen post-descent:
    - Increasing tissue partial pressure of oxygen adjacent to bubble encourages nitrogen to diffuse out of the bubble.
    - Oxygen supplementation relieves tissue hypoxia due to vessel obstruction.
- Hyperbaric oxygen therapy:
    - Symptoms may resolve on descent or following administration of 100% oxygen at ground level.
    - Threshold to treat by recompression is now generally low, even if symptoms have resolved.
    - Hyperbaric oxygen therapy according to US Navy Table 6 or equivalent in hyperbaric chamber.
    - Table may be repeated or extended as required.
    - Intermittent oxygen therapy (risk of oxygen toxicity).
    - Manage circulatory collapse with intravenous fluids; consider high-dose corticosteroids.

8.8 POST-DESCENT COLLAPSE

- Rare – Risk is 1:2500 exposures >30,000 ft.
- Collapse usually occurs within 2 hr of descent.
- High mortality (30–40%).
- Virtually never occurs without prior symptoms at altitude.
- Clinical picture: Anxiety, frontal headache, nausea, malaise and apprehension; cold extremities; skin mottling; fever; abdominal pain; neurological signs; peripheral vascular collapse; coma.
- Raised haematocrit (55–65+) is consistent finding.
- Massive loss of plasma to extravascular compartment.

8.9 PREVENTION OF SUB-ATMOSPHERIC DCS

Principles of prevention:
- Limit reduction in pressure (e.g. wear pressure suit, use pressure cabin).
- Limit duration of exposure.
- Eliminate nitrogen prior to exposure (pre-breathe/preoxygenation/denitrogenation).
- Breathe 100% oxygen during exposure.
- Avoid hyperbaric exposure (diving) for 12–24 hr prior to flight.
- Avoid unnecessary physical activity during flight.
- Avoid repeated exposure.

8.10 PRINCIPLES OF DENITROGENATION

- Breathing 100% oxygen prior to ascent (preoxygenation) reduces nitrogen load in body.
- Neurological DCS reduced most by preoxygenation (lipid in neural tissue); less benefit on limb 'bends' due to slower denitrogenation of subcutaneous tissue.
- Preoxygenation effective during initial decompression/climb up until 16,000 ft.
- Effectiveness of denitrogenation enhanced by exercise during preoxygenation (used in some spaceflight applications).
- Denitrogenation of tissue may be perfusion limited or diffusion limited:
  - Perfusion limited when tissue inert gas pressure equals venous inert gas pressure.
  - Diffusion limited when tissue inert gas pressure higher than venous inert gas pressure.
  - Diffusion limited tissue slow to equilibrate (e.g. tendons, cartilage and joint spaces).
- Equilibration of inert gas pressures is exponential; different time constant for each tissue.

Preoxygenation time to reduce risk during exposure to 25,000 ft for 20–30 minutes is typically around 30 minutes; longer preoxygenation times for higher altitudes or more hazardous activities (e.g. rapid decompression, exercise).

8.11 AEROMEDICAL MANAGEMENT – FITNESS FOR FLIGHT

- Airline travel usually permissible a minimum of 72 hr after hyperbaric oxygen therapy.
- Most DCS has full recovery and no limitation to aircrew employment required.
- Following neurological DCS, screening for patent foramen ovale (PFO) may be considered:
  - PFO common (found in around a third of population); right-to-left shunt may occur at rest, or at end of Valsalva manoeuvre.
  - Likely only large PFO has clinically significant risk of neurological DCS.
  - If large PFO, consider altitude limitation or PFO closure.

8.12 WHITE MATTER HYPERINTENSITIES (WMH)

- Subcortical hyperintense areas seen on brain T2 weighted MRI scans.
- In general population (mainly elderly), WMH associated with clinical conditions, including cardiovascular disease and symptomatic cerebrovascular disease; may also be associated with diving, head injury and many other factors; count increased in all people over age 55.
- In aviation, associated with non-hypoxic hypobaric exposure; abnormally high number and volume of WMH found in USAF U2 pilots and hypobaric chamber attendants.
- WMH associated with a small (non-clinically significant) reduction in cognitive function in U2 pilots.
- No clear association between WMH and DCS.
- Causality, prevalence, exposure threshold and significance of WMH still under investigation.

Acute hypoxia and hyperventilation

Contents

Key Facts
- Hypoxic hypoxia in aviation is predominantly caused by ascent to above 10,000 ft without supplemental oxygen or a failure of cabin pressurisation.
- Hypoxic Ventilatory Response reduces expected drop in P_AO_2 by lowering P_ACO_2.
- Hypoxia and hyperventilation may cause similar symptoms.
- Shape of oxygen dissociation curve offers some protection against hypoxia up to 10,000 ft.
- At 33,700 ft breathing 100% supplemental O_2, inspired oxygen tension is equivalent to that at sea level breathing air.
- Symptoms of hypoxia can be exacerbated by a number of other factors, in particular with exercise.

9.1 WHAT IS HYPOXIA?

Hypoxia is an insufficient supply of oxygen reaching the tissues. Acute hypoxia refers to effects experienced over a few seconds to a few hours; chronic effects of hypoxia predominate over days to weeks.

There are four main forms of hypoxia:

- Lack of alveolar oxygen: hypoxic.
- Reduction in oxygen carrying capacity of blood: anaemic.
- Reduction in blood flow to tissues: ischaemic.
- Inability of tissue to use oxygen: histotoxic.

In the aviation environment, main cause of acute hypoxia is insufficient alveolar oxygen as a result of reduced atmospheric pressure – **Hypoxic hypoxia**. Hypoxia should not routinely be experienced in flight, and presence of hypoxia symptoms could indicate:

1. Ascent to altitude without supplementary oxygen.
2. Oxygen system failure.
3. Failure of cabin pressure.

Multiple types of hypoxia can coexist (e.g. pre-existing anaemic hypoxia caused by chronic illness can reduce threshold for hypoxic hypoxia symptoms to occur, impairing performance at a lower pressure altitude).

9.2 ALVEOLAR GAS EQUATION

Alveolar gas equation is used to calculate alveolar oxygen content:

$$P_AO_2 = FIO_2 \times \left(P_B - P_{H_2O}\right) - P_ACO_2 \times \left[FIO_2 + \frac{1 - FIO_2}{R}\right]$$

'Short' form :

$$P_AO_2 = PIO_2 - \frac{P_ACO_2}{R}$$

When $PIO_2 = FIO_2 \times \left(P_B - P_{H_2O}\right)$

where:

P_B	= Environmental pressure
PiO_2	= Partial pressure of inspired O_2
P_AO_2	= Alveolar partial pressure of O_2
P_ACO_2	= Alveolar partial pressure of CO_2
FiO_2	= Fraction of inspired O_2 (0.21 at sea level)
R	= Respiratory ratio (0.8 at rest with normal diet)
P_{H2O}	= Water vapour pressure at 37°C, this is constant at 47 mmHg

Ascent to altitude causes reduction in P_B and therefore P_AO_2 reduced; note that arterial partial pressure (P_aO_2) may be up to 8–10 mmHg (1–1.3 kPa) lower than P_AO_2 due to venous shunts from bronchial veins.

WATER VAPOUR PRESSURE

Alveolar water vapour pressure remains constant with ascent to altitude, and so becomes increasingly important component of alveolar content (see Figure 9.1).

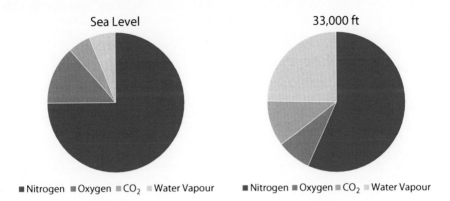

Figure 9.1 Chart showing increasing relative contribution of water vapour to the alveolar gas components from sea level ($P_B = 760$ mmHg) to 33,000 ft ($P_B = 196$ mmHg).

9.3 HYPOXIC VENTILATORY RESPONSE

Hypoxic ventilatory response (HVR) is a reflex which increases ventilatory drive in an attempt to maintain oxygen levels when P_AO_2 <55–60 mmHg (7.3–8.0 kPa):

- Fall in P_AO_2 detected in peripheral chemoreceptors (mainly carotid but also aortic body).
- HVR reduces P_ACO_2 through hyperventilation, enabling fractional concentration of O_2 within alveolus to increase.
- Subsequent fall in P_AO_2 is less than expected for given reduction in P_B (see Figure 9.2).

9.4 HYPERVENTILATION

Hyperventilation is defined as breathing in excess of metabolic needs, eliminating more carbon dioxide than is produced, to produce hypocapnia. Normal $P_ACO_2 = 35–45$ mmHg (4.7–6.0 kPa). CO_2 tension significantly influences the body's pH levels; there is a conflict between needing to maintain adequate P_AO_2 and normal acid-base balance. HVR is a normal response to hypoxia when P_AO_2 <55–60 mmHg (7.3–8.0 kPa); in aviation, hyperventilation may also occur in response to:

- Anxiety.
- Pressure breathing.
- Vibration.
- Motion sickness.
- Pain.

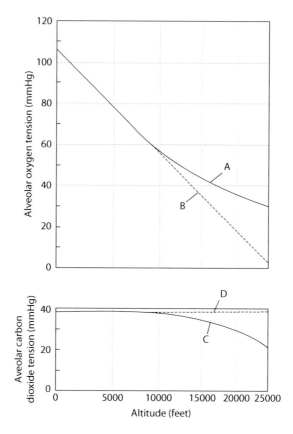

Figure 9.2 Ventilatory response to altitude; dotted line B = calculated reduction in P_AO_2 with ascent to altitude if ventilation is unchanged; solid line A is actual P_AO_2 seen as a result of Hypoxic Ventilatory Response; dotted line D = calculated P_ACO_2; solid line C is actual P_ACO_2 as CO_2 is off-gassed due to hyperventilation.

CEREBRAL BLOOD FLOW

Hypocapnia associated with hyperventilation causes cerebral vasoconstriction impairing cerebral perfusion.

- Cerebral blood flow (CBF) decreases by 2% for every 1 mmHg (0.13 kPa) decrease in P_ACO_2.
- At P_AO_2 above 45–50 mmHg (6–6.7 kPa) CBF is primarily determined by P_ACO_2.
- At P_AO_2 below 45 mmHg (6 kPa) cerebral hypoxic vasodilatation predominates (increasing CBF).
  - Therefore, CBF falls when breathing air up to around 15,000 ft but above this altitude CBF may increase.

SYMPTOMS AND SIGNS OF HYPOCAPNIA

Symptoms become apparent when P_ACO_2 falls below 25 mmHg (3.3 kPa):

- Dizziness.
- Paraesthesia.

- Muscle contraction.
- Hyper-reflexia.
- Visual impairment – flashing lights and hallucinations.
- Unconsciousness (<15 mmHg, 2 kPa).

Symptoms of hyperventilation can be similar to hypoxia – in the aviation setting, safest to assume symptoms may be due to hypoxia and to perform emergency drills.

9.5 PHYSIOLOGICAL RESPONSES TO ACUTE HYPOXIA

OVER SECONDS TO MINUTES

- Activation of carotid body chemoreceptors (see Figure 9.3).
- Increased pulmonary ventilation.
- Increased cardiac output.
- Peripheral vasodilatation (but little change in systemic blood pressure due to increased cardiac output).
- Increased cerebral blood flow (but nb influence of reduced P_ACO_2 may cause decreased central blood flow).
- Pulmonary vasoconstriction.

OVER MINUTES TO HOURS

- Switch from aerobic to anaerobic metabolism (impairment of mitochondrial respiration, increased anaerobic glycolysis).
- Upregulation of genes encoding glycolytic enzymes, erythropoietin, VEGF; mediated in large part by action of hypoxia-inducible factor-1 (HIF-1).

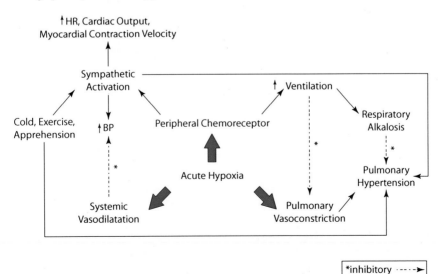

Figure 9.3 Physiological effects of acute hypoxia.

9.6 HAEMOGLOBIN

- Oxygen combines reversibly with haemoglobin (Hb) to form oxyhaemoglobin:
  - Each Hb molecule consists of four subunits, each containing a polypeptide chain (globin) attached to an oxygen binding haem group containing an iron atom.
- Normal sea level P_AO_2 is approximately 100 mmHg (13.3 kPa) and oxygen saturation (S_AO_2) 97%.
- Shape of oxygen dissociation curve (see Figure 9.4) favours oxygen uptake in the lungs and delivery to the tissues.
- Oxygen dissociation curve forms a plateau above about 60 mmHg (8 kPa) resulting in S_AO_2>90%:
  - Therefore, relatively little fall in S_AO_2 up to 10,000 ft PA (equivalent to 60 mmHg arterial oxygen tension).
  - Above 10,000 ft PA, steep part of curve causes large fall in S_AO_2 with increasing altitude.
- Raising P_AO_2 at sea level by hyperventilation or breathing oxygen can only add a small amount of dissolved oxygen.
- Hyperventilation may impair cerebral oxygen delivery because reduced arterial PCO_2 causes cerebral blood flow to fall (see 9.4).

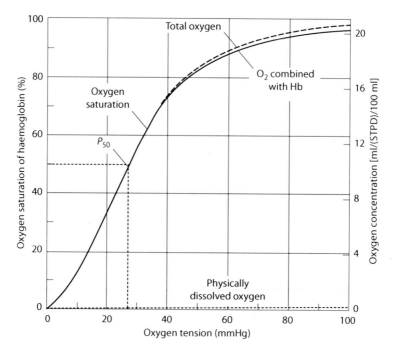

Figure 9.4 Oxygen dissociation curve of blood.

Bohr effect:

- Oxygen affinity of Hb reduced by:
  - Increased PCO_2.

- Increased [H+].
- Increased temperature.
- Increased 2,3 DPG.
- These changes occur in metabolizing tissues and aid oxygen unloading; changes reversed in lungs enhancing oxygen uptake.

9.7 TISSUE OXYGEN TENSION

- Tissue oxygen tension depends on oxygen tension in capillary blood.
- Shape of oxygen dissociation curve means that, at altitude, extraction of same volume of oxygen from blood causes a smaller fall in capillary oxygen tension than when at sea level (see Figure 9.5):
  - This minimises the arteriovenous oxygen tension difference.
  - Protects tissues from low oxygen tension.

9.8 SYMPTOMS AND SIGNS OF HYPOXIA

UP TO 10,000 FT

- Impaired light sensitivity (reduced acuity in low light).
- Performance of novel tasks may be impaired.

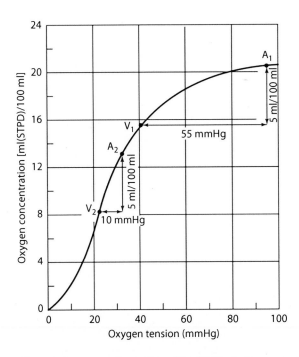

Figure 9.5 Oxygen dissociation curve. Extraction of 5 ml/100 ml of oxygen at 18,000 ft (A$_2$) results in a smaller arteriovenous difference (A$_2$-V$_2$) than at sea level (A$_1$-V$_1$), which is protective for tissues.

10,000–15,000 FT

- Physical work capacity reduced.
- Skilled tasks impaired.
- Headache.

ABOVE 15,000 FT

- Light intensity appears reduced.
- Narrowed peripheral vision.
- Loss of critical judgement.
- Impaired reaction time and coordination.
- Fatigue.
- Disinhibition.
- Personality change.
- Apprehension.
- Euphoria.
- Memory loss.
- Sensory changes.
- Air hunger.
- Nausea.
- Cyanosis (depending on skin pigment).
- Symptoms and signs associated with hyperventilation.

Above 20,000 ft breathing air, hypoxia may lead rapidly (see Section 9.10) to unconsciousness, hypoxic convulsions and ultimately death. At all altitudes, there is significant individual variation in symptom and sign presentation.

9.9 FACTORS INCREASING SUSCEPTIBILITY TO ACUTE HYPOXIA

- Higher altitude (see Chapter 13).
- Longer time.
- Greater rate of decompression (see Chapter 13).
- Increased exercise level (red blood cell transit time in pulmonary capillary reduced from 0.75 sec at rest to 0.25 sec on exercise; at altitude leads to failure to equilibrate with alveolar gas; alveolar-arterial oxygen tension difference increases from 8 mmHg at rest to 16–20 mmHg during exercise at moderate altitude).
- Increased cold (shivering increases O_2 requirement).
- Concurrent illness.
- Fatigue.
- Drugs/alcohol.
- Smoking (increased carbon monoxide level adversely affects blood oxygen carrying capacity).

9.10 TIME OF USEFUL CONSCIOUSNESS (TUC)

Period during which affected individual retains ability to take corrective actions.

Very large individual variation caused ventilatory response, age, physical fitness, degree of training to hypoxia, rate of decompression; figures should be used as a rough guide only due to very high individual variability (Table 9.1).

9.11 OXYGEN PARADOX

- Sudden restoration of alveolar oxygen tension may cause a transient worsening of severity hypoxia symptoms and signs for 15–60 sec.
- Usually mild; occasionally may produce clonic spasms and even loss of consciousness.
- Mechanisms undetermined:
  - Usually occurs in subjects who have become hypocapnic during hypoxia.
  - Accompanied by arterial hypotension.
  - May be related to fall in peripheral resistance on restoration of normal arterial oxygen tension.
- Training of aircrew to continue using O_2 despite apparent worsening of symptoms is important.

9.12 PHYSIOLOGICALLY EQUIVALENT ALTITUDES

Physiologically equivalent altitudes are those at which the inspired (tracheal) oxygen tension is equal. For example, the partial pressure of O_2 in the inspired gas when breathing air at sea level is the same as that at 33,700 ft when breathing 100% O_2, and under these conditions, the altitudes can be considered physiologically equivalent.

Table 9.1 Times of useful consciousness at various altitudes following a change from breathing oxygen to breathing air

PRESSURE ALTITUDE (ft)	TIME OF USEFUL CONSCIOUSNESS
25,000	3–5 min
28,000	2.5–3 min
30,000	1–2 min
35,000	30–60 sec
40,000	15–20 sec
43,000	9–12 sec
50,000	9–12 sec

9.13 OPERATIONAL SIGNIFICANCE OF HYPOXIA

Hypoxia generally recognised to be the most serious physiological hazard of flight at altitude, in part due to its insidious presentation. Hypoxia effects encountered at low altitudes (see Chapter 11), such as reduced visual acuity, contrast sensitivity and physical work capacity, can affect crew effectiveness.

10

Prevention of hypoxia

Contents

10.1 APPROACHES TO HYPOXIA PREVENTION

- Restrict permitted altitude of aircraft (e.g. balloons, light aircraft, gliders).
- Pressurise aircraft (e.g. most commercial aircraft).
- Use oxygen system (e.g. military fast jet in conjunction with pressurisation, aircraft conducting parachute drop).

10.2 USE OF OXYGEN SYSTEMS TO PREVENT HYPOXIA

- Oxygen supplied to crew from aircraft oxygen system, usually via oronasal mask.
- Proportion of oxygen in inspired gas must be increased on ascent to preserve P_AO_2.
- Ideal physiological target is for P_AO_2 to be maintained at equivalent of sea level value.
- This may be technically challenging: an acceptable degree of hypoxia is often tolerated (see next section).

MINIMUM ACCEPTABLE CONCENTRATION OF OXYGEN

- Inspired oxygen concentration required to maintain P_AO_2 equivalent to sea level breathing air ($P_AO_2 = 103$ mmHg; 13.7 kPa) is shown in Figure 10.1. Also shown are

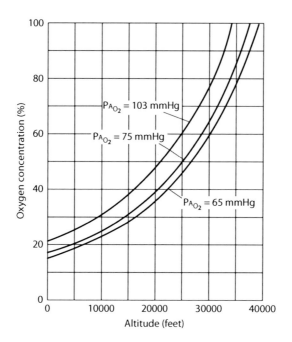

Figure 10.1 Inspired oxygen concentration required to maintain P_AO_2 equivalent to sea level ($P_AO_2 = 103$ mmHg; 13.7 kPa), 5000 ft ($P_AO_2 = 75$ mmHg; 10 kPa) and 8000 ft ($P_AO_2 = 65$ mmHg; 8.7 kPa) breathing air.

equivalents of 5000 ft ($P_AO_2 = 75$ mmHg; 10 kPa) and 8000 ft ($P_AO_2 = 65$ mmHg; 8.7 kPa).

- Note that 100% oxygen can only provide sea level equivalent up to 33,700 ft.
- Primary limitation preventing supply of O_2 to meet sea level P_AO_2 equivalent is aircraft capacity (i.e. amount of O_2 that needs to be carried). If P_AO_2 is less than sea level value, disadvantages are:
  - Mild degree of hypoxia associated with $P_AO_2 = 75$ mmHg (10 kPa) may still impair ability to recall recently learned procedures.
  - Significant performance impairment with mild exercise (e.g. aircraft rear crew duties) as P_AO_2 reduces.
  - Lower safety margin in event of mask leak:
    - If O_2 system designed to provide $P_AO_2 = 80$ mmHg (10.7 kPa, approximately 5000 ft equivalent) at 25,000 ft, inward leak equal to half pulmonary ventilation would reduce P_AO_2 from 80 mmHg (10.7 kPa) to 65 mmHg (8 kPa) – equivalent to breathing air at 8000 ft.
    - If O_2 system designed to maintain $P_AO_2 = 65$ mmHg (8.7 kPa, 8000 ft equivalent), then inward leak equal to half pulmonary ventilation would reduce from P_AO_2 to 40 mmHg (5.3 kPa) – equivalent to breathing air at 16,000 ft, causing significant hypoxia.
- Generally, oxygen system designed to deliver sea level P_AO_2 equivalent, or not below $P_AO_2 = 80$ mmHg (10.7 kPa).

- Protection above 33,700 ft breathing 100% O_2 will not provide sea level equivalent ($P_AO_2 = 54$ mmHg at 40,000 ft); positive pressure breathing required above these altitudes (see Chapter 13).
- In short-term use, P_AO_2 lower than sea level equivalent may be acceptable:
  - In military aircraft $P_AO_2 = 30$ mmHg acceptable for short-duration emergency use if 100% O_2 delivered within 2 sec.
  - For commercial flight crew $P_AO_2 = 75$ mmHg acceptable for emergency use for a few minutes; $P_AO_2 = 50$ mmHg acceptable for seated passengers.
  - In civilian parachute drops without supplemental oxygen up to 15,000 ft.
- In pressurised transport aircraft, crew and passengers are routinely exposed to up to 8000 ft (65 mmHg; 8 kPa).
- ICAO recommends oxygen use above 10,000 ft; however, national authority requirements may be less stringent (e.g. up to 14,000 ft permitted for up to 30 minutes without supplemental O_2).

MAXIMUM ACCEPTABLE CONCENTRATION OF OXYGEN

- In theory, possible to deliver 100% oxygen at all altitudes.
- Advantages:
  - Simple oxygen system.
  - Relatively cheap.
- Disadvantages:
  - Aircraft unlikely to be able to carry sufficient O_2.
  - 100% O_2 may cause respiratory tract irritation, delayed otic barotrauma, acceleration atelectasis (see Chapter 15).

OXYGEN SCHEDULE

- Aircraft oxygen system should automatically provide correct inspired oxygen (with remaining gas composed mainly of nitrogen) for cabin altitude – this is the oxygen schedule.
- Achieved by mixing with ambient air or control of oxygen generation concentration (see Chapter 11). Range of values permitted due to variations in systems and requirements; typical range of values permitted in oxygen schedule shown in Figure 10.2.

10.3 PERFORMANCE REQUIREMENTS OF OXYGEN SYSTEMS

Oxygen system must deliver adequate flow of breathing gas to prevent hypoxia and avoid other physiological consequences (e.g. hyperventilation). Main requirements relating to delivery of oxygen flow are:

PULMONARY VENTILATION

- Human pulmonary ventilation (minute volume of breathing gas) determined by metabolic rate; modified by hypoxia, excitement, anxiety, etc.
- Highest aviation pulmonary ventilation demands are related to running to aircraft (e.g. in emergency response aircraft), moving around in cabin (e.g. loadmaster) or physical exercise of anti-G straining manoeuvre (see Chapter 16).

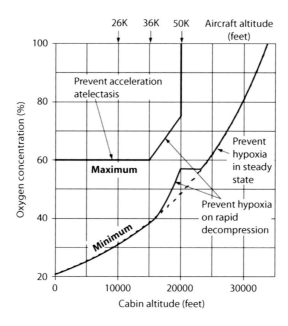

Figure 10.2 Example oxygen schedule found in fast jet aircraft.

- Seated active aircrew may require up to 50 L (atmospheric temperature and pressure, dry [ATPD])/min at sea level; system must be designed to meet this level for all crew members.
- Gas expansion at altitude means sea level gas delivery is usually most demanding application.
- Key implication is how much oxygen an aircraft needs to carry to meet demands of all crew (depends on expected altitude profile).

PEAK FLOW

- During breathing cycle, flow of gas in and out of respiratory tract changes very rapidly.
- Oxygen equipment must be designed to meet these changes while imposing minimum resistance to breathing.
- Speech, exercise and anti-G straining are the most demanding conditions (see Figure 10.3).
- In general, oxygen equipment should be designed to meet inspiratory peak flows of up to 200 L (ATPD)/min, with a maximum rate of change of 20 L (ATPD)/s/s at these peak flows.
- Oxygen systems which provide inadequate inspiratory flow may lead to inboard mask leakage and dilution of inspired oxygen; inadequate inspiratory or expiratory flow may increase breathing resistance and work of breathing leading to hyperventilation.

BREATHING RESISTANCE

- Increase in external inspiratory or expiratory breathing resistance may change rate and depth of breathing.

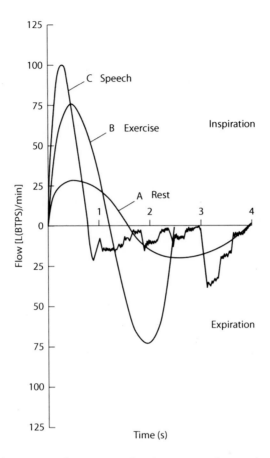

Figure 10.3 Typical respiratory flow patterns for aircrew seated at rest (trace A); aircrew moving about an aircraft (trace B); and aircrew speaking aloud while seated at rest (trace C). The flow throughout a single respiratory cycle is shown for each of the three conditions. (BTPS: body temperature and pressure, saturated with water vapour.)

- Much individual variation in response to increased breathing resistance.
- May result in hyper- or hypoventilation with hypo- or hypercapnia.
- Increases total respiratory work per minute.
- Decreases maximum ventilatory capacity.
- Can result in subjective disturbances (see Figure 10.4).
- To minimise effects, total changes of pressure in mask during respiratory cycle should not exceed:
    - 3.7 mmHg (500 Pa) during quiet breathing (peak inspiratory and expiratory flows of 30 L [ATPS]/min), or
    - 8 mmHg (1.1 kPa) during heavy breathing (peak inspiratory and expiratory flows of 110 L [ATPS]/min).

DEAD SPACE

- To avoid rebreathing of carbon dioxide, effective additional dead space imposed by use of an oxygen mask should be no more than about 150 mL.

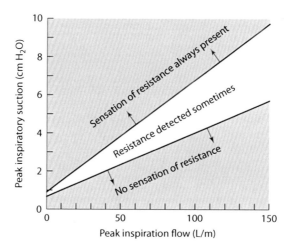

Figure 10.4 Relationship between peak inspiratory flow and peak inspiratory suction which gives rise to a sensation of breathing resistance.

- Following rapid decompression, amount of gas trapped in dead space must be small to prevent delay in inspiration of high concentration oxygen.
  - Any gas trapped with lower concentration of oxygen must be rapidly dispersed, not breathed.

10.4 AVIATION OXYGEN MASKS

REQUIREMENTS

- Stable and comfortable to wear for long periods.
- No skin irritation.
- Small.
- Low dead space.
- Fit a variety of facial sizes and shapes.
- Seal effectively against the skin of the face.

VALVES

- Inspiratory valve high up in mask to minimise obstruction by debris and to limit contact with moist expired air:
  - Ice-guard is fitted to its internal surface to provide further protection against debris and moisture.
- Expiratory (outlet) valve usually in lowest part to allow sweat and saliva to drain.
- External surface of expiratory valve can be protected against low temperature by an extension of the rubber facepiece trapping warm expired air just beyond the valve.

FUNCTIONS

- Provide breathing gas supply and remove expirate.
- Carry microphone for communication system.
- Protect face from bird-strike, canopy fracture and ejection windblast forces.

TYPES OF MASKS

- Passenger emergency mask:
    - For short-term use only, does not meet all the requirements listed above.
    - Supplied with continuous flow of oxygen.
    - Incorporates small reservoir bag (rebreathing or non-rebreathing) (see Figure 10.5).
    - May have simple inspiratory valve.
    - Usually stowed in overhead compartments.
    - Drops down automatically if the cabin altitude exceeds 13,000–15,000 ft.
    - Provides sufficient oxygen for most commercial aircraft decompression scenarios.
- Passenger therapeutic oxygen mask:
    - Simple continuous-flow systems, usually of the rebreathing reservoir type.
    - Pulsed-dose oxygen supply now sometimes used.
- Aircrew quick-don mask:
    - Oronasal emergency mask for quick-don by crew of pressurised large aircraft.
    - Usually uses inflatable straps for rapid use.
    - Provides access to 100% oxygen for emergency descent.
- Aircrew pressure demand mask:
    - For routine use in military fast jet, for example.
    - Able to accommodate breathing pressure above ambient (see Chapter 13) by compensation of back pressure on expiratory valve, to prevent inadvertent valve opening.
    - Achieved by pressure in the inlet port of the mask transmitted to the valve plate on the downstream side of the expiratory valve (see Figure 10.6).

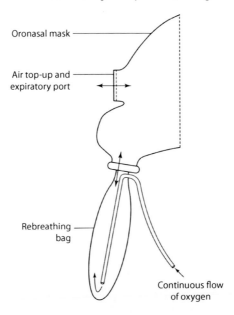

Oronasal mask

Air top-up and expiratory port

Rebreathing bag

Continuous flow of oxygen

Figure 10.5 Simple rebreathing reservoir oxygen mask. First portion of the expirate fills bag; contents of bag pass into the respiratory tract at the beginning of inspiration, followed by continuous flow of oxygen supplemented with air drawn in through the air inlet port.

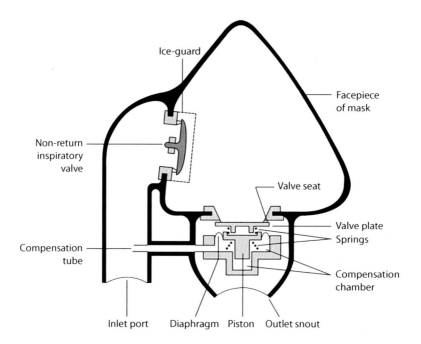

Figure 10.6 Valve system of a pressure demand oronasal mask. The inspiratory valve is a simple non-return device, with a mesh cover that acts as an ice-guard. The expiratory valve is compensated, the pressure of gas in the inlet port also being applied along the compensation tube and through a diaphragm and piston to the external surface of the expiratory valve plate.

- Anti-suffocation valve usually also fitted that opens when pressure within mask cavity falls to 9–13 mmHg (1.2–1.7 kPa) below ambient pressure, to prevent suffocation on gas supply failure or drowning on water entry.

10.5 ACTIONS ON EVENT OF SUSPECTED HYPOXIA

- Check all oxygen hoses and connections; toggle/tighten mask.
- Select 100% oxygen preferably from alternative gas source (to exclude contaminated supply); monitor flow and contents.
- Control rate and depth of breathing.
- Descend to below 10,000 ft cabin pressure altitude.
- Land as soon as practicable.

The pressure cabin and oxygen systems

Contents

11.1 FUNCTION OF PRESSURE CABIN

- Pressurisation of cabin helps to minimise:
  - Fall in alveolar PO_2 with ascent to altitude:
    - Slower reactions to novel tasks breathing air at 8000 ft pressure altitude.
    - Maximum permissible cabin altitude in commercial aircraft is 8000 ft, but often lower in modern aircraft (e.g. 6000 ft).
    - 8000 ft generally considered to be physiologically acceptable for passengers and crew.
    - Exposure to 8000 ft for prolonged period may present problems for travellers with cardiovascular disease.
    - Above 8000 ft cabin altitude, supplemental oxygen systems generally used.
  - Risk of decompression sickness:
    - See Chapter 8.
  - Expansion of gastrointestinal gas:
    - See Chapter 7.

11.2 HOW DOES IT WORK?

- Air drawn from outside aircraft, compressed, and delivered within cabin; desired pressure maintained by controlling air outflow from cabin.

- Modern aircraft have air recirculation systems to improve fuel efficiency; generally about 50% of air in commercial aircraft cabin recirculated.
- Risk of infectious disease minimised through high efficiency particulate air (HEPA) filters.
- Above 80,000 ft and in space pressurising gases must be carried within vehicle.

11.3 DESIGN OF PRESSURISATION SYSTEM

Design of pressurisation system should consider:

- Pressurisation schedule:
    - Ideally should maintain cabin at sea level pressure but impractical due to weight of equipment and power requirements.
    - Differential pressure – difference between the absolute pressure within aircraft and that of atmosphere immediately outside.
    - There is increasing risk of decompression injury with increasing differential pressure (see Chapter 12).
    - In commercial aircraft, for comfort and because risk of damage is low, high differential pressure cabin used (59.5–62 kPa [8.6–9 lb/in²]).
    - In combat aircraft, with increased risk of damage and need to minimise weight, low differential pressure cabin used (24–36.2 kPa [3.5–5.25 lb/in²]).
    - Pressure varies automatically with aircraft altitude (but may be set by crew in non-combat aircraft).
    - In combat aircraft, pressure schedule may include an unpressurised zone (below 8000 ft) and an isobaric zone (cabin pressure constant over a range of altitudes).
- Rate of change of pressure during ascent and descent:
    - In military aircraft, maximum permitted rate of 14 kPa (2 lb/in²)/min to prevent barotrauma.
    - In commercial aircraft, maximum recommended rate of 1.7 kPa (0.25 lb/in²)/min (approximately 500 ft/min) due to passenger inexperience.
    - Typical rate for commercial aircraft is 1 kPa (0.15 lb/in²)/min (approximately 300 ft/min).
- Magnitude of effects following cabin pressurisation failure:
    - See Chapter 12.
- Quality of cabin air:
    - Introduction of recirculating air has prompted interest in cabin air quality.
    - Infectious diseases most likely to be spread by close proximity; recirculation has negligible effect.
    - Low humidity may cause nasal dryness.
    - Concern over contaminants (atomised engine oils or other chemicals) raised but evidence not strong enough to link with disease.

11.4 OXYGEN SYSTEMS

Oxygen systems provide protection against some fundamental hazards of flight: may be for routine use (Primary system) or only used in emergency (Secondary system) depending on design and role of aircraft. Primary system usually has backup system to mitigate risk of failure. Oxygen systems comprise: oxygen source; contents indication gauge; pipework; breathing regulator; oronasal mask. International regulations govern conditions for use.

FUNCTIONS OF AN AIRCRAFT OXYGEN SYSTEM

- Prevention of hypoxia. Civilian aircraft oxygen requirements specified as tracheal inspired PO_2 (P_iO_2; easier to test); military requirement is alveolar PO_2 (P_AO_2; harder to measure but more accurate). P_AO_2 should be maintained between 60–103 mmHg; lower levels of P_AO_2 (but not below 30 mmHg) may be tolerated for short-term emergency use.
- Removal of expirate. Prevents build-up of CO_2 (potential physiological effects) and H_2O vapour (potential misting of visors, freezing of valves).
- Protection against smoke and fumes. Prevents inhalation of toxins in aircraft fire, may also provide eye protection.
- Protection against decompression sickness. Reduces risk through denitrogenation including preoxygenation.
- Protection during escape. Supplies adequate oxygen to prevent loss of consciousness during high-altitude escape. Some military naval aircraft also provide protection during underwater escape.

THRESHOLD ALTITUDE FOR OXYGEN USE

In low differential pressure cabin (e.g. military fighter), oxygen system typically used all the time from ground level (Primary system). In high differential pressure cabin (e.g. commercial passenger aircraft) oxygen system only used during failure of pressurisation or smoke and fumes (Secondary system). In civilian unpressurised aircraft, oxygen typically used above 10,000 ft; unpressurised military aircraft may use oxygen at lower altitudes for better human performance.

Commercial aircraft regulated by (for example) Federal Aviation Authority Regulations (FAR 25, 121 and 135) and European Aviation Safety Authority Certification Specifications (EASA CS 25, 121 and 135). These regulations require that:

- Oxygen equipment must be available in all commercial aircraft that fly above 10,000 ft PA.
- If pressurised aircraft is capable of maintaining cabin altitude below 10,000 ft, oxygen must be available to:
  - Supply all crew and passengers if pressurisation fails above 15,000 ft for a specified interval.
  - Supply all crew and 10% of the passengers if pressurisation fails below 13,000 ft.
- In unpressurised aircraft, oxygen must be carried for continuous use by all occupants above 12,000 ft, and for continuous use by crew and 10% of passengers if >30 minutes between 10,000 and 12,000 ft.

Non-commercial aviation regulated by similar standards (e.g. EASA part-NCO). Typically, oxygen required for flight above 13,000 ft or flight above 10,000 ft for >30 minutes.

Military regulations provided in NATO STANAGs and AFIC Air Standards to facilitate interoperability. Military transport aircraft tend to follow civilian standards but have additional oxygen requirements, for example, for deliberate decompression to release parachutists.

CLASSES OF OXYGEN SYSTEM

Open circuit. Most aircraft oxygen systems are open circuit. Most or all of expired gas exhausts to environment. Relatively wasteful of breathing gas, but simplicity of design is major advantage. Oxygen flows from source via breathing regulator to user (usually via mask).

Closed circuit. Used in spacesuits, aircraft smoke hoods, diving and anaesthesia. More complex than open circuit as CO_2 and H_2O vapour must be removed; exhaled oxygen is rebreathed, but oxygen concentration control more complex. Bulkier and heavier than open circuit, but conserves oxygen.

11.5 SOURCES OF OXYGEN

GASEOUS OXYGEN

- System:
  - Usually carried in a number of steel cylinders at a pressure of 1,800 lb/in² (12,411 kPa) with associated pressure reducing valves and pipes.
- Common uses:
  - Crew emergency oxygen supply in commercial aircraft.
  - Routine crew supply in simple military aircraft.
  - Therapeutic oxygen supply for commercial flights.
- Advantages:
  - Simplest technical solution.
  - Widely available (logistics).
  - Available immediately after charging.
  - Little gas loss in storage.
- Disadvantages:
  - Weight and bulk.
  - Limited supply available on board.
  - Explosion risk (cylinders can be wire-wound to reduce risk).
- Oxygen quality requirements:
  - 99.5% oxygen.
  - Odourless.
  - Virtually free of any toxic substances (e.g. carbon monoxide concentration must be <0.002%).
  - Water content must not exceed 0.005 mg/L at STP to prevent icing.

LIQUID OXYGEN

- System:
  - Aircraft converter consists of an insulated container (see Figure 11.1), control valves and connecting pipes.
  - Liquid oxygen (LOX) cooled to –183°C.
  - Container insulated to prevent excessive warming, evaporation and pressure build-up.
  - Stabilisation of LOX to prevent temperature stratification/uneven delivery usually required, by slight elevation of liquid temperature.

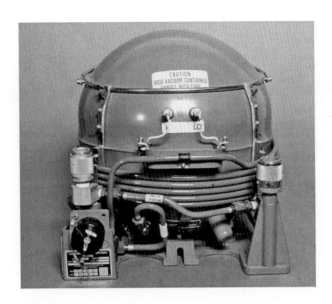

Figure 11.1 Typical liquid oxygen converter.

- Common uses:
  - Routine use in single and multi-crew military aircraft.
  - Routine use in military transport aircraft (e.g. by crew during parachute drops).
  - Becoming much less common due to the adoption of on-board oxygen generation.
- Advantages:
  - Light weight, low volume equipment.
  - 1 L LOX theoretically yields 840 L (NTP) gaseous O_2.
- Disadvantages:
  - 10% of supply lost every 24 hr through pressure relief.
  - Pressure fluctuations may affect gas delivery.
  - More complex logistics (LOX plant required).
  - LOX lost in transfer phases (less than 15% of O_2 transferred is available for use).
  - Potential for contamination by toxic materials from air used during compression and refrigeration; toxins do not evaporate at same rate as LOX (different boiling points) and can accumulate in LOX containers; contaminants may pass from container into breathing system in relatively high concentration.

ON-BOARD OXYGEN GENERATION (OBOG)

Two classes – air dependent, which needs flow of air from which to extract oxygen, and air independent which generates oxygen from other means without needing air source.

- Air independent OBOG:
  - Solid chemical storage (e.g. candle of $NaClO_3$ and Fe); exothermic reaction releases O_2. Typically used for passenger emergency supply or smoke-hood.

- – Advantages: Simple storage, unlimited shelf life, small bulk, no servicing requirement.
- – Disadvantages: Heat production, short duration of use.
  - Electrolysis of H_2O; produces hydrogen and oxygen (reverse fuel cell). Used in spaceflight. Large power requirement.
- Air dependent OBOG:
  - Pressure swing absorption technique used in molecular sieve oxygen generator (MSOC) (see Figure 11.2).
  - Zeolite beds absorb N_2; product gas contains maximum of 96% O_2 with 4% Ar.
  - Generator usually consists of two or more beds of molecular sieve material; engine bleed air passed through each in turn; one bed is depressurised and purged of nitrogen and other bed produces oxygen-enriched breathing gas; then alternates. Product gas supply continuous; small fluctuations minimised by use of plenum chamber.
  - Oxygen concentration of product gas controlled to match altitude requirement by varying cycle and purge time of bed in software.
- Common uses:
  - Single and multi-crew military aircraft.
  - Therapeutic oxygen on commercial aircraft.
- Advantages:
  - Small weight, volume, power requirement.
  - Unlimited source of oxygen.
  - Reduced need for ground oxygen logistics.
  - Reduced maintenance.
- Disadvantages:
  - Backup source of oxygen needed (in case of engine flameout or other fault).
  - 100% oxygen not produced.
  - Unable to respond to rapid changes in altitude (e.g. decompression).

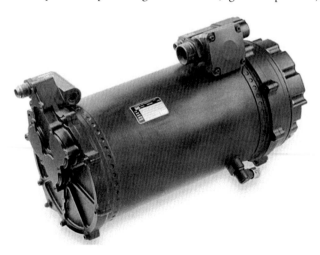

Figure 11.2 Advanced molecular sieve oxygen concentrator, in which three beds are arranged concentrically to reduce volume. (Photograph courtesy of Honeywell International Inc.)

- Water contamination can deactivate bed.
- Some concerns about hypoxia-like events in use; cause unknown.
- May not filter some contaminants (e.g. carbon monoxide) particularly if gas inlet pressure supply is low.

11.6 OXYGEN DELIVERY – CONSTANT FLOW SYSTEMS

- Types:
  - Direct flow: Regulator delivers O_2 from source to mask or nasal cannulae via hose. Mask has apertures through which cabin air drawn when the demanded inspiratory flow exceeds flow of oxygen from system. Very inefficient as oxygen flows to ambient during expiration (occupying 50–60% of total respiratory cycle time). Used for passenger therapeutic oxygen and simple bailout systems for combat aircraft.
  - Pulsed dose: Bolus of oxygen released when pressure fall (induced by inspiration) detected by regulator. Remainder of tidal breath met through inhalation of cabin air. Less wasteful than direct flow; can only respond to rate (not depth) of breathing. Used for helicopter, glider pilots and passenger therapeutic oxygen.
  - Rebreather: Oxygen is delivered continuously from regulator into reservoir bag. Mask has a single aperture with higher resistance than reservoir flow. At beginning of inspiration reservoir contents preferentially drawn into lungs before cabin air; first part of expirate (oxygen rich from dead space) fills reservoir. 50–70% less oxygen use with reservoir. Used for passenger emergency oxygen (2 L/min (NTP) is adequate for 20,000 ft) and therapeutic supply.
- Advantages:
  - Simple.
  - Low breathing resistance.
- Disadvantages:
  - Wasteful of breathing gas.
  - Unable to match varying breathing demand.
  - Unable to provide positive pressure breathing.
  - Risk of freezing.

11.7 OXYGEN DELIVERY – DEMAND SYSTEMS

- System:
  - Flow of gas from regulator varies directly with inspiratory demand of user.
  - Overcomes all the disadvantages of constant flow systems.
  - Flow of oxygen to mask from high-pressure supply is controlled by demand valve, which is held closed by demand valve spring. Reduction in pressure in demand chamber produced by inspiration displaces control diaphragm and opens demand valve.
  - Servo assistance allows miniaturisation.
  - Electronic regulators now available.
  - May be panel, seat or torso mounted.

- Air dilution:
  - For regulators with 100% gaseous oxygen or LOX supplies, air dilution (air-mix) mixes cabin air with oxygen to meet altitude requirement; adjusts automatically with altitude.
  - Suction or injection (Venturi) dilution techniques used.
  - Selector to provide 100% oxygen in emergency.
  - OBOG systems do not require air dilution (therefore simpler design).
- Pressure breathing:
  - Above 40,000 ft cabin altitude oxygen delivered above ambient pressure for adequate oxygenation.
  - Achieved by progressively loading control diaphragm of regulator (termed pressure demand regulator).

11.8 OXYGEN SYSTEM DESIGN CONSIDERATIONS

- Duplication – In low differential pressure cabins, alternative regulator and supply required in case of failure (standby not required where high-differential cabin pressure is primary source of protection).
- Automatic – All operation should be automatic (e.g. switch to emergency oxygen, pressure breathing).
- Gas temperature – Should be within 5°C of cabin temperature.
- Gas flow – Should be adequate for speech and anti-G straining in military fighter (e.g. up to 200 L/min).
- Concentration of N_2 should be sufficient to prevent acceleration atelectasis and oxygen ear (typically no less than 40% N_2).
- Safety pressure – Slight overpressure delivered to mask from ground level (OBOG systems) or 15,000 ft (conventional systems) to prevent inboard leakage from an inadequate seal to face.
- Press to test – Manually increases mask pressure (and counter-pressure garments) to assess mask seal and system integrity.
- Flow indication – Flow indicator ('doll's eye') used to diagnose system leaks and supply failure.
- Oxygen contents indication.
- Failure indication – Failure must be indicated immediately and clearly to user (e.g. by warning light or increase in breathing resistance).
- Compatibility of aircrew equipment – Breathing gas hose and mask should add minimum resistance to flow.

Loss of cabin pressure and rapid decompression

Contents

Key Facts

- Immediate decompression hazards:
    - Pulmonary barotrauma (with potential arterial gas embolism, pneumothorax, surgical emphysema).
    - Acute severe hypobaric hypoxia.
- Prolonged decompression hazards:
    - Decompression sickness.
    - Hypothermia, cold injury.
- Hazards depend on physics and time profile of pressure change; effectiveness of pulmonary ventilation; breathing gas composition before and after decompression.
- Ebullism may occur with decompression above Armstrong Limit (~63,000 ft).

Continued...

Continued...
- Rate of cabin decompression governed by:
  1. Pressure factor – Determined by ratio of initial cabin pressure to external ambient pressure.
  2. Dimensional factor – Determined by ratio of the cabin volume to area of decompression opening.
- Absolute differential pressure will determine severity of decompression with respect to gas expansion (e.g. risk of pulmonary barotrauma), worse with greater pressure difference.
- Absolute barometric pressure following decompression will determine physiological consequences (e.g. hypoxia, decompression sickness).

12.1 INTRODUCTION

- All cabin depressurisation needs immediate assessment and active management.
- Rapid/explosive cabin decompression is in-flight emergency:
  - Risk to life.
  - Risk of loss of air/space vehicle.
  - Needs immediate action.

Main hazards:

1. Pulmonary barotrauma.
2. Severe hypobaric hypoxia.
3. Decompression sickness.
4. Cold.

12.2 BACKGROUND

- Pre-planned, controlled decompression can be safe, providing effective protective measures and procedures used.
- Gradual, covert depressurisation may present insidious/progressive hypobaric hypoxia that risks cognitive impairment and loss of consciousness.
- Abrupt, rapid decompression threatens pulmonary barotrauma due to gas expansion and immediate profound hypoxia with loss of consciousness.
- Exposure to extreme hypobaria incompatible with life.

12.3 CAUSES OF AIRCRAFT CABIN DECOMPRESSION

- Intentional depressurisation.
- Failure of pressurisation systems.
- Loss of structural integrity.

DELIBERATE FULL DEPRESSURISATION/DECOMPRESSION

- High-differential cabins:
  - For high-altitude payload delivery (e.g. cargo, parachutists).
  - To purge cabin of smoke or fumes.

- As a precaution in event of cracked transparency.
- In response to threat of sabotage.
- Low-differential cabins: Explosive decompression upon ejection.

FAILURE OF PRESSURISATION SYSTEMS

- Reduced inflow:
  - Engine/compressor failure/flameout; engine 'idle' setting.
  - Inlet valves stuck closed or faulty.
  - Failure of pressurisation/conditioning systems.
  - Failure of control systems (e.g. computer failure).
- Excess outflow:
  - Failure to initiate cabin pressurisation (i.e. human error).
    - Helios Airways Flight 522; 14 Aug 2005; loss of Boeing 737–300; 121 fatalities; aircraft ascent with pressurisation system in 'manual' mode but assumed to be in 'automatic'; failure to respond to alarms or passenger mask 'drop down'.
  - Discharge valves stuck open or faulty.
    - Soyuz 11; 30 Jun 1971; pressure valve failure on re-entry at an altitude of 168 km; three fatalities.

LOSS OF STRUCTURAL INTEGRITY

- Leaking door, hatch and canopy seals.
- Loss or failure of door, hatch, window or canopy.
  - British Airways Flight 5390; 10 Jun 1990; BAC 1-11; windscreen failure with aircraft captain blown partially from the aircraft; no fatalities.
- External impact (e.g. bird strike, mid-air collision).
- Explosive damage (e.g. fuel system, oxygen cylinder, engine failure).
  - TWA Flight 800; 17 Jul 1996; Boeing 747-100; probable fuel tank explosion; 230 fatalities.
- Structural failure (mechanical fatigue, corrosion, excessive stress).
  - Aloha Airlines Flight 243; 28 Apr 1988; Boeing 737-297; loss of fuselage section due to metal fatigue with explosive decompression; landed safely with, remarkably, just a single fatality (flight attendant blown from aircraft).
- Sabotage or enemy action.
  - Pan Am Flight 103; 21 Dec 1988; Boeing 747-121; in-flight terrorist sabotage; 270 fatalities including 11 on the ground (residents of Lockerbie, Scotland).

12.4 LIKELIHOOD OF DECOMPRESSION

COMMERCIAL AIRCRAFT

- Global incidence of decompression of commercial passenger aircraft is low (30–40 events per year).
- Many instigated by crew as precautionary measure (e.g. smoke/fumes).

MILITARY AIRCRAFT

- More frequent decompression in military than in civilian flying.
- Typically 2–3 events per 100,000 flying hours.

PRIVATE AIRCRAFT

- Private aircraft (e.g. business jets and pressurised light aircraft) also vulnerable:
  - Learjet 24 accident; Dec 1988; overflew destination and crashed after entering Mexican airspace; two fatalities including Susan Reynolds, a NASA astronaut candidate.
  - Learjet 25 accident; Oct 1999; aircraft failed to respond to air traffic control and crashed after running out of fuel; six fatalities including professional golfer Payne Stewart.

12.5 PHYSICS OF RAPID DECOMPRESSION

During rapid decompression, pressure falls quickly at first and then more slowly as pressures equilibrate. Major factors influencing rate and time of decompression are:
  - Cabin volume – Larger cabin will take longer to depressurise.
  - Orifice size – Effective area of orifice may be less than geometric area.
  - Cabin absolute pressure at start of depressurisation.
  - Ambient absolute pressure external to cabin.
- The time of decompression is proportional to:
  - Ratio of cabin volume to defect area.
  - Ratio of initial cabin pressure to external barometric pressure.
- Rate of decompression can be predicted by:
  - Fliegner's Equation: Simplest model; gives good approximations for larger aircraft cabins.

  $$t = 0.22 \frac{V}{A} \sqrt{\frac{P-B}{B}}$$

- Haber-Clamann Model: More complex, but more accurate.

$$t_c = \frac{V}{AC}$$

$$t = t_c \left[1.68 \ln\left(\frac{P}{B}\right) + 0.27 \right]$$

where (all units imperial):
  t_c = time constant for cabin
  V = cabin volume
  A = area of opening
  C = speed of sound
  t = time of decompression
  P = initial cabin pressure
  B = external ambient pressure

12.6 RATE OF DECOMPRESSION

- Gradual decompression:
    - Most likely due to failure of environmental conditioning system.
    - Any suggestion of cabin depressurisation (e.g. ears 'popping' unexpectedly) should alert crew to possibility of covert hypoxia.
- Rapid decompression (see Figure 12.1):
    - Airliner: Explosive decompression requires catastrophic loss of structural integrity; most likely locations are doors, hatches and transparencies; passenger windows intentionally small to limit rate of cabin decompression.
    - Military fast jet: Loss of canopy due to damage or ejection; if defect faces direction of travel (e.g. after canopy bird strike), pressure inside cabin may be higher than external; if air flows across defect, may cause aerodynamic suction reducing cabin pressure below external barometric pressure.

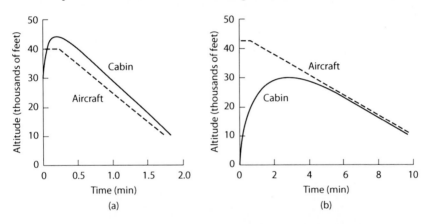

Figure 12.1 Effects of rapid descent of aircraft and pressure of aerodynamic suction on cabin altitude after failure of cabin pressurisation. (a) Decompression due to large defect (aerodynamic suction causes cabin altitude to exceed aircraft altitude). (b) Decompression through relatively small defect; descent of aircraft is started 30 sec after beginning of decompression.

12.7 HAZARDS OF RAPID DECOMPRESSION

- Pulmonary barotrauma (see Chapter 7).
- Profound hypoxia (see Chapter 13).
- Ebullism:
    - At 63,000 ft pressure altitude, ambient pressure (47 mmHg) approximates water vapour pressure at 37°C (human body temperature).
    - This altitude known as Armstrong Limit.
    - Liquid water boils at this temperature and theoretically so would body liquids.
    - In practice, body surfaces usually below 37°C and circulating blood at higher pressure due to haemodynamic pressure and hydrostatic pressure gradient.
    - Unprotected exposure to extreme altitude above Armstrong Limit should be anticipated to be rapidly fatal, although accidental human exposures and animal experiments indicate that brief exposure is survivable.

12.8 INADVERTENT DECOMPRESSION–IMMEDIATE ACTIONS (EMERGENCY DRILLS)

IMMEDIATE ACTION DRILLS FOLLOWING CABIN DECOMPRESSION

1. 100% oxygen.
2. Descent (ideally to ≤10,000 ft equivalent pressure altitude).
3. Recover the aircraft.

COMMERCIAL AIRLINERS

- Flight deck crew required to be able to access emergency oxygen within 5 sec.
- Usually via full-face, quick-don mask which automatically delivers emergency oxygen.
- Crew oxygen supply will be sufficient to ensure that elevated terrain may be crossed safely without risk of cognitive impairment.
- Passengers receive emergency oxygen from drop-down masks; the duration of supply is limited but is intended to maintain consciousness during emergency descent to safe transit altitude.

MILITARY TRANSPORT AIRCRAFT

- May be decompressed intentionally at altitude.
- Will be equipped with oxygen systems for crew to enable denitrogenation to prevent decompression sickness, and prevention of hypoxia.
- Decompression rate will be controlled to avoid any risk of barotrauma.

MILITARY FAST JET AIRCRAFT

- Equipped with life support systems that should automatically deliver emergency 100% oxygen (± positive pressure breathing) in event of cabin decompression.
- Immediate descent reduces hypoxia risk and need for pressure breathing (below 40,000 ft).
- At very high altitudes (approaching 60,000 ft) maximum breathing pressures using partial pressure assemblies limited to 72 mmHg by neck discomfort and fatigue.
- Above 60,000 ft altitude full pressure suits required to provide protection (e.g. U2 aircraft).

CHAPTER 13

High-altitude protection

Contents

13.1 PROFOUND HYPOXIA

- Abrupt decompression and consequent gas expansion cause an almost instantaneous fall in partial pressure of gases within the lung.
- Delivery of 100% oxygen immediately upon decompression (under positive pressure if above 40,000 ft) essential for preservation of consciousness (Figure 13.1).
- Loss of consciousness likely if P_AO_2 falls below 30 mmHg (4 kPa) (see Figure 13.2).

BREATHING GAS REQUIREMENTS

- Rapid decompression from 8000 to 40,000 ft over 1.6 sec while breathing air results in loss of consciousness within 20–25 sec.
- Even immediate delivery of 100% oxygen at the moment of decompression may be insufficient to prevent cognitive impairment.
- To protect against profound hypoxia, a sufficiently high concentration of oxygen must be present in breathing gas prior to decompression.
- At high cabin altitudes, this means oxygen concentration in inspired gas will be higher than that required to prevent hypoxia under steady state conditions (see Figure 13.3).

SEVERITY OF HYPOXIA FOLLOWING DECOMPRESSION

Severity of hypoxia experienced following rapid decompression will depend on:
- P_AO_2 prior to decompression:
  - Initial cabin pressure altitude.
  - Initial fractional inspired oxygen concentration.
- Final cabin pressure altitude:
  - Altitude range over which decompression occurs.
- Time course of decompression:
  - Rate of change of ambient pressure.

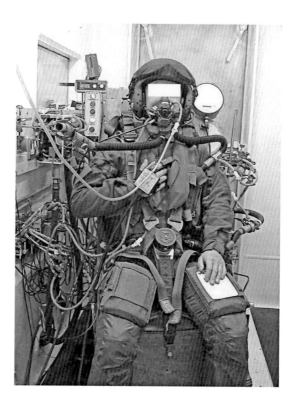

Figure 13.1 Volunteer research participant instrumented in preparation for rapid decompression to high equivalent pressure altitude in a decompression (hypobaric) chamber for the purpose of life support system test and evaluation.

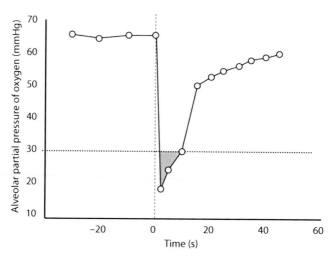

Figure 13.2 Alveolar partial pressure of oxygen following rapid decompression to high altitude. Following decompression at time 0, there is a precipitous decrease in alveolar oxygen tension; any fall in alveolar partial pressure of oxygen below 30 mmHg (4 kPa) threatens loss of consciousness; if the integral of the curve below this threshold (shaded) exceeds 140 mmHg/s, then loss of consciousness is very likely.

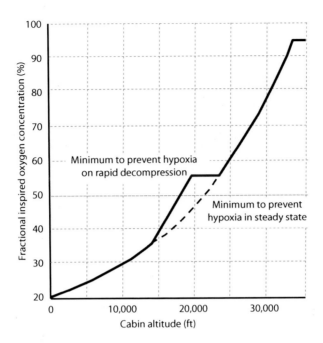

Figure 13.3 Inspired oxygen concentration requirement against cabin altitude for a generic fast jet aircraft; 'notched' area of schedule represents increased oxygen concentration needed to prevent unacceptable hypoxia in the event of rapid cabin decompression.

- Time taken to deliver 100% oxygen to lung.
- Time taken to deliver pressure breathing for altitude protection (PBA).

Delivery of 100% oxygen for the earliest breaths following decompression requires system 'dead space' to be purged rapidly of gas still containing nitrogen. Post-decompression severity of hypoxia will be determined by lung volume and effectiveness of pulmonary ventilation to eliminate alveolar nitrogen – deep breaths essential even when breathing against PBA; hypoventilation will delay alveolar oxygenation and could cause severe hypoxia.

13.2 PRESSURE BREATHING FOR ALTITUDE PROTECTION (PBA)

PHYSIOLOGICAL REQUIREMENT

- At 40,000 ft breathing 100% O_2, P_AO_2 is 54 mmHg (7.2 kPa), equivalent to 10,000 ft breathing air.
- To prevent hypoxia above 40,000 ft, oxygen system must be capable of delivering breathing gas to respiratory tract at pressures greater than ambient.
- Ideally oxygen should be supplied at pressure sufficient to maintain absolute intrapulmonary pressure at 141 mmHg.
- Pressure breathing delivery should be no more than 2 sec after decompression.

Exposure to 40,000 ft is an emergency situation only, as aircraft cabin usually pressurised. PBA is delivered following decompression to protect crew against hypoxia. However, elevated intrapulmonary pressure has significant physiological consequences.

PHYSIOLOGICAL CONSEQUENCES OF PBA

- Increased breathing effort:
  - Normal breathing cycle reversed; inspiration passive and expiration active.
  - Causes respiratory fatigue.
  - Trained individuals can tolerate breathing pressure of up to 30 mmHg (4 kPa) for some minutes.
  - Speech very difficult.
- Increased pulmonary ventilation:
  - Tidal volume and respiratory rate increased (especially in inexperienced individuals).
  - PCO_2 may fall to 25–30 mmHg when breathing at 30 mmHg (4 kPa).
- Distension of lungs and chest:
  - Lungs fully distended by breathing pressure of 20 mmHg (2.7 kPa).
  - When lungs supported by thoracic cavity, up to 80 mmHg (10.7 kPa) can be tolerated without damage.
  - Above around 80 mmHg, theoretical risk of lung parenchymal damage with risk of arterial gas embolus.
  - Respiratory counter-pressure used to reduce this risk.
- Soft tissue distension:
  - Discomfort in face and neck.
  - Eye discomfort, air escape via nasolacrimal ducts.
  - Splinting of tympanic membrane.
- Raised intrapleural pressure:
  - Intrapleural pressure rises with intrapulmonary pressure during pressure breathing.
  - If lung distension occurs, rise in intrapleural pressure will be less than applied intrapulmonary pressure.
  - Rise in intrapleural pressure determines the degree of pressure applied to the heart and great vessels.
- Respiratory counter-pressure:
  - Usually provided by inflatable garment worn around thorax, may include support to abdominal wall.
  - Inflated to same pressure as breathing pressure.
  - Reduces effort and fatigue associated with PBA.
  - Reduces risk of lung over-distension.
- Cardiovascular effects:
  - Central venous pressure increased, impeding venous return and cardiac output.
  - Blood pools in extremities and reduces circulating blood volume.
  - May lead to loss of consciousness (pressure breathing syncope) if pressure breathing is maintained for more than a few minutes.
  - Lower limb counter-pressure applied using anti-G trousers will limit pooling of blood in capacitance vessels of legs helping to maintain cardiac output.

BREATHING PRESSURE LIMITS

- Maximum pressure breathing with mask alone usually 30 mmHg (4 kPa); short-term protection to 50,000 ft.
- Maximum pressure breathing with mask, counter-pressure to trunk and lower limbs usually 72 mmHg (9.6 kPa); short-term protection to 60,000 ft.
- Maximum pressure breathing with pressure helmet, counter-pressure to trunk and lower limbs usually 110 mmHg (14.7 kPa); theoretical protection to above 80,000 ft but limited to lower altitude by ebullism risk; full pressure suit needed for protection above 65,000 ft.
- PBA is usually only used for a short time to permit aircraft descent to safe altitude.

13.3 FULL PRESSURE SUITS

- Suit may be worn unpressurised and pressurised in emergency, or worn electively for extra-vehicular activity in space.
- To reduce risk of decompression sickness, absolute pressure in suit generally greater than 282 mmHg (37.6 kPa) (equivalent of 25,000 ft) but can be less for short-duration exposures, especially with denitrogenation regime.
- Heat can be delivered with hot air/electric heating/liquid conditioning garment.
- Cooling system may also be required using heat exchange system.
- Care needed in design to avoid freezing of valves, misting of visor.
- Body mobility affected by inflation pressure and suit articulation design.
- Suit should provide noise and glare protection, communications.
- For use in space, pressure suit requires closed-circuit system to remove CO_2, water vapour, heat and odour, and to add O_2; limited radiation and micrometeorite protection also required.

Cosmic radiation

Contents

> **Key Facts**
> - The effect of radiation depends on the LET.
> - Radiation in space is of higher LET and higher risk than at aviation altitudes.
> - The amount and type of radiation depends on solar weather, which varies on an 11-year cycle.
> - True impact of cosmic radiation on aircrew is not clearly known.
> - In astronauts, cosmic radiation may result in an increased risk of malignant disease and potentially acute radiation sickness during SPE.
> - Radiation carries a greater risk to children, women and pregnant aircrew.
> - Solar radiation can also cause harm through damage to flight critical infrastructure and equipment.

14.1 INTRODUCTION

- Cosmic radiation poses a potential hazard to aircrew and astronauts relative to dose and exposure.
- Cosmic radiation (gamma rays, protons, neutrons) can ionize atoms and transfer energy to material.
- Effects of radiation on the body are complex and depend on type of radiation, dose, body tissue.
- For aircrew, measurement and avoidance are protective; for astronauts, more research needed for future interplanetary missions.

MAIN HAZARDS

1. High dose – acute radiation injury.
2. Low, recurrent dose – potential for malignant disease.
3. Failure of electronic systems including avionics and GPS.

14.2 BACKGROUND: COSMIC RADIATION AND SPACE WEATHER

- Cosmic radiation may originate from the sun (solar radiation) or from outside our solar system (galactic cosmic radiation).
- Most radiation at aviation altitudes is from galactic sources except in periods of solar maximum.
- Linear energy transfer (LET) measures amount of energy transferred from ionizing particles to surrounding environment.
  - In space, high LET particles cause secondary effects through collision with molecules in the spacecraft or astronaut.
  - At aviation altitudes, radiation has a low LET due to Earth's atmosphere and magnetosphere, which act as a shield against cosmic radiation.
    - Protection increases with distance from magnetic poles and with decreasing altitude.
    - Background radiation at equator is <50% of that at temperate latitudes; exposure at 39,000 ft is twice that at 26,000 ft.
- Solar radiation varies with an 11-year cycle (space weather); at solar maximum there are increased solar particle events (SPE) associated with coronal mass ejections (CME).

14.3 UNITS OF MEASUREMENT AND EXPOSURE

- Sievert (symbol: Sv) is a unit of ionizing radiation dose (in SI) and is derived to provide a measure of the health effect of low levels of ionizing radiation on the human body; rem also used, where 1 Sv = 100 rem. Table 14.1 shows typical radiation doses.

Table 14.1 Doses of radiation from a variety of sources

NAME	mSv
Chest x-ray	0.014
Transatlantic flight	0.08
CT scan of head	1.4
Typical background dose	2–3
Space Shuttle mission (8 days)	5.6
Long-haul aircrew additional yearly radiation	6
CT whole spine	10
Apollo 14 mission (9 days to moon)	11.4
Blood cell changes seen [single dose]	100
ISS mission (6 months)	160
Skylab 4 (87 days)	178
Acute radiation sickness [single dose]	1000
Estimated Mars mission (3 months)	1200
50% mortality at 1 month [single dose]	5000

14.4 EFFECTS OF COSMIC RADIATION

- Deterministic effects occur above a threshold radiation level; caused by significant cell damage or death. Physical effects occur when cell death burden is large enough to cause functional impairment of a tissue or organ (e.g. cataracts, sterility, radiation sickness). Offspring may be affected by exposure during pregnancy – risk is highest between 3 and 8 weeks (during organogenesis).
- Stochastic effects occur without a threshold, but effect increases with dose. Mutation of tumour suppressor genes or oncogenes may result in cancerous transformation; young children more susceptible.
- In aircrew, numerous confounding factors lead to varied results across studies (population required to power a study into effects of 1 mSv/yr estimated to be 500 million people).
  - One multinational study over two decades reported no significant difference in aircrew from population levels of female breast cancer, leukaemia and brain cancer; study indicated a reduction in fatal radiation-related cancers in male cockpit crew.
  - Meta-analysis showed increase in risk of breast cancer in female aircrew; one study found increased risk of bone cancer.
  - Increase in malignant melanoma noted in male cockpit crew, attributed to lifestyle related sun exposure.
- Young age and female sex are main non-modifiable risk factors.
- During SPE, exposure of aircrew and astronauts may increase; 20 mSv has been estimated during a severe event, equivalent to the annual occupational limit, with risk of fatal cancer increased by 0.1%.
- Ionization of electronic circuits during solar storms can damage aviation infrastructure:
  - Solar storm in 2003 caused the loss of GPS function in UK aerospace.
  - Backup equipment and drills are required in case of electronic system failure on ground and in air during a solar storm.

14.5 LEGISLATION

- Due to a lack of direct evidence, risk calculations for aircrew extrapolate data from high-dose single exposures; regulations are cautious to allow for lack of data.
- International Commission on Radiological Protection (ICRP) recommend effective dose limits for aircrew of 20 mSv/yr averaged over 5 years (100 mSv in 5 years).
- European Union member states require assessment of aircrew exposure via computer modelling when it is likely to be more than 1 mSv/yr.
  - Prevention through rota planning is required if predicted annual dose is >4 mSv/yr.
  - 6 mSv/yr is do-not-exceed level – if breached, then records must be kept for 30 years or until 75 years of age.
  - For aircraft flying >49,000 ft, crew must be individually monitored, and aircraft must carry active radiation sensors to aid decisions on descent during extreme solar weather.
- Regulation for pregnant aircrew varies between military and civilian authorities and takes into account additional health and occupational factors.
- NASA utilises a career exposure limitation for its astronauts who may not exceed a 3% risk of exposure-induced death (REID).

14.6 SPACEFLIGHT

- Astronauts receive significantly higher doses of higher LET radiation than aviators.
  - Reports of flashing streaks of light with closed eyes.
  - Pitting in astronauts' polycarbonate helmets from cosmic ray strikes.
- Dose and spectra of radiation dependant on mission profile.
  - Missions in low Earth orbit (e.g. ISS) receive protection from Earth's magnetic field.
  - Interplanetary missions will expose astronauts to direct solar and galactic radiation.
    - Lifetime REID from fatal cancer for a female astronaut on a 21-month Mars mission would increase from around 1-in-5 to 1-in-4, excluding previous missions (Table 14.2).
- Shielding may offer some protection for astronauts, but technology is challenging, and protection varies with particle type; shielding most effective for prevention of radiation exposure from SPE. Radio-protective drugs also have a role, but more basic research into cancer caused by charged particles needed.

Table 14.2 % Risk of exposure-induced death from fatal cancer in 40-year-old astronauts

MISSION	MALE (40yo)	FEMALE (40yo)
180-day Lunar mission	0.68%	0.82%
600-day Mars mission	4.0%	4.9%
1000-day Mars exploration	4.2%	5.1%

Acceleration physiology

Contents

> **Key Facts**
> - G is produced when an aircraft turns, or a rocket increases speed.
> - Force felt by aircrew/astronauts is in opposite direction to applied acceleration.
> - G exposure causes hydrostatic pressure gradient in blood vessels down body.
> - This leads to a fall in head level blood pressure and blood pooling in legs.
> - Fall in retinal blood pressure leads to grey-out and blackout.
> - Fall in head level blood pressure leads to G-induced loss of consciousness.
> - Baroreceptor reflex offers some protection but takes 7 to 10 sec.
> - Functional oxygen reserve means 4 to 5 sec delay before grey-out/blackout/ G-LOC occurs.
> - At high G onset rate, no grey-out seen before G-LOC (i.e. no warning).
> - At increased G it is harder to breathe in (inspiratory capacity reduced).
> - A large ventilation-perfusion mismatch develops, leading to arterial desaturation.
> - Acceleration atelectasis (lung collapse at bases related to oxygen use and G) may cause symptoms and desaturation.
> - G exposure has a profound effect on lung function; however, rarely presents a problem in aviation due to relatively short G exposures involved, and healthy participants.

15.1 WHAT IS G?

BACKGROUND

- G is term used to describe magnitude of forces to which aircraft and spacecraft occupants are exposed.
- It is a measure of acceleration not force, despite its common language usage.

ACCELERATION

- Acceleration is a change in *speed or direction*.

FORMS OF ACCELERATION

- Linear acceleration:
  - Change of speed without change in direction.
  - For example, aircraft takeoff, spacecraft re-entry.
- Radial acceleration:
  - Change in direction without change in speed.
  - For example, aircraft in level banked turn.
- Angular acceleration:
  - Change in speed and direction (angular velocity).
  - For example, when centrifuge starts to spin until it reaches constant rpm.

DEFINITION OF G

Represents acceleration that pilot or astronaut is exposed to:

$$G = \text{applied acceleration} / g$$

Where g is acceleration due to gravity, sometimes called standard gravity, equal to 9.81 ms^{-2}.

PHYSICS OF AN AIRCRAFT IN A TURN: CIRCULAR MOTION

- A force is responsible for change in direction.
- Acceleration causing change in direction is called centripetal acceleration.
- Occupants of an aircraft feel sensation in opposite direction (sometimes called centrifugal force) (see Figure 15.1).

ACCELERATION PRODUCED BY CIRCULAR MOTION

$$a = v^2 / r$$

where *a* is acceleration, *v* is velocity and *r* is radius of turn. As velocity component is squared, a unit change in velocity will have a greater effect on resulting acceleration than a unit change in turn radius.

ACCELERATION TERMINOLOGY

- Term G used to describe magnitude and direction as applied to human body.
- Direction is related to human (z axis aligned with spine), not aircraft (see Figure 15.2).

+	7	**Gz**
direction	magnitude	axis

- Acceleration most commonly encountered in high-performance aircraft is +Gz, because aircraft's wings produce lift force that will change aircraft's direction.
- As crew sit upright, this is a headward acceleration that results in a +Gz acceleration (forcing pilot downwards into their seat).
- In spaceflight, crews lie down for launch and re-entry, resulting in +Gx acceleration.

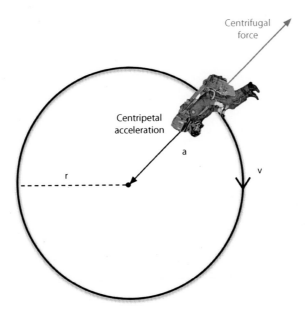

Figure 15.1. Acceleration of circular motion.

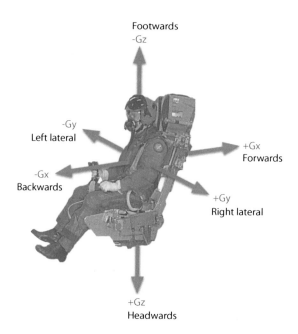

Figure 15.2 Notation used to describe direction of applied acceleration and inertial reaction.

GRAVITY

Acceleration due to gravity must also be included, for example in an aircraft performing a vertical loop:

- If aircraft's wings produce +3 Gz, then pilot will experience +4 Gz at bottom of loop (+1 Gz from gravity also included).
- At top of loop, if wings still producing +3Gz, then pilot will experience +2 Gz (aircraft is inverted, acceleration due to gravity acting in opposite direction with respect to pilot) (see Figure 15.3).

G ONSET RATE

- Describes how rapidly G is applied (or removed = offset rate).
- Usually expressed in $G \cdot s^{-1}$, and is a function of time taken to reach a particular G level.

15.2 SUBJECTIVE EFFECTS OF ACCELERATION

WEIGHT

- Pushed down in seat; body feels heavy, difficulty in moving limbs.
- Mass of head/helmet makes head movements difficult.
- Standing up impossible at greater than +3 Gz (so no unassisted escape from aircraft).

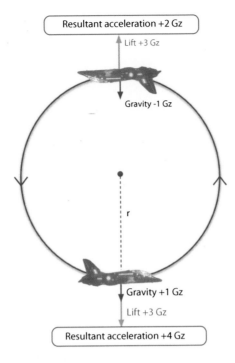

Figure 15.3 Forces acting on an aircraft in a loop.

VISION

- Loss of peripheral vision (grey-out, tunnel vision).
- Complete loss of vision (called 'blackout').
- Visual changes occur after approximately 4 sec.
- If not using any G protection, usually:
  - Grey-out threshold around +3.5 Gz.
  - Blackout threshold around +4.0 Gz.
  - Range is wide: grey-out threshold can be +2.7 Gz to +5 Gz.

UNCONSCIOUSNESS

- G-induced loss of consciousness (G-LOC) after approximately 4 sec.
- Without G protection:
  - G-LOC threshold around +4.5Gz.
  - Range is wide, G-LOC as low as +3 Gz in some normal individuals.

15.3 CARDIOVASCULAR EFFECTS OF ACCELERATION

HYDROSTATIC PRESSURE

Pressure exerted by column of blood determined by height, density and acceleration:

$$P = h \times \rho \times g$$

where:

P   is hydrostatic pressure

h   is height

ρ   is density and g is acceleration

If heart to head distance is 30 cm, density of blood is 1.06 times water, then:
For every +1 Gz increase in acceleration, head level blood pressure falls by about 23 mmHg.

VENOUS POOLING

Pressure across vein wall (transmural pressure) increases causing:

- Blood volume increase in lower limbs.
- Decreased venous return.
- Decreased stroke volume and cardiac output.

BARORECEPTOR REFLEX

- Reduction in neck level blood pressure under G reduces output of carotid baroreceptors.
- Baroreceptor reflex promotes:
  - Increase in peripheral resistance through arterial vasoconstriction.
  - Increase in heart rate and stroke volume.
- Resulting increase in blood pressure is relatively small, equivalent to no more than 1G.
- Rise in blood pressure not effective until 7 to 10 sec after G is applied.

RETINAL CIRCULATION

- Under increased +Gz acceleration, retinal artery blood pressure falls.
- Normal intra-ocular pressure (IOP) is 10–20 mmHg (average 15.5 mmHg).
- Therefore, greater arterial pressure required to perfuse retina than cerebral circulation, so for same acceleration level, retinal blood flow will cease before cerebral blood flow.

STANDARD GREY-OUT PATTERN THOUGHT TO OCCUR BECAUSE

- Retinal artery is an end artery.
- Retinal vessels branch from fundus, number of branches of periphery greater, blood pressure correspondingly lower in periphery.

CEREBRAL BLOOD FLOW

Cerebral blood flow preserved under increased +Gz acceleration; flow occurs at very low pressure, because:

- Active cerebral vasodilation.
- Possible venous siphon (hydrostatic gradient affects arteries and veins equally, maintains arteriovenous pressure difference).
- Reduction in cerebrospinal fluid pressure due to G.

FUNCTIONAL OXYGEN RESERVE

- Retinal and cerebral tissues have 'functional oxygen reserve'.
- After blood supply is abruptly stopped (e.g. by G exposure), tissues continue to function for around 3–5 sec.
- Implication: If high G is suddenly applied, there will be a delay of 3–5 sec before G-LOC.

'G MEASLES' OR PETECHIAL HAEMORRHAGE

- High capillary pressure in lower limbs causes petechial haemorrhage in skin.
- Fade after 24 to 48 hr.
- Benign.

CARDIAC RHYTHM

- Benign cardiac dysrhythmias seen during and after G exposure in centrifuge, also recorded in flight:
  - Commonly premature ventricular contractions.
  - Rarely premature supraventricular contractions.
  - Sinus bradycardia, brief atrioventricular dissociation sometimes seen after G exposure.
- Rhythm changes possibly related to large changes between sympathetic and parasympathetic tone.

G TOLERANCE

Definition: G level at which individual experiences grey-out or G-LOC. Large variation in G tolerance between individuals (range +2.7 Gz to +7.8 Gz, mean +4.7 Gz in one large study).

In research, tolerance is usually taken as G level where non-straining individual experiences 60° of light loss/grey-out.

G tolerance and G symptoms depend on G onset rate:

- At low G onset rate:
  - Head level blood pressure falls slowly.
  - Grey-out appears first, then blackout, then G-LOC.
  - Can act as an early warning to pilot to strain or reduce G.
  - Baroreceptors have time to act, may improve tolerance.
- At high G onset rate:
  - Head level blood pressure falls rapidly.
  - G-LOC occurs without preceding grey-out or blackout; functional oxygen reserve in retinal and cerebral tissues is used up simultaneously.
  - No early warning for pilot.
  - G tolerance is worse as baroreceptors do not have time to act (see Figure 15.4).

15.4 NEGATIVE G

NEGATIVE G (-GZ) EXPERIENCED IN OUTSIDE LOOP OR 'BUNT'

- Effects of negative G:
  - Negative G causes unpleasant sensation, including facial engorgement due to headward displacement of blood volume.

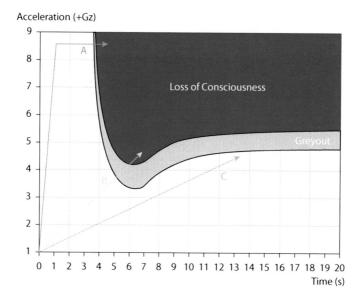

Acceleration (+Gz)

Figure 15.4 G-induced loss of consciousness vs time graph (after Martin and Henry, 1951). Line A loss of consciousness without warning at high G onset rate; line B progressive visual symptoms before loss of consciousness; line C improved G tolerance at lower G onset rate following baroreceptor activation.

- Red-out appears in textbooks but is not often experienced; no satisfactory explanation for condition exists. *NOT* due to retinal haemorrhage!
- Little risk of cerebral haemorrhage as cerebral capillary transmural pressure does not rise.
- Cardiovascular effects are opposite to +Gz:
  - Profound rapid onset bradycardia with a few heartbeats.
  - Vasodilatation.
  - Reduced cardiac output.
- Exposure to even brief negative G reduces tolerance to subsequent +Gz:
  - Sometimes called 'push–pull effect' after aircraft control column movement.

15.5 G-INDUCED LOSS OF CONSCIOUSNESS

- Occurs when there is insufficient cerebral perfusion during G exposure.
- Results in alteration of conscious state.
- Divided into two phases:
  - Absolute incapacitation:
    - Unconscious, with loss of muscle tone.
    - Mean duration 10 sec.
  - Relative incapacitation:
    - Impaired consciousness, recovering.
    - Mean duration 15 sec.
- Symptoms during recovery from G-LOC include dreamlike thoughts, confusion, light-headedness, involuntary muscle spasm, amnesia (in up to 50% of cases on centrifuge).

- Risk of G-LOC higher at high G onset rate as no visual warning signs first.
- 'Almost' loss of consciousness (A-LOC):
  - G-related incapacitation without overt loss of consciousness.
  - Occurs at G level just below that causing G-LOC but after greyout and blackout have occurred.
  - Sensory abnormalities, amnesia, confusion.
  - Disconnection between cognition and ability to act.

15.6 RISK FACTORS FOR G-LOC: G AWARENESS

Multiple factors can influence aircrew risk of G-LOC. Some of these can be controlled by aircrew – promotion of 'G awareness' in aviators is very important.

Main risk factors are:

- Hydration.
- Nutrition.
- Fatigue.
- Infection.
- Physical fitness.
- Temperature.
- Alcohol.
- Hyperventilation.
- Hypoxia.

- Body morphology.
- Time off from flying.
- Preceding –Gz exposure.
- Duration of G exposure.
- Vestibular influence.
- Experience.
- G training.
- Distraction.
- Anti-G suit.

15.7 PULMONARY EFFECTS OF ACCELERATION

LUNG VOLUME

- Vital capacity:
  - Vital capacity is (VC) reduced under increased G due to increased weight of the chest wall.
- Diaphragm descends under +Gz acceleration:
  - Caused by increased weight of abdominal contents and diaphragm.
  - Diaphragm descent causes increase in functional residual capacity unless G suit worn (then no diaphragm descent).
- Supine position (+Gx):
  - Applies to spaceflight.
  - Weight of chest wall greatly increased.
  - Chest pain and difficulty in breathing at +8 Gx.
  - Large reduction in VC: VC = tidal volume at +12 Gx.

VENTILATION/PERFUSION

- Ventilation gradient increases down lung:
  - Pleural pressure gradient from lung apex to base becomes steeper under increased +Gz acceleration.
  - Leads to a ventilation gradient due to elastic properties of lung tissue.
  - Ventilation reduced at apex and increased at base.

- Basal airways close:
  - Pleural pressure at bases exceeds airway pressure leading to collapse of small airways; gas is trapped in alveoli which do not take part in ventilation.
- Perfusion gradient increases down lung:
  - Same hydrostatic effect as systemic circulation, but vascular pressures are lower and distances shorter.
- Normal ventilation/perfusion mismatch is increased:
  - Upper portion of lung is ventilated but not perfused, lower portion of lung perfused but unventilated.
  - This causes shunting as O_2 tension in closed alveoli falls rapidly:
    - At +5 Gz, up to 50% of cardiac output shunted and arterial pO_2 falls to around 85% after 1 minute.

ACCELERATION ATELECTASIS

- G causes closure of basal alveoli.
- If little N_2 is present (>60% O_2), all alveolar gas in closed alveoli will be absorbed.
- Alveolar walls held together by surface tension forces and will remain collapsed on return to +1 Gz.
- Minimum conditions for development of acceleration atelectasis:
  - > +3 Gz.
  - Breathing >60% O_2 for at least 15 min.
  - Wearing an anti-G suit.
- Clinical features:
  - Dry cough.
  - Substernal discomfort.
  - May be implicated in hypoxia-like events.
- Management:
  - Usually cleared by cough or deep inspirations.
  - If not cleared, persists for 24–36 hr – no treatment indicated but be aware of possible risk during further flights made within this period.
- Physiological significance:
  - Vital capacity reduced by up to 60%.
  - Right-to-left shunt can be 25% of cardiac output.
  - Shunt causes fall in arterial pO_2 (be aware of importance during altitude exposure, physical work).
- Prevention:
  - Minimum N_2 concentration of 40% in breathing gas; recent studies suggest more N_2 may be needed for prevention in certain flight conditions.

16

Prevention of G-LOC

Contents

Key Facts
- Anti-G straining manoeuvre (AGSM) gives up to 3 G protection but must be learned, is fatiguing and carries a G-LOC risk if aircrew fail to carry it out adequately.
- AGSM acts by increasing peripheral resistance, reducing venous pooling and increasing heart level blood pressure.
- Anti-G suit improves G protection by 1 G (5 bladder suit) or up to 2.5 G (full coverage anti-G suit).
- Anti-G suit acts by increasing peripheral resistance and improving venous return.
- G protection of AGSM and anti-G suit are additive.
- Positive pressure breathing for G protection may augment or replace the AGSM Valsalva for improved tolerance at high G levels.

16.1 ANTI-G STRAINING

BACKGROUND

- G-LOC risk reduced by:
  - Voluntary straining manoeuvres.
  - Anti-G systems and flight clothing.
  - Avoiding G exposure – low risk if:
    - <3.5 Gz.
    - <4 sec exposure.

ANTI-G STRAINING MANOEUVRE (AGSM)

- Physical voluntary manoeuvre to elevate heart level blood pressure and minimise fall in head level blood pressure under increased G.
- May give up to around 3 G improvement in G tolerance.
- Combination of muscle tensing and Valsalva performed rhythmically every 3–4 sec:
  - Muscle tensing:
    - Leg muscles, abdominal muscles, gluteal muscles.
    - Muscle contraction sustained throughout G exposure.
    - Mechanical pressure on arteries and arterioles reduces vessel diameter, so increasing peripheral resistance and arterial blood pressure:

$$Blood\ Pressure = Cardiac\ Output \times Total\ Peripheral\ Resistance$$

    - Mechanical pressure on veins reduces venous pooling.
  - Valsalva manoeuvre:
    - Forced expiration against closed glottis.
    - Increased intrathoracic and intra-abdominal pressure.
    - Direct transmission of pressure to heart and great vessels.
    - Arterial blood pressure increased, but after 3–4 sec high intrathoracic pressure leads to reduced venous return (see Figure 16.1).
    - Muscle tensing essential to support venous return under G.
- AGSM may give up to around 3 G improvement in G tolerance.
- AGSM should be anticipatory and proactive:
  - Muscle tensing starts before G starts.
  - Valsalva at the moment G is applied.
  - Aircrew should not use grey-out as cue to start straining:
    - High G onset rate may remove visual cues.
    - Unrecoverable fall in head level blood pressure may have already occurred.

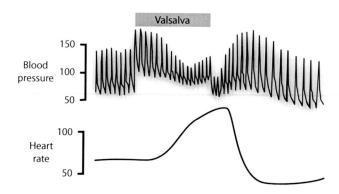

Figure 16.1 Blood pressure and heart rate during Valsalva manoeuvre.

G WARM-UP

Consists of two or three sustained exposures at increasing G levels before the start of air combat to:

- Raise awareness of G and rehearse anti-G straining.
- Assess personal G tolerance for the day.
- Test anti-G system is working.
- Raise circulating stress hormone levels (only lasts 3–5 minutes).

16.2 ANTI-G SUITS

FIVE BLADDER ANTI-G SUIT

- Most common design (see Figure 16.2).
- Five non-circumferential bladders inflated to uniform pressure with compressed air automatically by the anti-G valve.
- Provides 1.0 to 1.5 G increase in relaxed +Gz tolerance.
- Mode of action similar to muscle tensing, increasing peripheral resistance and decreasing venous pooling.
- Abdominal bladder of anti-G suit:
    - Prevents descent of heart which would otherwise increase head-heart distance.
    - Improves venous return by creating venous pressure gradient between abdominal cavity and thorax.

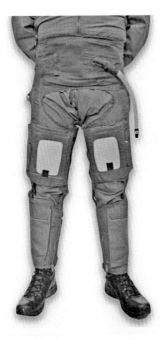

Figure 16.2 Five bladder anti-G suit.

FULL COVERAGE ANTI-G SUIT

- Developed in response to increasing aircraft performance.
- Increased surface area cover of lower body:
  - Standard five bladder anti-G trousers around 25% bladder cover.
  - Full coverage anti-G trousers around 90% bladder cover (see Figure 16.3).
- Circumferential bladder:
  - More efficient application of pressure.
- Provides 2 to 2.5 G increase in relaxed +Gz tolerance.
- Increased bulk may influence thermal stress, mobility in garments, cockpit interactions (e.g. stick, ejection path).
- Anti-G valve performance must be suitable to fill larger gas volume sufficiently quickly.

ANTI-G VALVE

- Senses +Gz acceleration and supplies required pressure to anti-G suit.
- Usually no inflation until above +2 Gz to prevent distraction in turbulence.
- Typical performance requirement for inflation rate is 90% anti-G suit inflation within 1 sec.
- Mechanical or electronic operation.

POSITIVE PRESSURE BREATHING FOR G PROTECTION (PBG)

- PBG supplied under increased G to:
  - Maintain head level blood pressure.
  - Reduce mechanical work of breathing.
- Typical pressure schedule starts supplying PBG above +4 Gz, rising at 12 mmHg/G to 60 mmHg (8 kPa) at +9 Gz.

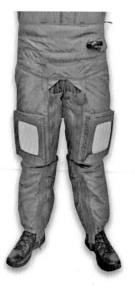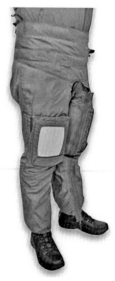

Figure 16.3 Full coverage anti-G suit.

- Raises intrapleural pressure to act on heart and great vessels to increase arterial blood pressure.
- Pressure reduces venous return to thorax, so anti-G suit essential.
- Full coverage anti-G trousers provide better support of venous return than five bladder anti-G trousers using PBG.
- Wide variation in G tolerance with PBG, but for many aircrew +8 to 9 Gz possible with reduced straining; Valsalva component of AGSM not always required.
- Evidence suggests use of PBG is safe without need for respiratory counter-pressure (unlike pressure breathing at +1 Gz for altitude protection).

16.3 HIGH G TRAINING

- Training objectives:
    - Awareness of potential for G-LOC.
    - Anticipation and recognition of symptoms.
    - Develop efficient and effective AGSM.
- Usually conducted on a human centrifuge for safety and optimal training delivery.
- Mandatory in most air forces for aircrew flying aircraft capable of +7 Gz or more.
- Often required for aircrew flying aircraft capable of +5 Gz or more.
- Should be completed prior to flying the aircraft (sometimes a pass/fail requirement); many air forces require refresher training.
- Human centrifuge design:
    - Rotating arm with gondola, actively powered cabin pitch and roll.
    - High G onset rate (up to 10 $G \cdot s^{-1}$).
    - Use of flight simulation improves training fidelity.
    - Centrifuge acceleration and deceleration produces extraneous accelerations not found in flight.
    - Vestibular effects (predominantly Coriolis) due to short radius turn and gondola roll can distract from training and cause nausea.

16.4 OTHER METHODS TO IMPROVE G TOLERANCE

- Pharmacological methods investigated, but side effects not acceptable for flight.
- Reclined seats:
    - In theory, >65° angled seat required to improve G tolerance significantly, but poor visibility.
    - 30° reclined seat (e.g. F-16) improves comfort (except neck) and may give up to 0.5 G improvement at +9 Gz.
    - Fully reclined seat used in space flight: tolerance to +8 Gx generally good without protection; above this level breathing becomes difficult.

16.5 MUSCULOSKELETAL INJURY AND CONDITIONING

- Neck and back pain occur in high G flying:
    - Career prevalence in fighter aircrew around 70 to 90%.

- Predisposing factors: high +Gz acceleration, high G onset rate, heavy helmet equipment, high flight hours, being unprepared for the manoeuvre (i.e. not pilot in control).
- Helmet mounted displays increase helmet weight and have unfavourable centre of mass/balance.
- Cockpit factors include head position, head movement.
- Mechanism of injury usually muscle strain/ligamentous injury.
- Cervical disk bulge, annular tear, compression fracture, fractured spinous process, facet joint dislocation occasionally reported.
- Chronic degenerative changes (disk degeneration, osteophytes) also reported but evidence mixed.

- Physical conditioning to reduce the risk of neck and back injury:
  - Evidence of efficacy limited due to small numbers.
  - General acceptance of conditioning as protective providing safe exercises are conducted.
- Physical conditioning to improve G tolerance:
  - Evidence of longer time to fatigue (30–50% improvement), but wide individual variation.
  - Many air forces recommend a high G fitness program, and there are general health benefits.

17

Short-duration acceleration

Contents

Key Facts

- Short-duration acceleration occurs during an impact event; time course is extremely short, typically 0.1–0.5 sec duration.
- Injury occurs when a person is exposed to forces of a critical magnitude for a brief period of time.
- Degree of injury is related to magnitude, duration, rate of onset and direction of the applied forces.
- In general, the longer the duration of the impact pulse, the lower the acceleration level that can be tolerated.
- Short-duration acceleration can be considered as mainly mechanical and transitory.
- Human tolerance to short-duration acceleration depends on structural strength of body and overall velocity change.
- Kinetic energy of a crashing aircraft can be absorbed by crushing and deforming of aircraft structure.
- Impact injuries can occur by: compression–tension load, fore–aft bending, left–right bending, fore–aft shear, left–right shear and clockwise–anticlockwise torsion.
- Injury can result from a direct blow to the body by a solid object or from indirectly transmitted force.

17.1 MECHANICS OF IMPACT

- When an aircraft impacts the ground, the aircraft experiences opposing forces of very short duration. Accelerations acting during ground impact are determined by:
  - Friction with ground resisting aircraft's velocity.
  - Collision with stationary objects.
  - Length of time over which force acts (peak magnitude of opposing forces higher with short duration).
- If crashing aircraft crushed or deformed progressively, then overall deceleration profile relatively smooth, as kinetic energy absorbed.
- If parts of aircraft plough into the ground, velocity is reduced rapidly and high magnitude peaks of abrupt decelerations produced; highest peak values occur when aircraft strike solid objects.
- Crashworthy design features can be used to allow structures to collapse progressively in a controlled manner; this increases chances of crew survival.
- Effects of short-duration acceleration related principally to structural strength of body part on which they act and overall velocity change induced in the body; stresses can be considered as mainly mechanical and transitory.

17.2 HUMAN TOLERANCE

- Impact injury results from disruption of biological tissue caused by a short-duration physical event.
- Short-duration acceleration forces can be separated into three categories:
  - Tolerable – forces may produce minor superficial trauma, such as bruises and abrasions, which do not incapacitate.
  - Injurious – forces result in moderate to severe trauma, which may or may not incapacitate.
  - Fatal – injuries result in death.
- Defining human tolerance levels to short-duration accelerations is complex due to variability of individual response and need to state level of injury that is considered acceptable.

In broad terms, Table 17.1 lists the accelerations that are considered the threshold for severe injury.

Table 17.1 Threshold for severe injury

AXIS	SEVERE INJURY THRESHOLD
$+Gz$	25 G
$-Gz$	15 G
$+Gx$	50 G
$-Gx$	45 G
$\pm Gy$	12 G

GX IMPACT

- Tolerance of occupant to a forward facing impact depends on effectiveness of support provided to front of body by restraint harness.
- Head flung down onto chest; arms and legs thrown forward at right angles to body.
- Without restraint, occupant will continue forward at their initial velocity until they strike a solid object such as an instrument panel.

GY IMPACT

- Significant lateral (±Gy) accelerations do not occur under normal flight conditions.
- Significant ±Gy accelerations can occur in crashes, particularly to seated occupants of sideways-facing seats (e.g. helicopters).

GZ IMPACT

- Significant +Gz acceleration can occur in crashes associated with a high sink rate, particularly in helicopters.
- Tolerance to accelerations in this axis is influenced by seat-back angle, sitting platform and posture of occupant.
- −Gz accelerations are reacted through any restraint harness and may occur during inverted crashes or following a rollover.

17.3 PHYSICAL BASIS OF INJURY

- Forces that could be involved in impact include:
    - Compression (axial) – tension loading.
    - Fore–aft bending.
    - Left–right bending.
    - Fore–aft shear.
    - Left–right shear.
    - Clockwise–anti-clockwise torsion.
- Bending of a tissue structure results in a number of internal stresses and will place one side in tension and other in compression.
- Shear stress is produced by a non-aligned force couple; tends to produce slip.
- Torsion is produced by axial rotation and can produce tension, compression and shear locally in tissue.

ANATOMICAL INJURIES

- An understanding of the sequence of events in an aircraft accident, including an assessment of probable kinematics of the occupant, will allow determination of most likely injury mechanism.
- Injury can result from a direct blow to the body by a solid object or from an indirectly transmitted force.

SKELETAL INJURY

- Damage to bony skeleton (including joints) is most common injury in crash environment.

- Injuries to upper and lower extremities are particularly common, primarily due to presence of solid objects within flail envelope.
- Direction of forces and rate at which they are applied, together with an estimation of the loads involved, may be obtained from radiological examination of fracture pattern.

JOINTS

- Application of forces that stress a joint beyond its normal range of motion results in failure of ligaments, tendons and joint capsule.
- Joint disruption can result in an unstable joint or a joint in which the range of movement has become restricted or hyper-mobile.

ABDOMINAL CAVITY

- Force of a blow to any part of the abdomen can be transmitted to all organs and structures within abdominal cavity virtually unchanged.
- Rupture of diaphragm, liver or spleen can occur from blunt trauma to any part of abdomen.
- Damping of pressure waves generated by an abdominal impact can occur through compression of gas in intestines and stomach.
- Blunt trauma can result in abdominal injury by several mechanisms, such as pressure-wave transmission, compression and shear forces.

CHEST

- Impact injuries to chest are often rapidly fatal, as all major contents of the chest are vital to life.
- Disruption of circulatory system with potentially fatal decreases in blood volume can result from blunt trauma to chest.
- Non-penetrating cardiac injuries (rupture of myocardium, cardiac septa, pericardium and valvular apparatus) and rupture of aorta frequently seen at post-mortem examinations of victims of aircraft accidents and high deceleration impacts.

SPINE

- Back injuries resulting from an aircraft crash may involve the musculoskeletal structures of vertebral column and/or the spinal cord itself.
- Response of thoracic vertebrae to impact is modified by presence of ribs.
- Increasing size of lumbar vertebrae and orientation of facet joints lead to increased stability of lower vertebral column.
- Forces required to cause fractures or fracture dislocations of thoracolumbar spine are very large due to the size of vertebral bodies and supporting ligaments but are typical in high +Gz impacts.

CHAPTER 18

Restraint systems and escape from aircraft

Contents

> **Key Facts**
> - Restraint system should attenuate crash dynamics and restrict movement of occupant to avoid impacts with aircraft structure.
> - Restraint system must be comfortable, have easy adjustment and must protect occupant from injury arising from multidirectional forces.
> - Aircraft assisted escape systems must eject the occupant clear of the aircraft at all speeds and provide sufficient ground clearance to enable full deployment and inflation of main parachute before ground impact.
> - Ejection seats expose aircrew to forces that may be at limits of human tolerance.

18.1 FUNCTION OF RESTRAINT SYSTEMS

Restraint systems are used to:

- Keep aircrew within their in-flight workspace so control of aircraft is maintained.
- Attenuate the crash forces during impact and restrict flailing by limiting movement of occupant to avoid impact with aircraft structures.

18.2 PROPERTIES OF A RESTRAINT SYSTEM

Restraint system is designed to resist motion of seat occupant: It should apply deceleration in most appropriate direction, and at sites over human body that are most suitable to take the load, minimising injury risk.

- Restraint system must be comfortable to wear, have easy adjustment and must protect occupant from injury arising from multidirectional forces.
- Harness anchor points should be capable of taking the maximum expected loads.
- Forces over the body should be distributed and should not lead to harness-related injury.
- System must be easy to put on and release.
- Single-point release mechanism is ideal with single-handed operation being possible.
- It should be possible to operate in restricted vision.
- Inadvertent operation should be preventable with two sequenced operations being incorporated to avoid accidental opening.
- System should allow the occupant to carry out all flight and emergency tasks.

18.3 TYPES OF RESTRAINT SYSTEMS

LAP BELTS

- Simplest restraint system.
- Typically used in passenger aircraft.
- Requires two anchorage points, positioned either side of the body on seat.
- Provides minimum restriction to occupant, so in order to increase survivability a good brace position needs to be adopted.
- Submarining: If belt rises up over iliac crests across the front of the abdomen, 'submarining' can occur as torso slips forward; abdominal and lumbar spine injuries may result.

THREE-POINT HARNESS

- Typical automobile harness.
- Good restraint for frontal impacts, but restraint in vertical and side impacts are less optimal.
- Submarining can occur (see above).

FOUR-POINT HARNESS

- Comprises lap restraints with straps across each shoulder.
- Provides better restraint than three-point harness as there is a larger spread of loading.
- Submarining can occur.

FIVE-POINT HARNESS

- Similar to four-point but additionally provides a negative-G strap which prevents submarining (see Figure 18.1).
- Negative-G strap also prevents upward movement out of seat during negative-G aerobatic manoeuvres.

AIRBAGS

- Common feature in automobiles, increasingly used in aircraft.
- Can supplement the protection afforded by restraint harnesses.
- Airbags can be cockpit or instrument panel mounted, as in automobiles, or integral with restraint harness straps.

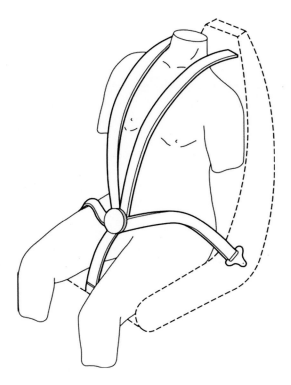

Figure 18.1 Five-point harness.

18.4 AIRCRAFT ASSISTED ESCAPE SYSTEMS (EJECTION SEATS)

Aim of an ejection seat is to permit aircrew to escape before aircraft crashes into ground. Ejection seats which have zero-zero capability (zero forward speed and zero altitude) will allow aircrew to eject safely from stationary aircraft on the ground.

- Ejection sequences vary depending on aircraft and ejection seat type, but all have broadly similar functions.
- Ejection initiation typically occurs by manual initiation by pulling the seat firing handle.
  - STOVL variant of F-35 Lightning II aircraft also has an automatically initiated ejection in case of lift fan failure.
- Cockpit canopy must be cleared before escape, achieved by:
  - Canopy destruction (fragmentation).
  - Physical removal (jettison).
  - Through-canopy ejection (the seat and occupant to punch a pathway through the canopy).

18.5 EJECTION SEQUENCE

1. Activation of the seat firing handle fires initiation cartridge and from this point onwards ejection sequence should be automatic with no further inputs required by the aircrew (see Figure 18.2).

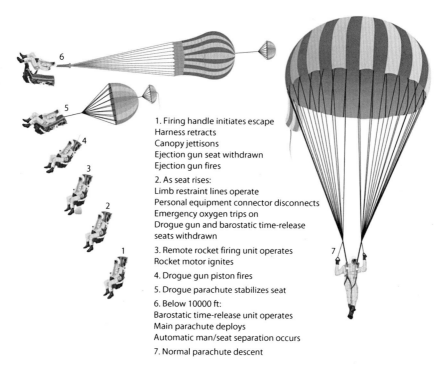

1. Firing handle initiates escape
Harness retracts
Canopy jettisons
Ejection gun seat withdrawn
Ejection gun fires

2. As seat rises:
Limb restraint lines operate
Personal equipment connector disconnects
Emergency oxygen trips on
Drogue gun and barostatic time-release
seats withdrawn

3. Remote rocket firing unit operates
Rocket motor ignites

4. Drogue gun piston fires

5. Drogue parachute stabilizes seat

6. Below 10000 ft:
Barostatic time-release unit operates
Main parachute deploys
Automatic man/seat separation occurs

7. Normal parachute descent

Figure 18.2 Sequence of events in a typical high-speed, low-level ejection from a fast jet aircraft.

- Some ejection seats have a rocket motor fitted to the base of the seat-pan to augment thrust of catapult, increasing escape velocity, and may give the seat a zero-zero capability.
2. Gases generated from ejection gun primary cartridge pressurise ejection gun tubes to initiate upward seat movement.
3. Secondary cartridges fire as the seat accelerates up the guide rails; these increase ejection thrust to increase the seat's upward velocity to give sufficient velocity to clear the aircraft tail-fin.
4. Emergency oxygen supply selected automatically as the seat is disconnected from aircraft's main oxygen supply.
5. Leg and arm restraint lines are activated.
6. Rocket motor initiator cartridge is fired, timed to occur immediately prior to gun separation from the aircraft, so that seat continues to accelerate away.
   - Rocket motor is designed to deliver sufficient height for the main parachute canopy to deploy in zero-zero ejections. Without a rocket pack, zero-zero ejections could only be achieved by delivering very high peak and high onset rate accelerations from the ejection catapult.
7. As the seat separates from the aircraft, it may still have a high forward speed which must be reduced before main parachute can deploy safely – a drogue parachute system stabilises and decelerates the seat to a safe speed for main parachute canopy deployment.

8. Following a possible short time delay if ejection occurs above height set by the altitude sensor of the Barostatic Time Release Unit, the locks securing the occupant's harness to the ejection seat are released automatically.
9. Once main parachute canopy is deployed, occupant is decelerated rapidly, and then descends beneath the parachute canopy.
10. On landing, parachute should collapse and aircrew can then release themselves from the parachute harness by unfastening the quick-release fitting.

18.6 EJECTION ENVELOPE

- Ejection seats are designed to function within certain limits which include maximum and minimum altitude, air speed, pitch, roll and descent rates.
- If ejections take place within such limits, then the ejection is said to have occurred within the safe ejection envelope, and aircrew should survive.
- Ejections occurring outside the safe ejection envelope are likely to result in very severe or fatal injuries.
- Ejections are extremely dynamic events, and even if injuries are sustained this does not necessarily indicate the system has malfunctioned; ejections expose aircrew to forces that may be at the limits of human tolerance, and typical ejection injuries may result.

18.7 EJECTION INJURY

Each phase of ejection sequence can result in specific injuries, even in normal operation. Injury patterns are relatively predictable unless a failure of an element of the ejection sequence has occurred. The following injuries may occur in each phase:

- Escape pathway clearance:
  - Miniature Detonation Cord (MDC) splatter burns.
  - Canopy jettison rocket motor flash burns.
  - Cervical spine, head, shoulder, sternum and limb injury (if there is through-canopy ejection).
- Ejection gun firing/rocket motor firing:
  - Spinal fractures – typically anterior wedge compression fractures.
  - Femoral fracture from contact of lower limb with seat-pan.
- Seat separation from aircraft:
  - Windblast flail injuries – typically upper and lower limb and cervical spine.
  - Impaired consciousness from helmet impact with headbox.
- Drogue parachute deployment:
  - Spinal injury from drogue parachute opening shock load.
- Main parachute canopy deployment:
  - Spinal injury from main parachute opening shock load.
  - Head/cervical spine injury from helmet and parachute rigging line interaction.
- Parachute landing (see Chapter 4):
  - Lower limb fractures.
  - Spinal injuries.

CHAPTER

19

Human physiology and the thermal environment

Contents

Key Facts
- For aircrew, consequences of being unable to cope with thermal stress range from discomfort and subtle decrements in performance to illness and death.
- To maintain stable body temperature, heat exchange with environment by conduction, convection, radiation and evaporation must be balanced with metabolic heat production.
- Behavioural responses to hot and cold have a greater impact on heat balance than physiological responses.
- Significant imbalances in heat balance lead to a range of illnesses and injuries.
- Cold water immersion is an important thermal risk in aviation.

19.1 BODY HEAT BALANCE

- Critical to maintain temperature of brain and vital organs (core temperature, T_C) within a narrow range (37 ± 2–$3°C$).
- Extreme thermal environments (hot or cold, natural or built) challenge our ability to maintain T_C through physiological and behavioural defence mechanisms.

- Factors that determine body heat content are expressed in the equation:

$$M - W \pm K \pm C \pm R - E = S \left(units - watts, W\right)$$

where:

M = metabolic rate (~100 W at rest)
W = external work
K = conduction
C = convection
R = radiation
E = evaporation
S = resultant heat gain/loss (0 in heat balance); see Figure 19.1

- In heat imbalance, S will increase (heat storage or $\uparrow T_C$) or decrease (heat debt or $\downarrow T_C$).
- Physical exercise and clothing exert a significant impact on body heat balance.

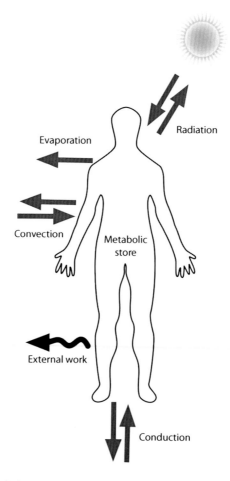

Figure 19.1 Body heat balance.

19.2 METABOLIC COST OF AIRCREW TASKS

- Metabolic cost of aircrew tasks is diverse but relatively modest: from 'Low' (50–175 W) for piloting during routine flight to 'High' (around 500 W) for piloting during combat manoeuvres/aerobatics, and rear crew activities (e.g. trooping and fast roping).

19.3 THERMAL ENVIRONMENT

- Aircrew are routinely exposed to extreme thermal environments in air and occasionally in water.
- The following physical parameters are relevant to heat exchange:
  - *Surface (solid) temperature*, relevant to K & R.
  - *Air temperature*, relevant to C (note that air temperature decreases 1°C per 150 m increase in altitude).
  - *Water temperature*, relevant to K & C.
  - *Air velocity*, due to wind and body movement, relevant to C & E.
  - *Water velocity*, due to waves/currents and body movement, relevant to C.
  - *Radiant temperature*, relevant to R.
  - *Humidity*, relevant to E.
- The following environmental measurement techniques are used:
  - *Air temperature*, measured when shielded from radiation by dry-bulb temperature.
  - *Radiant temperature*, estimated by a sensor placed in the centre of a metal sphere (globe temperature).
  - *Humidity*, expressed as relative humidity, wet-bulb temperature or water vapour pressure.

19.4 PHYSIOLOGICAL PARAMETERS

- *Core temperature* is the primary input to physiological thermoregulation and influences core-to-skin heat transfer.
- *Mean skin temperature* is a modulator of physiological thermoregulation, the site of heat exchange with environment and influences core-to-skin heat transfer; dictates water vapour pressure at skin.

19.5 HEAT EXCHANGE

INTERACTION OF PHYSICAL AND PHYSIOLOGICAL THERMAL FACTORS

- Heat exchange occurs within body (by K and C) and between body and environment (K, C, R and E), mainly at the skin surface (see Table 19.1 for details).
- Heat is gained from environment by convection when air temperature exceeds around 31°C.
- Evaporative heat loss reduced as environmental humidity increases.
- Greater air velocity enhances evaporative losses and convective gains and losses.

Table 19.1. Key features of heat exchange pathways

PATHWAY	MECHANISM AND MEDIUM	EQUATION (W) +/−=HEAT GAIN/LOSS (GRADIENT)	NOTES
Conduction (K)	Via direct molecular contact. Occurs within the body ($T_C–T_{SK}$), and between skin and solid surface in contact with skin ($T_{SK}–T_S$).	$K = h_K \times$ $(T_S–T_{SK})$	Important in contact heat exchange, but usually minor role in whole-body human heat exchange. Conductivity 24 times greater in water than air.
Convection (C)	Via a moving fluid. Occurs within the body by blood ($T_C–T_{SK}$), and between the skin (T_{SK}) and ambient air (T_A) or water (T_W).	$C = h_C \times$ $(T_A/T_W–T_{SK})$	Important heat loss pathway in cold, especially in wind or turbulent water. Much greater heat loss in water than air at same temperature.
Radiation (R)	Via electromagnetic waves. Occurs between skin (T_{SK}) and radiant sources (e.g. sun, hot/cold surfaces) (T_R).	$R = h_R \times$ $(T_R–T_{SK})$	Predominant heat loss pathway at rest. Solar radiation responsible for 'green-house effect' in cockpit.
Evaporation (E)	Energy absorbed when a liquid (e.g. sweat) changes to a gas.	$E = h_E \times$ $(P_{SK}–P_A)$	Predominant and potentially only heat exchange pathway in a hot environment.

Note: Physical parameters are identified in blue and physiological parameters are shown in grey. Pathways are quantified by temperature (*K*, *C* and *R* – 'dry' pathways) or water vapour pressure gradient (*E*), and a heat transfer coefficient (*h*). T_S = Surface temperature, T_A = Air temperature, T_W = Water temperature, V_A = Air velocity, V_W = Water velocity, T_R = Radiant temperature, P_A = Water vapour pressure, T_C = Core temperature, T_{SK} = Mean skin temperature

EFFECT OF CLOTHING

- Fabric and air trapped by clothing impose a thermal and evaporative resistance to heat transfer and create a microenvironment remote from the outside (macro) environment (Figure 19.2).
    - Key heat exchange surface is outer clothing layer which will be at a temperature (T_{CL}) between T_{SK} and T_A/T_R.
- Aircrew clothing and equipment may present considerable thermal and evaporative resistance:
    - Clothing with high thermal resistance ('insulation') is beneficial in cold and reduces the rate of dry heat gain in very hot environments (when $T_{A/R} > T_{SK}$).
    - Clothing with high evaporative resistance results in a humid microenvironment impairing sweat evaporation (a problem in heat) causing wet skin and under-clothing, leading to discomfort and reduced insulation (a problem in cold).

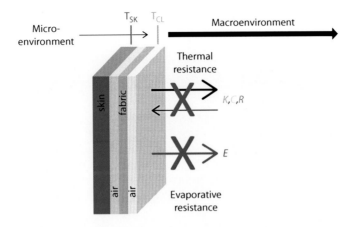

Figure 19.2 Thermal and evaporative resistance of clothing.

● Clothing should be worn in layers to match activity/environment requirements, and clothing designs should incorporate features to alter ventilation.

19.6 THERMOREGULATION

● Thermoregulation comprises physiological and behavioural/technological systems which are interrelated (see Figure 19.3).

PHYSIOLOGICAL THERMOREGULATION

● Body tries to regulate T_C. T_{SK} modulates the responses, particularly during initial stages of exposure.
● Receptors sensitive to 'warm' and 'cold' located in skin and core; these relay information to integrating controller in the hypothalamus, which instigates corrective mechanisms if there is a deviation from the reference thermal signal.
● Skin and core warming – 'Warm' receptors activated leading to vasodilatation, increased skin blood flow and sweat secretion:
   ● Increases T_{SK}, heat transfer to skin and increased potential for dry and evaporative heat loss.
● Skin and core cooling – 'Cold' receptors activated leading to vasoconstriction, decreased skin blood flow and thermogenesis (including shivering):
● Decreases T_{SK} and potential for dry heat loss, decreases transfer of heat to skin via blood-borne convection (increasing tissue insulation); increases metabolic heat production.

BEHAVIOURAL THERMOREGULATION

● Includes adding or removing clothing and moving faster or slower, initiated primarily by the activation of peripheral 'warm' or 'cold' receptors; T_{SK} is key determinant of thermal sensation and thermal comfort.
   ● Particularly important in cold (more cold than warm thermoreceptors in skin). Reduces need for physiological adjustments (which have disadvantages).

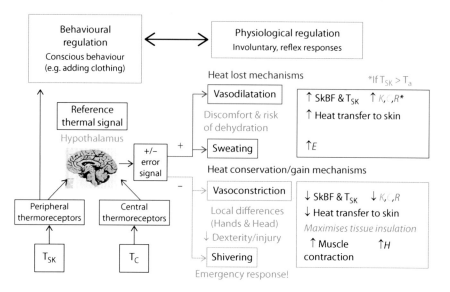

Figure 19.3 Physiological and behavioural thermoregulation.

19.7 COLD STRESS

BACKGROUND

- Usually possible to control cockpit environment to prevent cold stress:
  - Exceptions include some unpressurised aircraft operations, operating with doors open.
- Cold stress mainly a problem following emergency egress from aircraft on land or in water (see Chapter 22).
- Whole-body thermal balance usually not a problem in cold air, but in water immersion, cold shock and hypothermia are high risks due to greater cooling power of water. Therefore, immersion protection is a key element of aircrew clothing.

HAZARD

- Extremities vulnerable in cold air, with intense vasoconstriction causing discomfort, impaired manual performance (strength and dexterity) and risk of local cold injury:
  - Scalp, forehead and neck have limited vasoconstriction and are most comfortable regions in cold but must be insulated to prevent heat loss.
- Local cold injury may be classified as:
  - Freezing cold injury (FCI) due to sub-zero T_A and high V_A, ranges from superficial/reversible frostnip to frostbite.
  - Non-freezing cold injury (NFCI) due to prolonged exposure to cold and wet/damp conditions.

INDICES

- Cold stress quantified by Windchill Index (WCI) (see Chapter 22).

19.8 HEAT STRESS

BACKGROUND

- Combination of ambient temperature, aircraft heat sources and aircrew survival clothing may lead to heat stress in normal operations.
- As T_A increases, thermal balance usually maintained over wide ambient temperature range termed the zone of compensable heat stress (CHS).
  - As skin-to-environmental temperature gradient narrows, heat balance is achieved by increasing contribution from sweat evaporation.
- When the evaporative requirement exceeds evaporative potential of environment, thermoregulatory compensation is not possible (termed uncompensable heat stress, UCHS), leading to a progressive increase in T_C:
  - For routine piloting (around 140 W workload), onset of UCHS is at T_A of around 44°C.
  - At metabolic heat production compatible with rear crew activities (around 400 W), UCHS occurs at a T_A of approximately 38°C.
- Calculations are based on lightweight sports clothing; clothing with higher thermal/evaporative resistance (e.g. aircrew clothing) will narrow CHS zone further.

HAZARD

- Problems in hot environments include: discomfort, impaired physical and cognitive performance and heat illness (heat exhaustion, heat stroke):
  - Problems unlikely if $T_C < 38°C$, but profuse sweating increases risk of dehydration (can impair thermoregulation and performance).
  - Aircrew clothing may result in higher skin blood flow which can cause cardiovascular strain.
  - Head is most uncomfortable region in heat, so an ideal location to cool for comfort.

INDICES

- Environmental heat stress quantified by wet-bulb-globe temperature (WBGT) (see Chapter 22).

CHAPTER
20

Aircrew equipment – General

Contents

20.1 BACKGROUND

- Aircrew equipment is provided to aircraft occupants to support life and reduce risk of injury during flight, crash and emergency abandonment.
- Aircrew equipment sometimes termed aircrew equipment assembly (AEA) or pilot flight equipment (PFE) to cover scope of its composition and function.
- Aircrew equipment can be considered as personal protective equipment (PPE) and falls within the boundaries of national legislative controls. These typically require the employer to:
  - Provide the equipment.
  - Ensure it is fit for purpose.
  - Ensure it is fitted and maintained.
  - Provide training as required.
- The employee in turn must:
  - Use the equipment correctly.
  - Look after the PPE.
  - Inform the employer if equipment is damaged or functioning incorrectly.
- PPE in aviation is often used to reduce risk (the likelihood of harm) from a hazard (the potential to do harm). It is the last resort within a hierarchy of control measures which, in order of preference, would: eliminate; substitute; enclose or manage exposure to a hazard prior to considering PPE.

20.2 HAZARDS, RISKS AND MITIGATIONS

- Table 20.1 lists some common items of aircrew equipment and the hazards they mitigate.
- Aircrew equipment must 'integrate' with occupant, aircraft and the other protective equipment.
- Some items of equipment may be advantageous for more than one hazard but can also impose a burden on the user, so risks from the hazard must outweigh the risks in using the equipment. For example:
  - Aircrew helmet reduces risks from impact and noise but increases risk of musculoskeletal injury to neck.

Table 20.1 Aviation hazards and aircrew equipment intended to mitigate risk

AIRCREW EQUIPMENT	NOISE	SUSTAINED ACCELERATION	HEAT	COLD	HYPOBARIC HYPOXIA	TOXIC FUMES	DROWNING	BALLISTIC	ELECTROMAGNETIC RADIATION	IMPACT
Helmet (shell)	✓			✓						✓
Visor, goggles or glasses			✓					✓	✓	✓
Oronasal oxygen mask			✓	✓	✓	✓				
Flame retardant coveralls			✓	✓					✓	
Immersion suit			✓	✓			✓		✓	
Body armour			✓	✓				✓	✓	✓
Smoke hood/mask						✓				
Life preserver							✓			
Anti-G trousers		✓	✓	✓						
Boots			✓	✓						
Gloves			✓	✓					✓	
Headset	✓									

Table 20.2 Commonly used aircrew equipment, including main function and potential disadvantages

ITEM	DESCRIPTION	FUNCTION	OTHER CONSIDERATIONS
Anti-G Suit	Five-bladder or full coverage trousers that inflate to provide protection from Gz acceleration or as an adjunct for altitude protection.	Compresses lower limbs and abdomen, increasing peripheral vascular resistance and improving venous return.	Increased bulk, reduced comfort but increased thermal protection (heat and cold).
Life Vest	Waistcoat or jacket with integral survival aids, pockets and flotation collar.	Provides flotation in water. Carries location aids. Integrates with escape system in ejection seat aircraft.	Increased bulk, reduced comfort, decreased head and neck mobility, reduced visual field of regard, impaired egress. Provides thermal protection (fire) but increases thermal burden (heat).
Helmet	Rigid helmet with open face that incorporates face visor, ear cups and chin strap.	Provides impact protection and mounting platform for communications, oxygen mask, clear and tinted visors, laser eye protection, display systems and night vision enhancing equipment.	Increased head-mounted mass, decreased comfort. Provides some ballistic protection; improves speech intelligibility and preventing hearing loss (see Chapter 24). Provides protection from heat (flame) and cold.
Immersion Suit	Single piece overall with wrist and neck seals plus socks or integral boots. Constructed from Ventile fabric (fine weave cotton) or laminate containing a moisture vapour permeable membrane.	Dry suit for water immersion. Increases survival time and reduces cold shock risk.	Increased bulk, reduced comfort and mobility. Provides some additional in-water buoyancy. Provides protection from heat and cold but increased thermal burden in non-emergency setting.
Body Armour	Usually tabard type vest of soft armour to which hard plates can be added (front, back and loin). Survival aids pockets, weapons and ammunition are also attached.	Provides ballistic protection and carriage of equipment for war fighting or escape and evasion.	Significant weight and bulk, which increases physiological burden and reduces mobility. Issues with safe operation of aircraft, crash survival and escape/abandonment.
Flying Clothing	Comprises a base and shell layer. Base layer provides insulation and comfort and is usually a long-sleeved vest and long johns made from a lightweight woven fabric (cotton or Kermel viscose). The shell layer is either long-sleeved jacket and trousers or a single piece coverall. Often made from fire retardant aramid fabric.	Provides protection from heat and cold (including flame exposure), carriage of personal effects and small items such as maps.	To function effectively for fire protection, a complete shell and base layer must be worn (omitting base layer decreases protection by up to 50%). Thermal burden in hot weather from base layer must be balanced against fire risk.

  ◦ Fire protective clothing reduces risk of burn injury from flame exposure (see
    Section 20.3) and protects the skin from mechanical abrasion, UV light and
    other irritants but imposes a thermal and physical burden on the wearer.
- Table 20.2 shows the main categories of commonly used aircrew equipment, high-
  lighting main function and potential disadvantages.

20.3 PROTECTION FROM FIRE

- Fire risks in aviation are small, but consequences are significant as burn injuries cause
  high morbidity and mortality; even small burns may result in scarring that causes a
  loss of function and employment.
- Fire occurs in all aircraft types but is most frequent in rotary platforms; a fast jet
  ejectee may land in crash site; multi-engine aircraft may have on-board electrical fire,
  smoke and fumes.

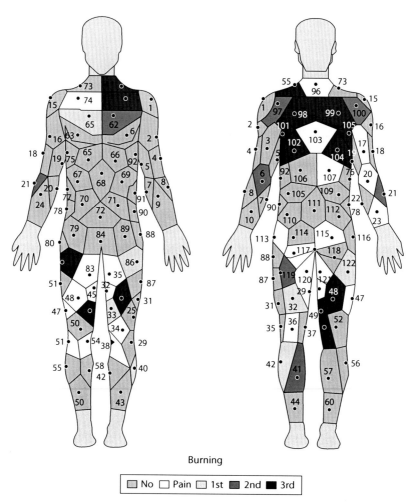

Burning

No ☐   Pain ☐   1st ☐   2nd ■   3rd ■

Figure 20.1 An example of a prediction of burn injury using an instrumented mannequin.
(BTTG Fire Technical Services, BTTG Ltd Group.)

- Many aircraft feature fire suppression systems, auto shutoff valves and crashworthy fuel tanks to reduce fire risk.
- Clothing systems are used when the residual risk of burns from fire remains intolerable:
  - Typical standard for clothing system flash fire protection is 4-second exposure to flame source simulating aviation fuel fire.
  - Following fire exposure, clothing equipment should not continue burning, exhibit molten drip or propagate flame.
  - Predicted severe burn injuries must remain below 30% (see Figure 20.1).
- Smoke hoods and masks can provide protection from toxic fumes and thermal environment.
- Fire-fighting equipment carried on board wide-bodied aircraft includes breathing systems, fire gauntlets and additional clothing.
- Aircrew gloves allow the wearer to grasp a hot surface during escape but are inadequate for burn protection. Fire-fighting gauntlets provide adequate protection but are too bulky for routine flight duties.

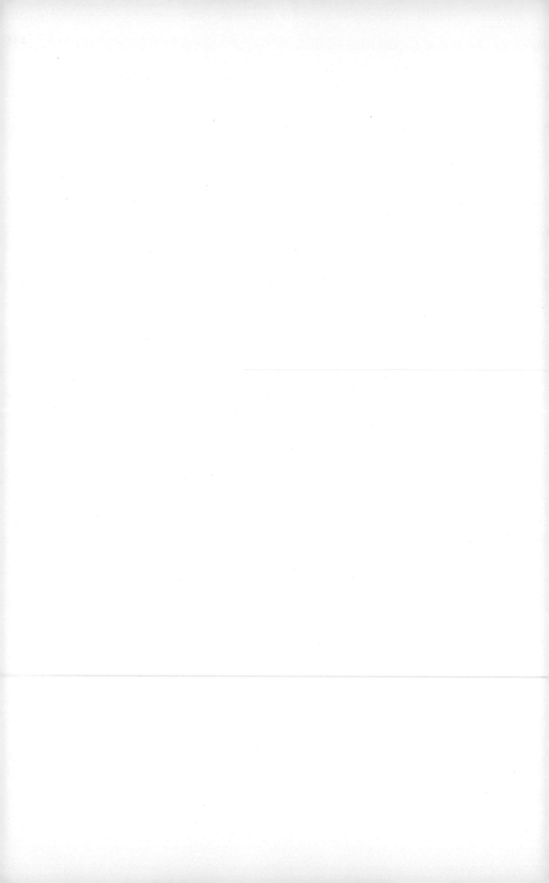

CHAPTER

21

Aircrew equipment – Head injury and protection

Contents

Key Facts
- Head injury is common in all aircraft accidents.
- Head protection can improve survivability by preventing severe head trauma and by limiting disturbances of consciousness, permitting aircrew to escape from a crashed aircraft.
- Head injuries can be classified into three categories: skull fractures, focal brain injuries and diffuse brain injuries.
- Head impact acceleration often made up of linear and rotational components.
- A helmet protects the head by distributing the impact load to reduce soft-tissue injury and prevent deformations of the skull.

21.1 TYPES OF HEAD INJURY

- Head injuries encountered in aviation can be classified as:
  - Skull fractures.
  - Focal brain injuries.
  - Diffuse brain injuries.
- These injury types result from static and dynamic mechanical loading. Static loading, where force is applied to the head very slowly, is rarely seen in aviation. Dynamic loading is characterised by a rapid input to the head and can be of two types:
  - Impulsive loading – occurs when the head is set in motion or the moving head is arrested without being struck.

- Impact loading – results from a combination of contact forces and inertial forces. Impact loading is most frequently seen type; inertial forces can be minimal in impacts where the head is prevented from moving.

21.2 MECHANICS OF HEAD INJURY

SKULL INJURY

- When the head is subjected to a heavy blow, skull bones break in a characteristic way to absorb energy:
  - If struck by a discrete object, skull can fracture over an area corresponding closely with shape of the striking object; secondary fissures radiate outwards into surrounding bone along lines dictated by architecture of skull.
  - If struck by a broad impact, multiple fissures radiate away from site of the blow; fissures turn downwards towards the skull base and are directed into channels between thicker buttresses and skull floor.
  - A heavy blow directed from underneath may lift the cervical spine such that it breaks away from its ring-base attachments.
- Brain and covering membranes underlying impact are commonly injured, resulting in contusions or lacerations; these are known as coup injuries and occur at the point of primary impact.
- Breaking strength of facial and cranial bones has been determined from cadaveric studies:
  - 30 G for nose.
  - 40 G for jaw.
  - 50 G for zygomatic arch.
  - 100 G for front teeth.
  - 50–100 G for temporo-parietal bone.
  - 100–200 G for frontal bone.

BRAIN AND VASCULAR INJURY

- Inertial load leads to rapid movement of the head and can cause functional and structural damage.
- Differential movement of skull and brain occurs because brain is free to move within the skull and momentarily lags skull movement due to inertia.
- Skull and dura move relative to the brain surface and parasagittal bridging veins may tear.
- Rotational head motion may tear membranes and cause intracranial haemorrhage:
  - Blood accumulates in epidural, subdural or subarachnoid spaces according to source.
  - Injured person may appear initially dazed or temporarily concussed but unconsciousness can occur after a latent period as intracranial pressure increases due to blood accumulation.
- In a head strike, skull decelerates rapidly while semi-fluid brain continues moving towards the impact point:
  - Severe contusions opposite the impact point can occur where the brain glides over the jagged contours of the skull's inner surfaces.

- These contra-coup injuries can be more severe than corresponding coup-type contusions.
- Head motion may also produce strain within brain parenchyma itself, leading to classical cerebral concussion, diffuse axonal injury and associated tissue-tear injury.

CHARACTERISTICS OF HEAD ACCELERATION

- Impact acceleration can consist of two components:
  - Translational acceleration, which occurs when the centre of mass of the head is accelerated in a straight line; pure translational acceleration is uncommon.
  - Rotational acceleration, which occurs when the head is rotated around its centre of mass.
- Anchoring of the head by the neck results in angular acceleration as the head centre of mass angulates about a point in the mid or lower cervical region:
  - Angular acceleration considered most injurious in causing concussion, diffuse axonal injury and subdural haematoma.
  - Virtually every known type of head injury can be produced by angular acceleration.

HEAD INJURY TOLERANCE

- Wayne State Tolerance Curve (WSTC) derived from cadaveric and other studies to produce plot of head acceleration against impact duration to provide an indication of impact tolerance.
- Head Injury Criterion (HIC) later derived from WSTC for use in automotive industry but does not address rotational acceleration.
- Model predicting tolerance to both linear and rotational injuries yet to be fully developed due to complexity.

21.3 PREVENTION OF HEAD INJURY

- Aim is to eliminate potential head impacts:
  - Restraint harnesses, airbags and provision of adequate space in the cockpit can minimise head contact with aircraft structures.
  - Aircrew protective helmet is the standard method of reducing head injury risk.

AIRCREW HELMET DESIGN

- Two basic energy-absorbing systems can be used in protective helmets:
  - Glass fibre shell that breaks up on impact; each time a glass fibre ruptures or is pulled out of its resin matrix, energy is absorbed inelastically. This technique requires a strong, rigid shell.
  - Rigid foam layer beneath the shell; crushes on impact to about 40% of its initial thickness. Provision of a finite stopping distance reduces peak acceleration imposed. In this design, a lighter shell can be employed.
- Helmet protuberances should be minimised or designed to break away at a non-injurious force level, and the helmet surface should be smooth, to increase tendency for helmet to slide along a surface and reduce rotational acceleration.

HELMET STANDARDS

- Level of head protection provided by helmets is determined by helmet construction, liner/suspension characteristics, sizing and accessory attachment features.
- Many helmet impact test standards available; choice of test standard should be tailored to hazard and type of injuries anticipated.
  - For example, rotary crew helmet may require greater front and side impact protection from crash forces, whereas fast jet helmet may require greater rear (occipital) protection from ejection sequence.
- Aspects of helmet performance specified include:
  - Shock absorption – test to assess transmitted force (e.g. no more than 300 G transmitted through helmet to head form of impact test rig).
  - Helmet retention – test to assess whether a helmet may be lost during impact.
  - Penetration resistance – test to assess penetration by conical point; not included in recent standards as penetration impacts unlikely in most aircraft accidents.

ADDITIONAL FUNCTIONS OF AIRCREW HELMET

- Additional functions of aircrew helmet are described in Chapter 20.
  - Ballistic protection is technically difficult to achieve in an aircrew helmet without increasing the overall mass substantially.
  - Fast jet aircrew helmets also need to provide windblast protection during high-speed ejections and bird strike protection.
  - Helmet noise attenuating ear cups can offer additional impact protection without any increase in helmet weight.
- Helmet mounted display systems add mass and should be mounted so that the centre of gravity of the helmeted head is not unduly displaced from its normal position:
  - Heavier objects mounted in front of the eyes (such as night vision goggles) are sometimes counterbalanced by placing components such as batteries at rear of helmet.
  - Goggles should separate from helmet before ejection or impact to reduce injurious forces on the neck.
- Helmets should not be uncomfortable or impair aircrew performance.

Aircrew equipment – Thermal protection and survival

Contents

> **Key Facts**
> - Aviation heat strain risk can be predicted using heat stress indices.
> - Pre-takeoff phase may be the most thermally stressful.
> - Most insulation from cold weather clothing comes from air trapping.
> - Heat loss is much greater in water than air; a dry immersion suit is required whenever there is risk of ditching in cold water.
> - Training improves effectiveness of general principles of survival: protection, location, water, food.

22.1 HEAT

- Heat strain is a risk in air operations. Risk depends on heat production by individual, aircrew equipment worn, air temperature, humidity, radiant heat load (see Chapter 19).
- Sources of heat include: pilot's metabolism (0.06 kW); aerodynamic heat load (9 kW); avionics (1.2 kW); solar radiation (2.5 kW).
- Other stressors may be additive, including dehydration, noise, vibration, G, motion illness and confinement.

IDENTIFYING THOSE AT RISK

- Risk factors for heat illness in aircrew include:
  - Lack of acclimatisation.
  - Poor hydration status.
  - Body size (mass, skinfold thickness); heat stroke 3.5 times more prevalent in overweight.
  - State of training/sudden increase in training, low aerobic fitness (>12 min for 1.5 mile run) and high body mass index (>26 kg·m^{-2}); 9-fold greater risk of heat illness.
  - State of health (intercurrent disease).
  - Sleep deprivation.

ASSESSING THE ENVIRONMENT

- Environment assessed using one of the heat stress indices (e.g. Wet-Bulb-Globe Temperature [WBGT] index):

$$WBGT = 0.1T_{db} + 0.7T_{wb} + 0.2T_{g}$$

where:

T_{db} = dry-bulb temperature
T_{wb} = wet bulb temperature
T_{g} = globe temperature

The weightings emphasise the importance of humidity for heat stress (see Chapter 19).

- WBGT metres are relatively inexpensive. To reduce chance of heat injury in lightly clothed individuals, the following limits are recommended:
  - 26.5–28.8°C: Use discretion, especially if untrained or unacclimatised.
  - 29.5–30.5°C: Avoid strenuous activity in the sun.
- WGBT of limited applicability to aviators as it relies on sweating which may not be effective wearing aircrew clothing; may not reflect cockpit thermal conditions.
- Fighter Index of Thermal Stress (FITS) developed using ambient WBGT values to predict thermal strain in fast jet pilots during low-level flight; now of limited utility due to changes in aircrew equipment design and flight profiles.

EFFECT ON PERFORMANCE

- Literature conflicting, but WBGT above 26.7°C associated with negative effects on attentional, perceptual and mathematical processing tasks.
- Heat may also affect physiological performance (e.g. sweating and vasodilation can reduce acceleration tolerance by 1 G [see Chapter 16]).

PREVENTION/PROTECTION

- In the preflight phase:
  - Allow time for crews to acclimatise if starting to operate in hot environment (can take 10 days).
  - Provide air-conditioned buildings and transport.

- Cover aircraft/use shade wherever possible; wet or spray cabin cover; use mobile air-conditioning units.
- Minimise walk-round or have someone else perform it.
- Allow sufficient recovery time between flights.
- In the flight phase:
  - Use Environmental Conditioning System (ECS) of aircraft to provide cockpit cooling (bleed air from engine cooled through ram-air heat exchangers, and Cold Air Unit).
  - Minimise ground cockpit standby and taxi times due to inefficiency of ECS cooling when engines at idle thrust.
  - Consider use of personal conditioning garments worn next to skin:
    - Air cooled type relies on evaporative cooling (i.e. sweating) and is less comfortable; high volume of air required.
    - Liquid cooled type relies on removing heat by convection through coolant pumped through tubes in elastic garment, supplied by an aircraft vapour cycle refrigeration system or portable ice bottle plus battery-powered pump.
    - Personal conditioning garments rarely used in aviation due to practical difficulties, bulk, hoses, thermal load when not in use, practicality.
    - Liquid conditioning garment forms an essential part of spacesuit design for EVA (see Chapter 6).

22.2 COLD

- Cold stress not usually a problem in the cockpit unless operating with doors open (e.g. transport aircraft or helicopter); convective cooling by airflow may increase risk.
- Cold threat occurs mainly on the ground before/after flight or following abandonment.
- Risks include hypothermia, cold injury and cold shock/drowning.
- Water represents a greater threat because of its higher thermal conductivity and specific heat.

ASSESSING THE ENVIRONMENT

- Cooling power of the environment is the result of air temperature, air movement or movement through air.
- These factors combined into the wind chill index (WCI), which illustrates the cooling effect of temperature and wind on bare skin, predicting danger of freezing cold injury.
- WCI of little use in predicting time to hypothermia or clothing requirements.
- Required Clothing Insulation Index (IREQ) can be used to calculate acceptable time of environmental exposure (includes effect of clothing).

PREVENTION/PROTECTION

- Acclimatisation: debate about practical extent to which humans can acclimatise to cold. Hazardous initial responses to cold water immersion can be reduced by 50% following five 2-minute immersions in cold water (habituation may last for months).

- Protective clothing for cold should:
  - Prevent heat loss from body by insulation.
  - Provide insulation by trapping a large volume of dry air in small sections; minimise internal convection and cold air ingress (windproof).
  - Enable adjustments in insulation to cater for increased/decreased metabolic heat production (use of layers, openings).
  - Wick moisture away from body.
  - Be vapour permeable to prevent accumulation and condensation of moisture under the clothing which reduces clothing insulation.
  - Include head protection (due to the absence of cold constrictor fibres in blood vessels of scalp).

22.3 PRINCIPLES OF SURVIVAL

- Following emergency, aircraft occupants may be required to survive in hostile environment.
- Survival training greatly enhances chances of survival.
- Priorities of survivor (in order) are:
  - Protection – principally clothing and shelter (see below for protection from water immersion).
  - Location – includes filing a flight plan, use of personal locator beacons, pyrotechnic and other visual aids such as strobes and brightly coloured clothing.
  - Water – intake can be reduced to 110–220 mL per day under ideal conditions for short period; reverse osmosis pumps, desalination kits and solar still may be used to source water.
  - Food – intake can be reduced to 600–1,400 calories for a short period; use of survival rations (primarily carbohydrate) and survival skills enhances preservation of function.

22.4 WATER IMMERSION

- Hazards of water immersion can be considered in three phases: Cold Shock, Underwater Escape, Swim Failure.

COLD SHOCK

- Sudden immersion in cold water (<15°C) causes cold shock which results in:
  - An inspiratory gasp.
  - Severe hyperventilation.
  - Hypertension.
- Breath hold time significantly reduced and in untrained individuals is probably less than 15 sec.
- Diving reflex may also be triggered by cold water stimulation to face, causing bradycardia and apnoea.
- Sympathetic/parasympathetic conflict between the two reflexes may lead to incapacitating arrhythmias.

UNDERWATER ESCAPE

- Following a helicopter ditching, occupants must escape while disorientated, with potential entrapment or obstruction from crashed structure.
- Escape time from an immersed, inverted helicopter takes between 15 and 30 sec.
- Loss of life following ditching can occur from cardiac shock or drowning due to inadequate breath hold capacity.

Table 22.1 Characteristics of life preservers used in aviation

CHARACTERISTIC	WHAT	WHY
Inflation	Automatic for ejection seat aircraft. Manual for all others. Compressed gas cylinder with standby oral inflation valve.	Automatic inflation prevents unconscious ejectee from drowning. Manual inflation allows the survivor to delay activation until required, as inflation within a ditched helicopter cabin would delay or prevent escape.
Self-Righting	Ability to turn a floating survivor face up within 5 sec.	Prevents weak or unconscious survivors from drowning if turned face down by a wave.
Freeboard	The amount the stole holds lowest part of airway (usually mouth) above water (typically around 120 mm).	Prevents drowning of unconscious survivors from splashes.
Flotation Angle	The angle at which an unconscious survivor is supported in the water (optimally 45°).	45° offers best compromise between freeboard and self-righting and provides good wave riding stability.
Visibility	Bright orange or yellow with reflective tapes. Water activated lights often embodied.	Allow survivors to be seen in water.
Location	Whistles for attracting attention in poor visibility. Electronic beacons with satellite technology to provide rapid global location.	Allow rapid location and recovery of survivors.
Recovery	Lifting beckets and jacket harness system.	Allow retrieval of survivors from the water; note risk of postural hypotension if lifted vertically from water.
Survival Aid Pockets	Pockets for beacons and survival aids.	Allows survivors to assist rescuer in location and recovery or, if required, to escape and evade.

- These risks can be mitigated by:
  - Immersion suit to reduce cold shock.
  - Helicopter underwater escape ('dunker') training to reduce escape time.
  - Short-Term Air Supply System (STASS), underwater breathing apparatus (30 sec) to manage reduced breath hold time.

SWIM FAILURE

- Rapid cooling of the limbs results in nerve and muscle contraction failure, reducing dexterity and swimming, making water inhalation more likely. Shivering also interferes with swimming.
- Hypothermia (cooling of body core) occurs after around 30 minutes, increasing drowning risk.
- Swim failure can be reduced by use of:
  - Immersion suits and thermal insulation – suits designed for protection against immersion are defined as 'wet' or 'dry'. Dry suits preserve insulation properties of dry clothes and may provide some flotation.
  - Life rafts.
  - Life preservers – inflatable stole to provide flotation (see Table 22.1).

CHAPTER

23

Noise, hearing and vibration

Contents

Key Facts
- Noise is a significant aeromedical occupational hazard.
- Key components of noise include frequency, intensity and duration.
- Aircrew and flight line personnel should be enrolled in a hearing conservation program, including surveillance (both site and medical), audiometric testing, employee training, engineering controls, hearing protection and record-keeping.
- Hearing loss may be conductive, sensorineural or mixed; temporary or permanent.
- Whole body vibration entails risks to health and safety of aircrew.
- Sources of aircraft vibration include engine, transmission, aerodynamic forces and wind, mission equipment, others.
- Vibration is associated with deleterious health effects and performance degradation.

23.1 NOISE

SOUND: SENSATION FROM STIMULATION OF AUDITORY MECHANISM

- Requirements:
  - Source that vibrates, explodes or impacts.

- Medium (e.g. air).
- Receiver (e.g. human ear).
- Travels in waves with cyclic pressure changes of compression and rarefaction; frequency quantified as cycles per second or hertz (Hz) (see Figures 23.1 and 23.2).
- Speed: depends on medium (more dense = faster).
  - Air = 335 m/s (1100 ft/s).
  - Water = 1372 m/s (4500 ft/s).

COMPONENTS

- Frequency: number of cycles per second.
- Intensity: physical level of sound; describes strength of sound wave:
  - Objectively expressed in units of decibels (dB).
  - Ear can perceive extremely large pressure range; logarithmic dB scale used.
  - Multiple scales to measure sound pressure level (SPL):
    - dB SPL – measuring physical pressures.
    - dBA SPL – measuring subjective pressures that are adjusted to represent response of human ear (A-weighted scale on a sound level metre).
    - dBP SPL – measuring the maximum sound pressure of impulse.
  - Loudness is subjective perception of intensity.

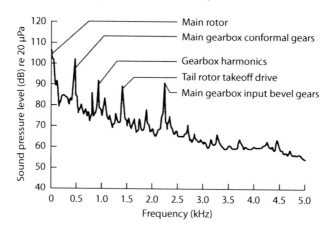

Figure 23.1 Cabin noise spectrum of a helicopter with a single rotor (Lynx), showing the various aircraft components contributing to the cabin noise levels.

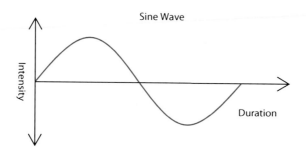

Figure 23.2 Properties of sound wave.

- Temporal characteristics:
  - Steady-state.
  - Blast overpressure.
- Duration:
  - Important consideration for judging sound's potential for damaging hearing, quantified by 'noise dose'.
- Mathematically key behaviours:
  - Doubling distance from source (steady-state or impulse) decreases the level by 6 dB (outdoors only).
  - Doubling the noise source:
    - Combination of two different noise sources of equal loudness will increase intensity by 3 dB (e.g. steady-state noise source 'A' is 93 dBA and noise source 'B' is 93 dBA, combined result is 96 dBA).

HAZARDOUS NOISE

- Continuous/steady-state noise:
  - Nations have various standards for occupational noise exposure.
  - Action level (exposure level at which hearing testing, health education training and availability of hearing protection are required) typically 85 dB over an 8-hour time period.
  - Maximum exposure level above which employees cannot be exposed is 115 dB(A) in the United States, Exposure Limit Value is 87 dB(A) in Europe.
- Impulse noise:
  - Hazardous level is ≥140 dBP SPL.
- What makes noise unsafe?
  - Hazard depends on overall exposure, intensity and duration.
  - Long-term exposure to hazardous steady-state noise can cause gradual hearing loss.
  - Exposure to hazardous impulse noise can cause immediate permanent hearing loss.
  - Large inter-individual variability.

23.2 HEARING

RANGE AND SPEECH

- Audible range: 20–20,000 Hz at birth.
- Intensity range for impulse noise:
  - 140 dB SPL – threshold of pain.
  - 180 dB SPL – threshold of tissue damage.
  - 200 dB SPL – threshold of death (estimated).
- Speech frequency range: 250–4000 Hz.
- Consonants:
  - Soft, low energy, high frequency.
  - Convey 80% of meaning of speech.
- Vowels:
  - Loud, high energy, low frequency.
  - Convey 80% of energy of speech.

ANATOMY OF HEARING

- See Figure 23.3.
- Outer ear – cartilage and soft tissue:
  - Pinna – focus energy to localize the direction.
  - External ear canal – connects the pinna to eardrum; resonator making sounds louder and deeper.
- Middle ear:
  - Ossicles – small bones behind eardrum (malleus, incus and stapes).
  - Eardrum – transmits vibrations via ossicles through middle ear to inner ear.
  - Eustachian tube – connects middle ear to posterior oropharynx for pressure equalization.
- Inner ear:
  - Cochlea
    - Fluid-filled tube divided into three cavities (scala media, scala tympani and scala vestibuli).
    - Basilar membrane forms a partition between the scala media and scala tympani, contains the Organ of Corti.

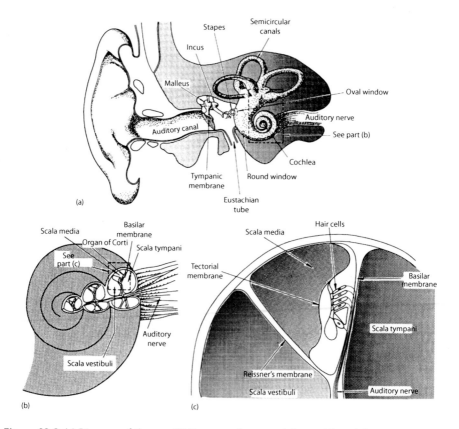

Figure 23.3 (a) Diagram of the ear. (b) Cutaway diagram of the cochlea of the inner ear. (c) Cross section of the basilar membrane and the organ of Corti, the hair cells of which are stimulated by movement of the tectorial membrane relative to the basilar membrane.

- Organ of Corti contains approximately 20,000 hair cells; hair-like projections (stereocilia) attached.
    - Hair cells respond based on sound frequency; create signals that become nerve impulses.
  - Vestibular system:
    - Utricle, saccule, three semicircular canals.
    - Semicircular canals respond to angular acceleration; utricle and saccule respond to linear acceleration (control posture and balance).
- Acoustic nerve (VIII CN) carries the nerve impulses through brainstem to auditory processing centres in brain.

HEARING LOSS

- Conductive:
  - Occurs within outer and/or middle ear.
  - May be amenable to medical or surgical correction.
  - Sound not conducted efficiently through outer/middle ear to inner ear; reduction in sound level heard or ability to hear soft sounds.
  - Causes may include fluid in the middle ear, eardrum perforation, impacted earwax, ear infection or auditory tube dysfunction.
- Sensorineural hearing loss (SNHL):
  - Occurs when inner ear is damaged; usually permanent.
  - Reduces ability to hear faint sounds (e.g. consonants).
  - Speech may sound unclear or unintelligible even if loud enough to be heard.
  - Causes include illnesses, ototoxic drugs, aging, head trauma or unprotected exposure to hazardous noise.
- Mixed:
  - Conductive and SNHL in combination.
  - Damage in the outer or middle ear concurrent with inner ear.
- Noise-induced hearing loss (NIHL):
  - Permanent loss caused by exposure to hazardous noise or if hearing protection not worn properly.
  - One of the most common occupational diseases; may occur gradually or from single high impulse exposure.
  - Hearing difficult in noisy listening environments (e.g. combat, military vehicles and aircraft, weapons fire or industrial operations).
  - Loss may adversely impact communication and mission effectiveness.
  - Early stage usually associated with a high frequency SNHL.
  - Continued, unprotected exposures to hazardous noise can produce a marked loss in ability to communicate; inability to hear sound frequencies necessary for speech intelligibility.
  - Reduced job performance and quality of life.
- Temporary hearing loss:
  - Known as temporary threshold shift (TTS); usually abates within 48 hr but can last longer.
  - Symptoms include a temporary muffling of sound after hazardous exposure, a sensation of fullness in the ears, tinnitus and increased feelings of stress or fatigue.
  - Repeated TTS can result in permanent hearing loss; permanent threshold shift (PTS).

- Permanent hearing loss:
  - Loss from steady-state noise exposure occurring gradually, often over many years.
  - Usually no outward symptoms associated; individuals are often unaware of the gradual change until impairment.
  - Single impulse high-intensity noise may cause.
  - Initially results in hearing loss in the higher audiometric test frequencies (e.g. 3000–6000 Hz).
- Tinnitus:
  - Perceived ringing, buzzing or hissing sound; damage to inner ear from unprotected, high-intensity noise exposure.
  - May be temporary, serving as warning sign that overexposure has occurred; may also be permanent, with or without hearing loss.
  - Treatment (e.g. behavioural modification, sound therapy, hearing aid usage) may decrease level of annoyance but not curative.
  - Can be prevented by the regular use of hearing protection.
- Ototoxin exposure:
  - Exposure to certain chemicals, alone or in combination with hazardous noise, may result in hearing loss.
  - Organic solvents are the most commonly identified; others (e.g., metals, chemical asphyxiants, some classes of antibiotics) may also contribute.
  - Effects of noise and chemicals may be synergistic.

23.3 VIBRATION

VIBRATION BASICS

- Definitions:
  - Vibration – mechanical oscillation of a structure about an equilibrium point.
  - Resonant frequency – external forces induce oscillations at greater amplitudes at specific frequencies resulting in energy increase.
  - Damping – reduction in amplitude of an oscillation resulting from energy being drained from system.
- Units of vibration:
  - Frequency – repetition rate; measured in Hertz (cycles per second).
  - Amplitude – maximum displacement of oscillation; measured in inches or centimetres (root mean square).
  - Acceleration – rate of change of velocity of oscillation; measured in metres per second squared (m/s^2) or gravity (g).

VIBRATION THEORY

- Every object that has mass has a resonant frequency; different masses have different resonant frequencies.
- An object will vibrate (excite) when it receives energy input.
- Energy input near resonant frequency will be amplified.

- Damping will reduce vibration by reducing energy through suspension systems, shock absorbers or other energy-dissipating devices.
- Vibration can be introduced into airframe from engine components, rotor blades, wind, aerodynamic forces.

VIBRATION IN HUMANS

- Humans are made up of different 'components' with different masses and resonant frequencies (see Figure 23.4).
- Affected by vibration in three translational axes (X, Y, Z) as well as rotational.
- Low frequency vibration most harmful to humans (0.1–1,250 Hz):
  - Motion sickness, 0.1–0.5 Hz.
  - Whole body vibration (WBV), 0.5–80 Hz.
  - Hand arm vibration (HAV), 6–1250 Hz.
- Individual differences in resonance frequency:
  - Height, weight, body mass.
  - Posture.
- Key frequencies of interest for WBV:
  - Vertical vibration, 4–8 Hz.
  - Horizontal vibration, 1–2 Hz.
- Key frequencies of interest for HAV:
  - All directions, 6–350 Hz.

HAZARDS OF VIBRATION

- WBV hazards include visual disturbance, reduced tracking task performance, fatigue, hyperventilation, motion sickness, reduced coordination, musculoskeletal disorders, cardiovascular and gastrointestinal disorders.
- HAV hazards include loss of grip strength and reaction time, inflammatory changes, including carpal tunnel syndrome and vibration-induced white finger syndrome.

VIBRATION LIMITS

- International and military standards exist for exposure to WBV and HAV based on:
  - Frequency weighted acceleration (frequencies that are harmful).
  - Vector sum of vibration in all three axes.
  - 8-hr equivalent exposure.
- Some helicopter platforms found to approach or exceed vibration limits in certain crew seating positions.

PROTECTION AGAINST VIBRATION

- Attenuation of source through aircraft design or flight path selected.
- Dynamic vibration absorbers (e.g. in floor of Chinook helicopter).
- Vibration isolating seat.
- Active vibration damping (e.g. Merlin EH101 helicopter).

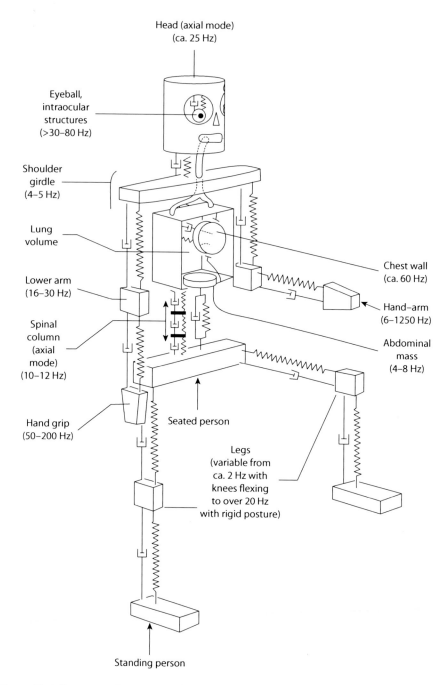

Head (axial mode)
(ca. 25 Hz)

Eyeball,
intraocular
structures
(>30–80 Hz)

Shoulder
girdle
(4–5 Hz)

Lung
volume

Chest wall
(ca. 60 Hz)

Lower arm
(16–30 Hz)

Hand–arm
(6–1250 Hz)

Spinal
column
(axial
mode)
(10–12 Hz)

Abdominal
mass
(4–8 Hz)

Hand grip
(50–200 Hz)

Seated person

Legs
(variable from
ca. 2 Hz with
knees flexing
to over 20 Hz
with rigid posture)

Standing person

Figure 23.4 Resonance frequencies of body parts.

CHAPTER 24

Hearing protection and communication

Contents

Key Facts
- Exposure to high noise over time will cause permanent hearing damage.
- High noise will reduce communications intelligibility and be of operational consequence.
- Exposure to high-level communications over time will cause permanent hearing damage.

24.1 EXPOSURE TO NOISE

BACKGROUND

- Exposure to aircraft noise may reduce speech intelligibility.
- Exposure to aircraft noise may cause noise-induced hearing loss (NIHL) – see Chapter 23.
- Communications signal can also cause hearing damage.
- Noise exposure is limited by national regulations, typically with mitigation priorities given as:
    1. Reduction of noise at source through engineering controls.
    2. Reduction of exposure through organisational measures.
    3. Personal hearing protection.

24.2 HEARING PROTECTION

CONVENTIONAL AIRCREW NOISE PROTECTION

- Flight helmets and communication headsets incorporating:
    - Circumaural earmuff assemblies (earshell, earseal, internal damping material) mounted on suspension system (in helmet shell) or headband.
    - Integrated telephone for communications.

NOISE ATTENUATION OF CONVENTIONAL PROTECTION

- Attenuation can be considered in three distinct regions:
    - Low frequencies (<400 Hz); attenuation controlled by movement of earshell against the head. Influencing parameters:
        - Earshell volume.
        - Stiffness of earseals.
        - Air volume.
        - Fit of earshell to head.
    - Intermediate frequencies (400 Hz–2 kHz); attenuation controlled by transmission loss of noise through earshell. Influencing parameters:
        - Type and mass of the earshell material.
    - High frequencies (>2 kHz); attenuation controlled by:
        - Type of earshell lining material.
        - Direct shielding of head by flight helmet shell.
- Other factors:
    - Structures within earshell (e.g. telephones), if not properly supported, can be detrimental to attenuation between 500 Hz and 2 kHz.
    - Different earshell suspension mechanisms in flight helmets can affect attenuation afforded around 1–2 kHz.

LIMITATIONS OF CONVENTIONAL PROTECTION

- In high-level noise, effective protection to outer ear is limited as noise is also transmitted to cochlea via the bony parts of the head, face and torso (bone-conducted noise) and can become the dominant source:
    - Bone-conduction transmission greatest around 1–2 kHz, where useful attenuation of conventional hearing protectors may be limited to around 45 dB.
    - Helmet shell and visor provide additional noise reduction at cochlea above about 4 kHz due to direct shielding of head.
- Typical attenuation afforded by earmuff devices is relatively poor at lower frequencies, increases steadily in the mid-frequency bands with high levels of protection >2 kHz (see Figure 24.1).
- Noise levels under a helmet peak around 250 Hz; to further reduce hearing damage risk, additional attenuation is required at these frequencies.

ENHANCED HEARING PROTECTION

- Active noise reduction (ANR) is a supplementary electronic system incorporated into earmuff to provide additional attenuation.

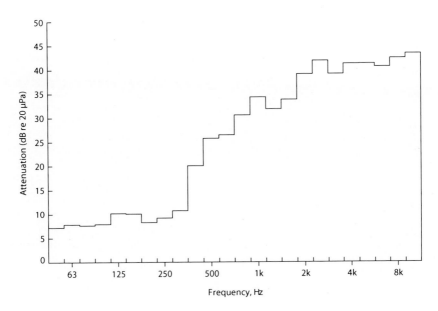

Figure 24.1 Typical attenuation afforded by earmuff devices.

- Current systems provide additional attenuation of about 8–14 dB(A) below 1 kHz by:
  - Sampling noise in earshell with microphone.
  - Inverting signal 180° out of phase.
  - Reintroducing inverted signal via telephone transducer causing destructive interference of acoustic field (see Figure 24.2).
  - Benefits ANR provides for reducing hearing damage risk vary due to different cockpit noise fields (see Figure 24.3).
  - ANR system requires power supply; provided directly from aircraft or via man-mounted pack.
- Earplugs (generic fit or personally moulded) are worn in ear canal underneath helmet, forming double hearing protection system:
  - Passive earplugs: attenuate both cockpit noise and communications signal.
  - In-ear communications devices (IECDs): include small transducers allowing communication signal to be introduced on occluded side of earplug.

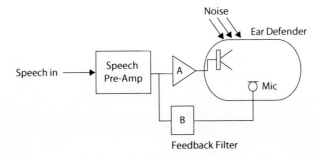

Figure 24.2 Block diagram of conventional feedback analogue active noise reduction.

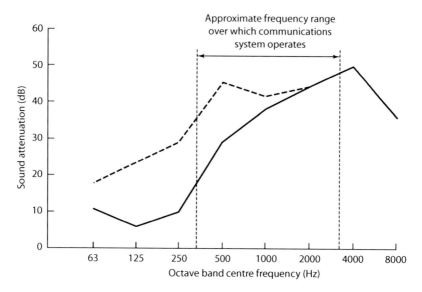

Figure 24.3 Attenuation of external noise provided by a modern protective helmet is shown in the lower curve. Note that the acoustic attenuation is poor at low frequencies (below 250 Hz). The upper curve shows the extra acoustic attenuation afforded by a well-designed active noise reduction system, with increased protection from below 63 Hz up to 1 kHz.

- ANR earplugs: include circuitry and provide similar levels of additional active attenuation as flight helmet ANR.
- Vented earplugs for high altitude: occlusion of external ear canal may cause pressure differentials across tympanic membrane which may be slow to equalize, particularly during explosive decompression.
- Overprotection: aircrew need to discriminate and locate critical audio cues within given cockpit environment, so the appropriate level of enhanced protection should be selected, along with optimal comfort and ease of use.

24.3 COMMUNICATIONS IN AIRCRAFT

TYPES OF COMMUNICATION USED

- Speech:
  - *Person to person*:
    - Aided: radios and intercom.
    - Unaided: direct face-to-face conversation.
  - *Person to machine*:
    - Speech recognition algorithms used to 'understand' contents of spoken message and activate avionic systems.
- Non-speech:
  - *Machine to person*:
    - Digitised verbal messages or audio warnings (e.g. Lyre Bird tones, klaxons) presented via communications headset or loudspeakers in cockpit.
    - Audio monitoring tasks (e.g. listening for sonar returns).

AIRCRAFT COMMUNICATION SYSTEM

- Requirement to relay speech/non-speech signals in aircraft clearly; intelligibility depends on:
  - Signal to noise ratio (SNR).
  - Quality of microphone and transducers.
  - Quality of transmission system.
  - Noise level at talker and listener positions.
- SNR will increase as noise levels decrease, by reduction in working noise environment or using ear protection, including enhanced hearing protection (e.g. ANR).
- Output from talker:
  - Speech (pressure wave) is converted to electrical signal by a microphone; common types used in aircraft are:
    - Mask mounted microphones (used in most fast jets).
    - Noise-cancelling boom microphones (used in rotary and transport aircraft).
  - Louder talkers produce higher SNRs.
  - As noise at talker's ear increases, talking levels tend to increase (Lombard effect):
    - Side-tone signals feed speech signal back to talker's ear, adjusted in level, to control voice output.
- Input to the listener:
  - SNR of 15 dB recommended for good speech intelligibility.
  - Satisfactory SNRs may be achieved by turning up intercom volume.
  - Raising intercom levels will add to risk of hearing damage caused by cockpit noise; speech >125 dB causes discomfort and pain and is a hearing damage risk.
  - Undesirable to present speech >100 dB so, for adequate intelligibility, ambient noise must not be >85 dB.

24.4 SPEECH INTELLIGIBILITY ASSESSMENT

AIDED COMMUNICATION

- To assess effectiveness of communications system, including noise attenuation, various intelligibility tests can be performed.
- Subjective tests include Harvard Phonetically Balanced (PB) list and Diagnostic Rhyme Test (DRT):
  - Participants listen to word lists in realistic noise over communication system under test and select from visual display the word they thought they heard.
  - Scoring mechanism, based on number of correct responses, allows communication system to be ranked for acceptability.
  - Require large numbers of talkers and listeners for statistically robust test; can be costly and time-consuming.
- Objective tests include Articulation Index (AI) and Speech Transmission Index (STI):
  - Offer predictive methods for assessing probable speech intelligibility from direct measurement of noise and speech signals.
  - Assess the relative contributions different parts of speech frequency spectrum make to overall intelligibility of the speech signal.

NON-AIDED COMMUNICATION

- To assess direct face-to-face communication, Preferred Speech Interference Level (PSIL) used to assess suitability of noise environment for communication:
  - Cabin noise levels measured in octave bands 500 Hz, 1 kHz, 2 kHz and 4 kHz.
  - Average level then compared with a set of figures that will indicate the level of communication possible.

CHAPTER

25

Vision

Contents

Key Facts
- Vision is most important sense in aviation.
- Small refractive errors should be corrected for flying.
- Abnormal colour vision limits employment in pilot role.
- Contact lenses are most popular refractive correction for flying.
- Corneal refractive surgery is allowed for aircrew.

25.1 VISION IN AVIATION

- Vision is most important sense needed for flying.
- Vision is only sensory means for orientation in space.

Brain processes visual information by:

- Focal system:
  - Concerned with object recognition/identification.
  - Requires high degree of resolution.
  - Relies on foveal and parafoveal areas of retina.
- Ambient system:
  - Concerned with orientation.
  - Generally works without conscious awareness.
  - Less reliant on resolution or brightness.
  - Uses larger pattern stimuli in peripheral visual field.
- With good aerial visibility and clear horizon, pilots use ambient vision to orientate; requires low-level conscious processing similar to process used in natural habitat.
- When visual cues degraded/absent (in cloud or at night), pilots must determine orientation from flight instruments using focal visual system; requires conscious effort which reduces aviator's overall capacity.
  - This 'unnatural' way of orientating is more prone to misinterpretation, increasing the risk of spatial disorientation.

25.2 VISUAL ACUITY

- Visual acuity (VA) commonly refers to clarity of vision.
- VA dependent on:
  - Sharpness of retinal focus within the eye.
  - Health and functioning of retina.
  - Sensitivity of interpretative faculty of the brain.
- Measurement of VA:
  - Resolving power of eye is the smallest angle of separation between two distinct points that allows the formation of two discernible images.
  - Empirically defined as 1 minute of arc in a normal subject.
  - Snellen Test type is most common chart used to measure VA:
    - Letters designed such that each component of the letter is separated by 1 min of arc when viewed at a specific distance; largest letter at 60 m, smallest letters at 4 m.
    - Subjects read chart at a distance 6 m, one eye at a time, with other eye occluded (do not press on eye).
    - Individual only being able to read the top letter described as having a VA of 6/60 (i.e. they can only see from 6 m what normal sighted subject could see from 60 m).
    - Many people with normal vision will be able to see better than 6/6.
- Measurement of near acuity:
  - Uniocular and binocular near acuity tested (with normal reading correction if used) using standard test types at 33 cm.

REFRACTIVE ERROR AND REFRACTIVE CORRECTION

- Refractive error means that focusing structures of eye (cornea and lens) do not focus light correctly, resulting in a blurred image.

Main types of refractive errors are:

- Myopia (short sightedness):
  - Refractive power of relaxed eye too strong for length of eye.
  - Light from far distance falls in front of retina.
  - Only near objects in focus.
  - Requires negative (minimising) lenses to correct (e.g. −2.25 dioptre sphere [DS]).
- Hypermetropia (long sightedness):
  - Refractive power of relaxed eye not strong enough for length of eye.
  - Focal point beyond back of retina.
  - Eye is out of focus at distance and near.
  - Low hypermetropia can be overcome by natural accommodation (focusing power) of eye.
  - Many young people with normal vision are low hypermetropes.
  - Requires positive (magnifying) lenses to correct (e.g. +2.5 DS).
- Astigmatism:
  - Refractive surface of the eye is not spherical, but rugby ball shaped.
  - Light focused to a different point depending on where it passes through the cornea/lens, leading to a blur circle.
  - Requires a cylindrical lens (Cyl) with power along one axis to correct (dioptre cylinder [DC]).
  - Can be negative or positive (e.g. +1.25 DC or −1.25 DC) but will always be written with angle alongside it (e.g. +1.25 × 90°).
- Presbyopia:
  - Ability of eye to focus (accommodation) gradually declines from birth.
  - Most people begin to have trouble focusing at normal reading distance by late 40s.
  - Myopes can overcome problem by removing glasses to read (as naturally in focus for near when eye relaxed).
  - Low hypermetropes need reading glasses at a younger age than emmetropes (people with no refractive error), as already use some of their accommodative effort for distance.
  - Presbyopia corrected using a positive (plus) correction for near tasks.
- A standard glasses refraction contains a spherical component and a cylindrical component:
  - Spherical component written first, then cylindrical component along with its axis.
  - For example, −2.25/−1.25 × 180 (myope), or +3.00/−1.50 × 165 (hypermetrope).

ACCEPTABLE VISUAL ACUITY FOR AVIATION

- National, civil and military standards vary.
- On selection, pilots generally require 6/6 uncorrected/corrected.
- Non-pilot aviation personnel have lower VA requirements.
- Refraction limits for pilots on selection typically: Sph = plano to +1.75, Cyl = +0.75.

MANAGEMENT OF REFRACTIVE ERRORS

- Corrective flying spectacles:
    - Must be suitably robust and integrate with flight equipment (e.g. helmet and mask).
    - Spare pair should be carried in flight.
    - Bifocal lenses permitted, but progressive power varifocal lens use limited due to edge distortion/blur risks.
- Aircrew contact lenses:
    - Usually daily disposable type preferred.
    - Dehydration from environment sometimes an issue.
    - Usually stable under increased +Gz acceleration.
    - Aircrew should be alert to risks of microbial keratitis.
- Refractive surgery:
    - Laser epithelial keratomileusis (LASEK); epithelial flap replaced after laser procedure.
    - Laser in situ keratomileusis (LASIK); stromal bed under epithelial flap ablated.
    - Risks include loss of contrast sensitivity, haloes and starbursts around light sources.
    - Wavefront-guided LASEK and LASIK generally considered safe for flying duties following 3–6 months grounding.

25.3 LIGHT/DARK ADAPTATION AND COLOUR VISION

RETINAL CELL TYPES

- Cone cells (three types):
    - Respond to bright, photopic light.
    - Predominate in fovea and parafoveal region; mediate fine detailed vision.
    - Each type has different maximum wavelength sensitivities in line with short (S-blue), medium (M-green) and long (L-red) wavelength part of light spectrum.
    - Perception of colour is complex; depends on overlapping factors such as hue colour brightness, contrast and degree of saturation.
- Rod cells:
    - Active at lower, scotopic, light intensities.
    - Mesopic vision is intermediate stage between photopic and scotopic vision where both rods and cones are functioning (e.g. night flying).
    - Maximum sensitivity at about 510 nm in blue/green part of spectrum (but do not contribute to colour perception).
    - Photopigment (rhodopsin) becomes desensitised in higher light intensities so rods cease to function.
    - 100 times more sensitive to light than cones but respond more slowly and so less able to sense temporal changes (such as quick-changing images).
    - Not present at high densities in macula; less detailed image than cones.

DARK ADAPTION

- Visual system is capable of operating over changes in ambient illumination of about 12 orders of magnitude; 100-fold change in luminance in daylight goes largely unnoticed by observer.

- Adaptation from scotopic to photopic conditions (dark to light) is relatively rapid, occurring over a period of about 5 minutes.
- Dark adaptation from photopic to scotopic conditions is slower and occurs in two stages. Cone dark adaptation takes approximately 9–10 minutes and rods 30–40 minutes (see Figure 25.1).

PURKINJE SHIFT

- Phenomenon where relative brightness of blue and red objects in daylight change in mesopic light conditions (dusk or dawn).
- Occurs as rod photoreceptors start to become active.
- Rods and cones have differing spectral sensitivities (see Figure 25.2); in mesopic conditions blue objects will seem brighter and red objects duller than photopic conditions.
- Can be troublesome for aviators as changing colour brightness can lead to misperceptions when judging depth.

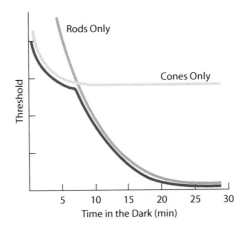

Figure 25.1 Dark adaption time of rods and cones.

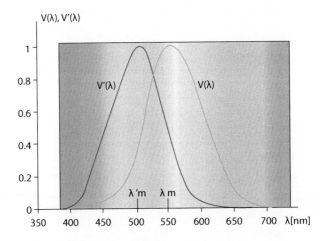

Figure 25.2 Spectral sensitivities of rods (V*(λ)) and cones (V (λ)).

25.4 ABNORMAL COLOUR VISION

CONGENITAL COLOUR VISION DEFICIENCY

- Genes coding for photopigments show little variability in most individuals (see Table 25.1).
- Approximately 8% of males and 0.5% of females have anomalous colour vision, mostly in red/green.
- 'Colour-blind' individuals have either:
  - Missing type of cone (protanopia – red, deuteranopia – green or tritanopia – blue), or
  - Mutated type of cone where sensitivity range is shifted (protanomaly, deuteranomaly or tritanomaly).
  - Deuteranomaly most common (6% of males, 0.4% of females); mutated form of medium-wavelength (green) pigment with sensitivity shifted towards red; reduces sensitivity to green.

Table 25.1 Prevalence of congenital colour vision deficiency

	MALES	FEMALES
DICHROMACY	2.4%	0.03%
Protanopia (red deficient: L cone absent)	1.3%	0.02%
Deuteranopia (green deficient: M cone absent)	1.2%	0.01%
Tritanopia (blue deficient: S cone absent)	0.001%	0.03%
ANOMALOUS TRICHROMACY	6.3%	0.37%
Protanomaly (red deficient: L cone defect)	1.3%	0.02%
Deuteranomaly (green deficient: M cone defect)	5.0%	0.35%
Tritanomaly (blue deficient: S cone defect)	0.0001%	0.0001%

ACQUIRED COLOUR VISION DEFICIENCY

- Tends to affect blue/yellow end of spectrum.
- Not routinely tested for by most aviation organisations in the past as testing difficult and defects usually associated with other problems.
- Occurs as a result of disease, toxicity or age (see Table 25.2).
- Reduction in cone function may also affect VA.
- Routine periodic testing now more viable with modern computer-based testing systems.

COLOUR DEFICIENCY IN AVIATION

- Electronic flight instruments use colour screens to increase the amount of information available but designed with redundancy built in; no critical information given by colour change only.
- A few older aviation signalling mechanisms do not have colour redundancy; individuals with congenital red/green colour vision deficiencies at risk of misinterpreting these signals as no other visual clues other than colour discrimination:
  - Precision approach path indicators (PAPIs).

Table 25.2 Causes of acquired colour deficiency

Disease	Macula – Blue/Yellow (e.g. Central Serous Retinopathy)
	Optic Nerve – Red (e.g. Optic Neuritis)
Drugs	Alcohol Tobacco Oral Contraceptive Pill Viagra 'Blue'
Age	Cataract Age-Related Macular Degeneration

- Air traffic control coloured flare-gun or lamp signals for aircraft that have lost radio communication.
  - Airfield traffic/taxi lights.
  - Aircraft navigation lights.
- Therefore, red/green colour deficient individuals unfit for many flying duties.
- Electronic flight instrumentation tends to use blues and yellows but potential for error with acquired colour vision deficiencies.
  - Displays feature colour redundancy but some military operators concerned about risks in intense aviation environments and have taken up routine colour vision testing for acquired deficiencies.

ASSESSMENT OF COLOUR VISION

- Screening conducted using Ishihara plate test.
- If plate test failed, lantern test (e.g. Holmes-Wright) can be used but most lantern equipment obsolete.
- Computer-based testing such as Colour Vision Assessment and Diagnosis (CAD) test or Rabin Cone Contrast Test becoming commonplace.

25.5 DEPTH PERCEPTION

A number of visual cues used simultaneously and unconsciously to give depth perception:
- Monocular cues:
  - Relative size.
  - Perspective: parallel lines to a point on horizon.
  - Overlapping of objects.
  - Position in visual field: object moving into distance appears to be closing in on horizon.
  - Aerial perspective: distant objects have more of a blue tinge than near objects, from Rayleigh scattering of atmospheric light.
  - Parallax: disparate movement of objects on head movement.
  - Motion parallax: as observer moves, nearer objects appear to move faster.
- Binocular cues:
  - Proprioceptive feedback from convergence and accommodation.

- Stereopsis: ability to perceive depth and three-dimensional structure by neurological processing and interpretation of disparity between images at each eye.
  - Coarse stereopsis used to judge stereoscopic motion in periphery; important, for example, when descending to land in an aircraft.
  - Fine stereopsis based on static differences; important for fine motor tasks such as threading a needle; form that is measured during aircrew selection.
  - Upper limit that stereopsis is effective is estimated as being only up to about 30 metres, only really relevant when taxing fixed wing aircraft or low-level/speed rotary flying.
  - Individuals with poor stereopsis often have other ocular problems (e.g. reduced vision in one eye).
  - Stereopsis ability important for use of biocular/binocular helmet mounted displays.

25.6 VISUAL FIELDS

- Visual field is portion of subject's surroundings that can be seen at any one time.
- Normal extent is 50° superiorly, 60° nasally, 70° inferiorly and 90° temporally.
- Equivalent concept for optical instruments is field of view (FoV).
- Binocular field is superimposition of two monocular fields; brain processes visual information binocularly in terms of right or left visual field rather than right and left eye.
  - Important when judging effects of pathology on aviators; clinician will monitor monocular visual fields, but aviation specialist is mainly concerned with binocular visual field function (not routinely measured in medical practice).

25.7 OCULAR MUSCLE BALANCE

- Ocular imbalance can result in a misalignment of eyes known as squint or strabismus.
- Visible squint described as a tropia; usually prefixed by a directional term (esotropia – eye turning in; exotropia – eye turning out; hypertropia – up; hypotropia – down).
- Most people's eyes will adopt a resting position that is not entirely straight if they are covered; this latent misalignment is called a phoria.
- Excessively large phorias can indicate extraocular muscle weakness or cranial nerve palsy; individuals with large phorias are at risk of developing a manifest squint.
- Tropias can be diagnosed using the cover/uncover test.
- Tropias and phorias can be measured by using hand-held prisms of various strengths while performing the cover tests until one is found where no movement of the eye behind the prism can be detected.
- Limits for acceptable tropias and phorias set for aircrew selection and periodic assessment.

25.8 FLIGHT HAZARDS TO VISION

GLARE

- Intrusive light source that can reduce visual acuity and contrast sensitivity.
- Veiling glare – for example, reflected image of map placed on instrument panel reduces contrast of outside world.

- Dazzle glare – bright glare source not on fovea (e.g. sun on horizon).
- Scotomic glare – bright light reduces retinal sensitivity (e.g. following a flash, or sun reflection).

SOLAR DAMAGE

- UV(A) exposure can cause cataract formation.
- Tinted visor or sunglasses used to protect eyes (10–15% transmission through tint).

LASER

- Light Amplification by Stimulation Emission of Radiation.
- Frequent use in aviation for targeting, also nuisance use from ground.
- Problems range from glare and distraction to retinal or corneal damage.
- Nominal Ocular Hazard Distance gives distance beyond which only temporary photo-stress results.
- Ocular filters are possible but can affect colour vision.
- Countermeasures include training not to look directly at beam.
- Amsler grid used to detect associated visual field defects.

EMPTY FIELD MYOPIA

- Occurs during flight at high altitude or over featureless terrain.
- Ciliary muscles unable to stay relaxed as no visual target.
- Far point becomes nearer (physiological myopia).
- Aviator unable to spot collision hazards at distance as out of focus.
- To avoid, focus regularly on wingtips or HUD.

HIGH-SPEED FLIGHT

- Pilot scan pattern of exterior view may take 5–10 seconds.
- Aircraft on reciprocal bearing have no relative movement at retina, so less likely to be detected.
- Foveal fixation required to see collision threat, not seen during saccades.
- At high speed, risk of not seeing collision hazard until very close (object size at retina related to square of distance).

CANOPY DISTORTIONS

- Distortions in canopy or windscreen can give false perception.
- Multiple reflections, dirt or oil staining may reduce visual performance.

Visual systems

Contents

Key Facts
- Visual and thermal imaging sensors used to augment vision in flight.
- Crew-mounted night vision goggles provide acceptable night vision with moon or starlight illumination.
- Aircraft-mounted thermal imaging sensors often displayed on helmet-mounted display.
- Significant challenges in effective integration of sensor image display with outside visual scene.

26.1 INTRODUCTION

- Airborne visual systems provide enhanced images of ground and other aircraft during darkness.
- Useful range of visual systems typically covers clear sky full moon (0.1–0.26 lux [lx]) to overcast moonless sky (0.001 lx).

VISUAL SENSORS

- Image intensifiers and low light electronic imaging sensors.
- Amplify light in visual (390–700 nm) and invisible near infrared (IR) waveband (700–900 nm).
- Small size, light weight and low power consumption.
- Used in night vision goggles (NVGs) typically attached to pilot's helmet.
- With sufficient illumination from moon or stars NVG image may be very good:
  - Below 10 mlx intensified images are visually noisy.
  - Unusable below approximately 2 mlx.

THERMAL IMAGING SENSORS

- Detect invisible radiation in short-IR (1.4–3 μm), mid-IR (3–8 μm) and long-IR (8–15 μm).
- Not dependent on environmental illumination; rely on thermal emissions of scene.
- Scene in thermal spectrum appears different to visual/near IR spectrum.
- Thermal radiation attenuated by cockpit transparencies and sensors too large to be man-mounted so must be installed in aircraft.

26.2 NIGHT VISION GOGGLES

- NVG comprises: optical assembly for each eye with an objective lens, an image intensifier and an eyepiece lens (see Figure 26.1).
- Each image intensifier is powered by a 3 V battery so NVG operates independently of the aircraft.
- Cockpit instruments are viewed directly by looking under eyepieces.

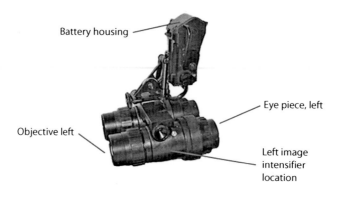

Figure 26.1 Night vision goggles.

- With NVGs misalignments between image and real scene (and latency between scene and image due to head movement) are not visible.

NVG COCKPIT LIGHTING COMPATIBILITY

- To achieve NVG compatible cockpit:
    - Displays and instrument lighting spectrally filtered to attenuate emissions at wavelengths above 650 nm.
    - Objective lens of NVG is filtered to block wavelengths below 650 nm (see Figure 26.2).

NVG LIMITATIONS

- Neck muscle fatigue: NVG mass typically 500–800 g; counterbalance weights may be fitted to rear of helmet to mitigate the forward moment.
- Reduced field of view (FoV): NVG FoV typically 40–47° (compared to over 200° for human visual system).
- Low light image quality: NVGs may not provide an acceptable image for several nights in every lunar cycle or when illumination from moon and stars is obscured by cloud or terrain.

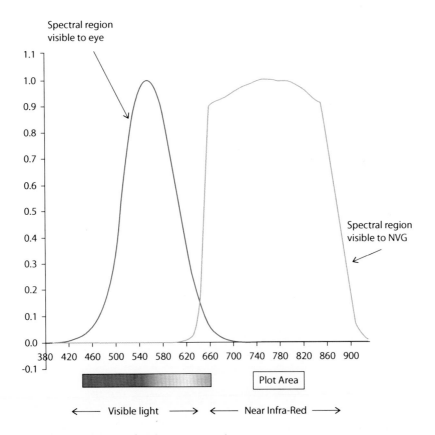

Figure 26.2 Spectral range of night vision goggles.

26.3 THERMAL IMAGING SENSORS

- Traditionally displayed on a screen within the cockpit but helmet-mounted display (HMD) systems can be used.
  - Sensor system must have an instantaneous FoV that matches HMD.
  - To minimise HMD mass, 40° is largest FoV typically used.
- Sensor system must be mechanically steered to follow the pilot's head with high accuracy and low latency; some systems use electronically combined images from multiple sensors.
- Accurate helmet tracking is necessary.
- Display system must be integrated with pilot's helmet without degrading impact protection or mass and balance.

26.4 VISUAL SYSTEM REQUIREMENTS

FIELD OF VIEW

- Most HMD/NVG systems provide 40°–47° FoV, limited by equipment size/mass constraints.
- Provides little peripheral vision (used by human visual system for motion cues).
- Exaggerated left/right head scan required to compensate for FoV reduction.

MONOCULAR/BIOCULAR/BINOCULAR

- Monocular – image presented to one eye (see Figure 26.3)
- Biocular – same image presented to both eyes (see Figure 26.4)
- Binocular – different image presented to both eyes (e.g. NVGs)

RESOLUTION/ACUITY

- Good visual acuity facilitates faster, lower flight with lower workload.
- NVGs do not provide optimal visual acuity:
  - VA at best around 6/9.
  - May be as low as 6/24 in low light.

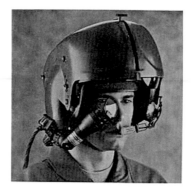

Figure 26.3 Integrated Helmet and Display Sight System (IHADSS) in AH-64 Apache is monocular.

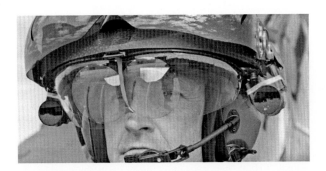

Figure 26.4 TopOwl HMD system can be either biocular, when connected to a single aircraft-mounted IR sensor, or binocular when displaying images from image intensifiers fitted to each side of helmet.

26.5 CHALLENGES OF INTEGRATING VISUAL SYSTEMS

DEPTH PERCEPTION AND HYPERSTEREOPSIS

- NVG binocular images provide stereo vision only at very short ranges compared with unaided eye.
- Hyperstereopsis occurs with HMDs that display a binocular image from image intensifiers fitted to each side of the helmet:
  - Causes distorted perception of depth.
  - Degrades estimation of distance to short-range objects.
  - Can affect ability to estimate hover height.

BIOCULAR/BINOCULAR ISSUES

- Biocular and binocular display channels must be aligned so that optical axes converge in far distance:
  - Required in order to match natural ocular vergence at distance.
  - Minimises differences between display image and visual scene.
- May be difficult to visually merge images from both channels if also concentrating on visible targets through visor:
  - Focus on targets closer to or further away than convergence distance of the optical channels will cause double image/ghosting.
- Slight vertical misalignments between optical channels can also affect ability to merge visually.

ACCOMMODATION AND EYESTRAIN

- HMD image appears to eye to be at a distance of several hundred metres ('infinity'); allows symbology to be read while overlaying real world scene.
- Eye piece of NVG adjustable to allow a preferred distance to be set (between 0.25 m and infinity).
- Any significant mismatch between focal point of display and visual scene outside helmet can lead to eye strain (asthenopia), headache and fatigue.

OCULAR DOMINANCE AND BINOCULAR RIVALRY

- Ocular dominance: tendency to prefer visual input from one eye to the other.
- Most monocular displays provide images to right eye.
  - Can cause discomfort in certain visual conditions for left eye dominant crew members.
- Binocular rivalry: results from presentation of dissimilar images to each eye (dichoptic viewing).
  - Can be induced by differences in image colour, resolution, field of view, motion, luminance or displacement.
  - Brain resolves this problem by suppressing one of the images, most commonly from non-dominant eye.
  - May be difficult to make necessary attention switch to attend to appropriate visual input.
  - Can lead to significant fatigue, especially during a long sortie or in situations where there is obvious system flicker or poor image quality:
    - Bright green phosphor in right eye, leading to difficulty in attending to a darker visual scene via left eye (e.g. cockpit).
    - Bright city lights causing difficulty in shifting view to HMD.
- 'Pulfrich effect': optical illusion where an object moving in parallel plane appears to approach and/or recede from viewer if there is significant luminance difference between the eyes:
  - Visual latency is shorter for brighter image.
  - Difference in processing times between eyes causes depth effect.

DISPLACED VISUAL INPUTS

- View point from imaging sensor presented on HMD may be several metres away from pilot's view point (see Figure 26.5).
- Can cause difficulties during close-range tasks (e.g. takeoff/landing/formation/low-level manoeuvre), as normal visual references from within cockpit are not present.

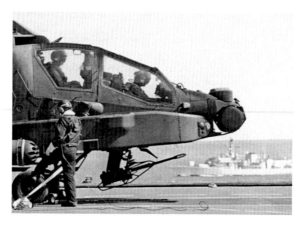

Figure 26.5 Forward, low position of Apache AH-64 imaging sensor compared to crew head position.

- Visual parallax errors are small with NVGs, as viewpoint (objective lens) is only 150 mm in front of normal eye view point.

LATENCY

- Time delays in helmet-tracking system, symbol generation and sensor control cause latency.
- Result is that sensor image lags pilot's head movements and stabilised symbols can move away from intended position.

SYMPTOMATOLOGY – PILOT SURVEYS

- In surveys of Apache pilots using monocular IHADSS system, 80–90% of users reported visual complaints, including 'visual discomfort', headache, blurred vision, disorientation and after images.
  - Symptoms sometimes persisted after flight.
  - Poor slope estimation, faulty height judgement, undetected aircraft drift and illusory drift also reported.

MASS, CENTRE OF GRAVITY, STABILITY, COMFORT

- Addition of display capabilities to aircrew helmet increases total mass.
- Centre of gravity often moved forward.
- Fitting system should be designed to counter forward rotation of helmet and minimise local pressure points in brow area.
- A forward centre of gravity may also lead to neck fatigue and musculoskeletal injury.

VIBRATION

- Tri-axial vibration (0.5–100 Hz) caused by rotary aircraft problematic for HMDs:
  - Compensatory eye movements are ineffective at image stabilisation with low frequency (<20 Hz) vibration leading to visual blur.
- Helmet slip with resultant image loss is possible with vibration but mitigated by careful helmet fit.

EQUIPMENT INTEGRATION

- HMD system must integrate with other equipment, including communications system, corrective spectacles, aircrew clothing and survival equipment.

Spatial orientation and disorientation in flight

Contents

> **Key Facts**
> - Pilot is disorientated if unaware of true attitude or position of aircraft.
> - Disorientation occurs because airborne environment is deceptive.
> - Inattention, visual and vestibular effects may cause spatial disorientation in flight.
> - In most accidents involving spatial disorientation, pilot was unaware of being disorientated.

27.1 WHAT IS SPATIAL DISORIENTATION?

- Spatial disorientation (SD) is a state characterized by an erroneous sense of position, attitude or motion in relation to a fixed, 3-D coordinate system defined by the surface of the earth and the gravitational vertical.
- Classified into Type 1 (unaware of sensory error) and Type 2 (aware of conflicting sensory inputs):
  - Type 1 occurs in up to 85% of serious SD accidents (military study)
  - Type 2 occurs with much greater frequency, but is less often identified as contributory to accidents.

- SD implicated in 10–45% of serious accidents:
  - All-cause aviation accident rate falling but SD resistant as a cause.
  - Highest risk in military operations.
  - Higher risk of fatality compared with non-SD accidents.
- Greatest risk to flight safety occurs when the disorientation is unrecognised (Type 1); in mildest form SD may reduce attentional capacity; at most severe may cause an accident.

27.2 MECHANISMS FOR NORMAL ORIENTATION

VISION

- Predominant mode for orientation.
- 80% of orientation input in good visual conditions.
- Ambient visual system is primary system for determining orientation (little effect on conscious processing).
- Distance, speed and height cues provided by detailed foveal vision and flight instrumentation.
- Dominance of vision system may suppress correct non-visual orientation cues (can allow a false visual orientation model to persist).

VESTIBULAR

- Otolith organs detect linear acceleration, including gravity.
- Semicircular canals detect angular acceleration associated with normal head movements or from changes to the aircraft in pitch, roll and yaw.
- Vestibular-ocular reflex stabilises retinal image in presence of moderate angular acceleration (usually head movements).

KINAESTHETIC

- Sensory endings in skin, joints, muscles and ligaments stimulated by forces acting upon body to provide 'seat of the pants' sensations.
- Cues provide an instinctive sense of accelerative change without diminishing attentional capacity, but notoriously inaccurate.

AUDITORY

- Aerodynamic and engine noise can be useful in detecting a change to aircraft configuration.
- However, hearing system is usually not regarded as primary sense for orientation.

27.3 CAUSES OF SPATIAL DISORIENTATION

INATTENTION CAUSES

- Distraction from principal flying task is most common contributory factor in disorientation incidents:
  - Preoccupation with something outside aircraft (e.g. acquiring a ground target) or within cockpit (e.g. surveillance equipment, map, radio).
- SD incidents and accidents often occur in good flying conditions when pilot pays insufficient attention to visual cues available:
  - Inattention was primary cause in 49% of serious military accidents.

- Human factor demands include high workload, inappropriate division of attention, low arousal states (fatigue, boredom, health/medication), distraction, expectancy of alternative (safer) outcomes.

VISUAL CAUSES

- Strong visual cues are compelling; what brain perceives it 'sees' is affected by surrounding objects; during flight can cause discrepancies between what the pilot thinks is seen and what is actually there.
- Scale illusions:
    - Distance of object determines apparent size, augmented by other depth cues (e.g. stereopsis, parallax, perspective, overlap).
    - In absence of visual information, assumptions made about size based on previous knowledge.
    - For example, pilot may assume that a forest of pine trees are full height, when in fact they are stunted or saplings, causing aircraft to fly at a lower height than expected.
- Shape constancy:
    - Shape of runway/landing site used to gain perspective of aircraft's position and distance (see Figure 27.1).
    - Sloping runway changes perspective and influences normal glide path.
    - For example, when landing on an upsloping runway, pilot may feel too high on approach and so may come in too low.
    - Similar issues arise when runway is a different width than expected (see Figure 27.2); especially at night, pilot may adopt a steep or shallow glide path as using runway width to determine correct landing approach angle; this may also affect height at which pilot flares the aircraft.

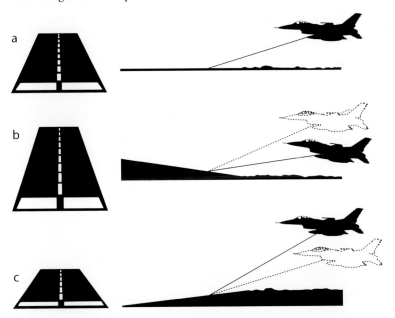

Figure 27.1 Effect of runway slope on pilot's image of runway and potential effect on glide slope.

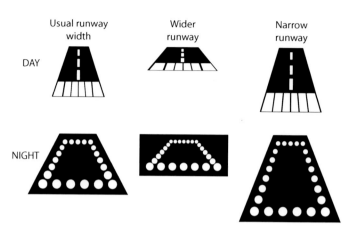

Figure 27.2 Effect of runway width on pilot's image of runway.

- False horizon:
  - When visual cues limited (e.g. above cloud, haze, night flying), pilot may develop a false interpretation of horizon and fly accordingly.
  - False cues may arise from outside the cockpit (e.g. sloping cloud bank [see Figure 27.3], mountainous terrain) or inside the cockpit (e.g. shaded sections on the helmet's visor).
- Black hole approach:
  - When approaching a landing site at night over featureless terrain, pilot has few visual references to judge approach angle, distance or rate of closure.
  - Typically pilot perceives aircraft is at a higher altitude than it actually is, and consequently makes a lower approach than necessary.
  - Illusion disappears once aircraft is close to runway/landing site; important to fly normal safe altitude approach and not to fly visually until that point.
- Vection illusion:
  - Movement of visual references within ambient vision can provide false sense of aircraft movement (e.g. particulates moving downwind in recirculation, grass or

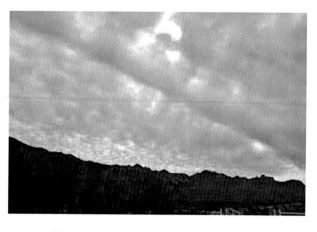

Figure 27.3 Sloping cloud bank.

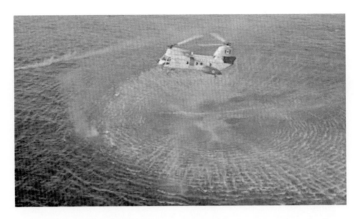

Figure 27.4 Water movement in helicopter downwash can lead to vection illusion.

  water ripples in helicopter downdraft or shadow of moving blades across cockpit
  [see Figure 27.4]).
  - Particular concern to helicopter pilots hovering at low level.
- Reflections:
  - Reflections may be misinterpreted when good visual cues scant (e.g. starlight
    confused with shipping).
  - Even in good visual conditions, inverted reflection from still water (e.g. moun-
    tainside seen off a still lake) can generate considerable difficulty with depth
    perception and level orientation.
- Lean on the sun:
  - When flying through thin cloud layer, cloud is brighter in direction of sun, even
    if sun not visible.
  - Pilot may attempt to orientate aircraft to keep sun directly overhead; alterna-
    tively, if brightness is to left or right, pilot may feel as though they are flying one
    wing low, even when flying straight and level.
  - If flying towards bright area, pilot may feel as though aircraft is nose up.
  - Pilot may 'correct' perceived aircraft position erroneously.
- Autokinesis:
  - Solitary light (star or aircraft light) seen against a black background will appear
    to wander.
  - Background visual information insufficient to inhibit normal involuntary move-
    ments of the eye; slow phase eye movements are then interpreted as movement of
    light source.

VESTIBULAR CAUSES

- Somatogyral effect:
  - False turning sensation following a prolonged turn (e.g. coordinated turn whilst
    orbiting, sustained roll during aerobatics or spinning).
  - Semicircular canals highly sensitive to onset of angular acceleration but insensi-
    tive if acceleration is sustained beyond 10–30 sec, particularly if operating in a
    degraded visual environment.

- Once habituated, semicircular canals will signal turn in opposite direction on cessation of the original turn (see Figure 27.5).
- This may make pilot resume original turn; aircraft descends during turn due to loss of lift, but as pilot thinks they are in wings-level descent, they add more stick back pressure; this tightens the spiralling turn, losing more altitude; this effect sometimes called 'Graveyard Spiral'.
- Vestibular-ocular reflex drives oculogyral effect in parallel with visual target displacement in same direction as somatogyral effect; marked nystagmus may hinder recovery in first few seconds.
- Somatogravic effect:
  - Development of false perception of attitude on exposure to a force vector which differs in direction and/or magnitude from normal gravitational force (see Figure 27.6).
  - Consequences are most important in fixed wing aircraft where significant thrust is delivered in Gx plane (e.g. acceleration on climb-out or go-around in cloud, encouraging dangerous forward stick movement).
  - Helicopters may only accelerate by changing pitch/roll first, and thus pilot does not perceive the same somatogravic effect from Gx acceleration.
    - Helicopter pilots may fail to recognise an attitude change and onset of drift whilst hovering from a negative somatogravic effect; in this instance alignment of resultant vector remains in longitudinal axis of body (see Figure 27.7).
  - Oculogravic effect complements the somatogravic effect, whereby visual targets move in same direction (e.g. appearance of upsloping runway on takeoff).

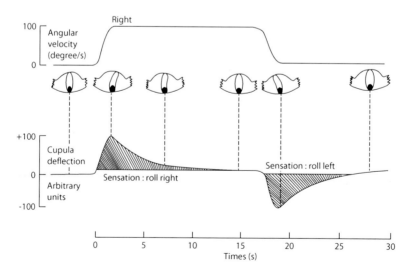

Figure 27.5 Response of semicircular canal and sensation of turning during prolonged rotation.

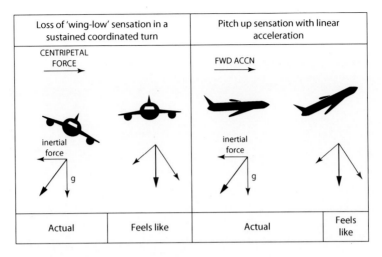

Figure 27.6 Examples of somatogravic effect.

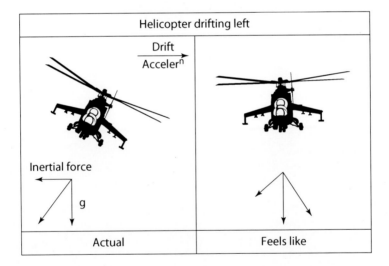

Figure 27.7 Somatogravic effect in helicopter drift.

- The leans:
  - False sensation of roll attitude.
  - Most commonly reported manifestation of spatial disorientation.
  - Often associated with recovery from a coordinated turn or roll error to level flight whilst flying in instrument meteorological conditions.
  - Pilot left with sensation that during actual recovery to level flight, they abruptly banked into a new turn (see Figure 27.8).
  - False sensation may persist for many minutes, draining capacity of even experienced pilots; leans are usually dispelled as soon as pilot regains unambiguous external visual cues.

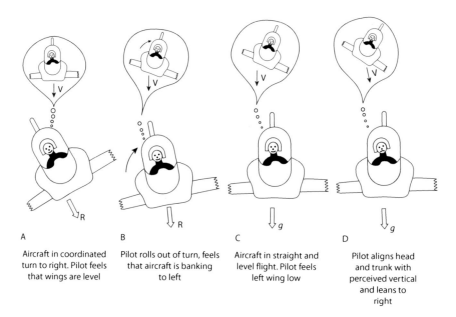

A	B	C	D
Aircraft in coordinated turn to right. Pilot feels that wings are level	Pilot rolls out of turn, feels that aircraft is banking to left	Aircraft in straight and level flight. Pilot feels left wing low	Pilot aligns head and trunk with perceived vertical and leans to right

Figure 27.8 Diagrammatic representation of one cause of 'the leans'.

- Sub-threshold drift:
    - Otoliths have a minimum threshold for detection which may allow mild but sustained linear acceleration to go undetected.
    - Particular problem for helicopter crews hovering in recirculation or degraded visual environment; has resulted in undetected drift over 50–100 m.
    - Whole body vibration in helicopters adds to background 'vibrational noise' and may reduce opportunity for early detection.
- Coriolis effect:
    - Occurs if semicircular canals are moved out of plane whilst accelerating in another plane (e.g. downward head movement for a radio-frequency change whilst conducting a prolonged turn).
    - So-called cross-coupled stimulation of semicircular canals can cause an abnormal sense of rotation, often quite unexpectedly and when busy with other tasks.
    - Effect may also occur in absence of head movement in high agility aircraft with vectored thrust.
- G excess effect:
    - Head movement when experiencing significant Gz may cause transient sensations of aircraft attitude change, commonly pitch up/down.
    - Probably caused by atypical stimulation of otoliths; often worse with quick head movements.
- Elevator illusion:
    - Change in magnitude of Gz force (e.g. sudden updraft) is correctly perceived by otolith organs, but visual field paradoxically also appears to move in the same direction.
    - May induce a false sense of pitch change and hazardous control inputs in opposite direction.

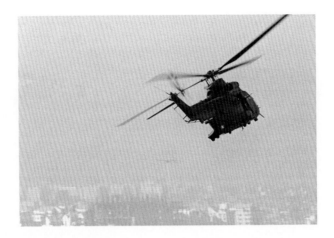

Figure 27.9 Loss of horizon due to smog.

- Pressure (alternobaric) vertigo:
  - May be caused by abrupt or asymmetric pressure changes within middle ear during ascent/descent.
  - Sensation is usually intense but short lived (10–15 seconds).
  - 10–17% of pilots report pressure vertigo at some stage in their flying career.
  - Mechanism is not fully known but may relate to transient deflection of cupula in semicircular canals when middle ear pressure is relieved.

INSUFFICIENT ORIENTATION CUES

- Reduced cues:
  - Conditions with limited visual cues increase likelihood of disorientation.
  - These include flying in cloud, degraded visual environments (low light, reduced visibility – see Figure 27.9, recirculation), flight over featureless terrain (desert, snow, water).
  - Pilots should be aware of these limitations and adapt aircraft profile or task to suit conditions.
- Bright light:
  - Glare from bright sunlight, NVG bloom or LASER dazzle (nuisance or hostile) reduces visual resolution and may distract aircrew from attending to their primary orientation cues (see Chapter 25).
  - Laser dazzle is a growing problem especially if close to ground; pilots are taught to look away in first instance but may suffer dazzle effects for several minutes.

CENTRAL CAUSES

- Break off:
  - Often described as a feeling of detachment from the aircraft.
  - Risk factors include solo flight, high altitude, lack of motion cues and boredom.
  - Usually relieved by diverting attention to another task.
- Giant hand:
  - False perception of external resistance to normal control inputs; often associated with a high-stress situation.

27.4 RISK FACTORS FOR SPATIAL DISORIENTATION (SEE TABLE 27.1)

Table 27.1 Risk factors for spatial disorientation

AIRCREW	AIRCRAFT	TASK	ENVIRONMENT
• Inexperience (500–1000 hr) • Infrequent flying • Sub-optimal crew resource management • Human factors (fatigue/alertness, concurrent illness +/– medication side effects, alcohol & recreational drugs) • Physiological stressors (thermal, altitude, etc)	• High performance • Whole body vibration • Reduced field of view • Cockpit design (head-down displays; size, clarity, position of avionics) • Lack of automation & stability control • Instrument failure	• High workload • Solo pilot operations • Low-level flight • Sustained acceleration • Hostile environment • Operational imperative (commercial, save life, etc)	• Degraded visual environment – light levels, poor visibility (cloud, mist, precipitation, particulates, recirculation) • Featureless terrain/over water • Indistinct horizon

27.5 PREVENTING SPATIAL DISORIENTATION

EQUIPMENT

- Visual displays:
  - Augment external visual cues whilst maintaining an eyes-out position (HUD or HMD).
  - Low light levels can be offset by image intensification or thermal imaging (see Chapter 26) but cannot overcome low visibility (particulates, moisture).
  - Longer wavelength systems (millimetre wave) have limited ability to see through atmospheric obscurants but suffer from range, fidelity and integration issues.
  - Synthetic vision systems (LIDAR) generate real-time 3-D images of visual field using laser.
  - Symbology (2-D or 3-D conformal) provides additional aircraft orientation information.
- Advanced Flight Control Systems (AFCS):
  - Coupled with precision navigation system and suitable sensors may allow hands-free operation and reduce reliance on visual cues.
- Audio cues:
  - Widely used in low height warning systems.

- Potential applications for 3-D audio as a proximity warning for obstructions, threat warning and terrain/collision avoidance.
- Tactile displays:
  - Make use of vibrating tactors to relay intuitive information to the skin about unrecognised drift and threats.
- Others:
  - Radar altimeter for accurate height.
  - Stick/yoke switches to encourage eyes-out operations.
  - Stick-shaker for stall warning.

TRAINING

- Aircrew taught to use instruments, not just in cloud but also when visual cues are poor or misleading.
- Standardised techniques and communication developed for high-risk phases (e.g. catapult launch, weather abort, brownout landing, overshoot from instrument approach).
- Effective crew coordination important part of multi-crew operations.
  - Enhances management of cockpit workload (less risk of inattention).
- Aviation medicine training for crew should focus on awareness and preventative strategies.
  - Mandated currency for many aircrew.
  - SD training may be augmented by use of disorientation simulators, mission simulators, in-flight demonstration or simple concepts such as the Barany chair.

CHAPTER 28

Motion sickness

Contents

Key Facts

- Motion sickness (MS) has multiple symptoms; operators should learn their own warning signs.
- Occurs commonly but with high variability among people.
- Is a threat to safety and performance during operations.
- Most strongly associated with non-transient vehicle acceleration that varies in magnitude and/or direction and is within 0.1–0.5 Hz frequency range.
- Usually exacerbated by head movement.
- Most effective countermeasures are motion adaptation and medications.

28.1 WHAT IS MOTION SICKNESS?

- Noxious symptoms elicited by motion outside one's normal experience.
- Caused by being unused to multisensory and/or sensorimotor orientation inputs (motion maladaptation); persists until adaptation has been acquired.
- Viewing a giant-screen movie or virtual environment also may induce symptoms, as moving fields act on the same brain centres that process real motion.

28.2 SIGNS AND SYMPTOMS OF MS

- Nausea and vomiting are most obvious.
- Other common symptoms shown in Table 28.1.

28.3 WARNING SIGNS OF MS

- Generalizations are best made within people, but some early symptoms common across people (see Table 28.2).

Table 28.1 Motion sickness signs and symptoms (X = non-shared symptoms across two different MS criteria)

GRAYBIEL'S ORIGINAL PENSACOLA DIAGNOSTIC CRITERIA FOR MS	KENNEDY'S EXPANDED CRITERIA (MS/ SIMULATOR SICKNESS QUESTIONNAIRE)
Stomach awareness/Discomfort`	✓ (Check = matches Pensacola criteria in Column 1 sufficiently)
Nausea	✓
Retching or Vomiting	✓
Increased salivation	✓ (Any change in salivation)
Cold sweating	✓ (Sweating)
Pallor	✗ (Not used in these criteria)
Drowsiness	✗ (Fatigue, difficulty focusing or concentrating and confusion)
Headache	✓ (Also fullness of head)
Flushing/Warmth	✗ (Not used)
Dizziness	✓ (Also vertigo)
(N.A.)	Eyestrain or blurred vision
(N.A.)	Digestive (Change in appetite, burping, desire to move bowels)
(N.A.)	Other (General discomfort, boredom, depression, faintness or awareness of breathing)

✓ = matches Pensacola criteria in Column 1 sufficiently
✗ = symptoms not shared between the diagnostic criteria

Table 28.2 Early signs and symptoms of motion sickness

Mild stomach symptoms (of any kind)
Dizziness
Headache
Thermoregulatory effects (warmth, flushing or sweating)
Pallor

- Knowing early indicators helps inexperienced to modify behaviour early to slow progression.

28.4 VEHICLE ACCELERATIONS THAT CAUSE MS

- Vary in magnitude and/or direction.
- Are within the 0.1–0.5 Hz frequency range of vehicle oscillation (see Figure 28.1).
- Are non-transient; acceleration-related MS exacerbated by head movements.

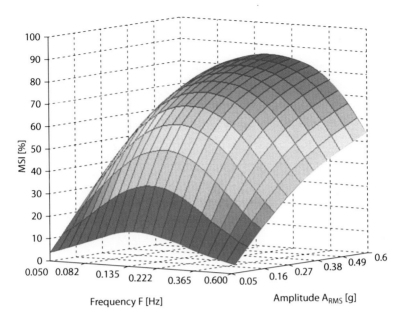

Figure 28.1 Matsangas's and McCauley's estimate of MS Incidence (MSI), i.e. % of people who vomit as a function of vertical oscillation frequency and acceleration amplitude (by permission).

28.5 WHY THE MS RESPONSE OCCURS

- No universally accepted theory of causation.
- Most popular theory is *sensory conflict* or *neural mismatch* (see Figure 28.2):
  - Intra- and/or multisensory inputs about motion/orientation conflict with relationships anticipated from sensory experience and previous outcomes of motor commands.
  - Explains sensory aspects of the disturbing situation but not why motion causes nausea and vomiting.
  - An additional hypothesis for why these responses occur: control of eye/head movements is perturbed by motion similarly to sensorimotor disturbances that arise when one ingests toxins (i.e. vehicle motion activates the body's ancient poison responses).

28.6 OPERATIONAL SIGNIFICANCE

- Occurs commonly and poses a challenge to sea, air and space operations (see Table 28.3).
- Over 40,000 cases of motion intolerance occur per year in the US Navy.
- Valuable time lost due to MS: during a 150-day frigate voyage, approximately 15 days of work were lost (due to time in sea states 5–7).
- Arises on land during cross-country armoured vehicle operations and training with virtual environments/simulators.
- Airsickness detracts from flight training and is one of the most frequent reasons for flying waivers.

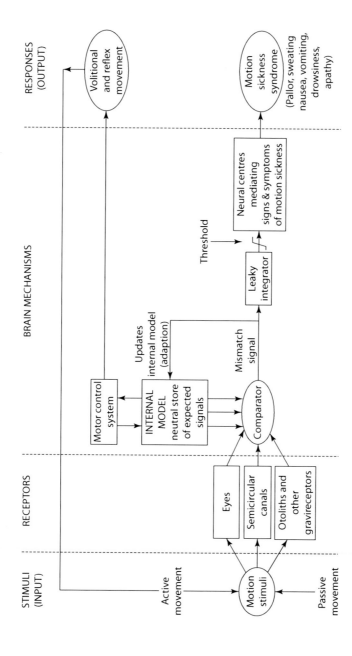

Figure 28.2 Diagrammatic representation of a model of motion control, motion detection and motion sickness compatible with the neural mismatch hypothesis. (Reproduced from Benson 1984.)

Table 28.3 Incidence of motion sickness in different situations

SICKENING SITUATIONS	INCIDENCE OF NOXIOUS SYMPTOMS	INCIDENCE OF SEVERE EFFECTS
Sea: Ship at Sea	70%	5–56%
Sea: Life Rafts	76–99%	≤55%
Aircraft: Pilots in Flight Training	10–50%	7–18%
Aircraft: Airborne Troops	10–75%	25%
Laboratory: Head Movement During Rotation	90–96%	(Majority: varies with defined testing end point)
Laboratory: Visual Surround Motion (e.g. Optokinetic Drum)	50–100%	20–42%
Simulators	10–90%	5%
Virtual Environments	60–80%	0–17%
Microgravity Spaceflight	67–70%	10–20%

Sources: Ernsting et al.; Lawson et al.; DeHart et al.

- Spaceflight extra-vehicular activity is delayed after entry into orbit, to avoid space sickness.
- Significant operational penalty when even one sick crewman: specialized job, few replacements.
- Assisted-breathing situations (e.g. high-altitude flight, extra-vehicular activity in space, diving or medical evacuation of a patient) much more hazardous when vomiting is possible.
- Inexperienced travellers or travellers exposed for long durations occasionally vomit without warning.
- Dehydration via fluid loss caused by sweating and vomiting.
- Nausea causes poor appetite, which contributes to physiological stress and low energy.
- Specific performance-related decrements associated with MS:
  - Less careful performance.
  - Decreased strength/coordination.
  - Decreased performance with self-fixed visual displays.
  - Decreased ability to estimate time.
  - Decreased ability to perform arithmetic.
- Additional performance decrements associated with motion-induced drowsiness (Sopite Syndrome):
  - Difficulty concentrating.
  - Decreased initiative or motivation.
  - Decreased communication.
- Incidence of MS will increase as combat vehicles become more manoeuvrable and greater reliance is placed upon electronic weapons systems, head-mounted displays and virtual interfaces. Driverless and tele-operated vehicles also cause MS (for passengers and operators, respectively).

Table 28.4 Motion sickness countermeasures (darker shading = more verification of efficacy needed for that category)

COUNTERMEASURE CATEGORIES	SPECIFIC EXAMPLES OF COUNTERMEASURES WITHIN EACH CATEGORY (EACH CELL =ONE COUNTERMEASURE)				
Dietary:	Protein is better than carbs	Avoid rich foods	Avoid large or no meal	Avoid alcohol	Stay hydrated
Alternative:	Ginger	Acupressure			
Behavioural Therapy:	Biofeedback	Relaxation	Breathing exercises	Hypnosis	Education
Selection:	(Note: Helps organizations rather than individuals)				
Behavioural Strategies:	Limiting head movement	Lying supine	Closing eyes or viewing horizon	Not reading inside vehicle	Taking control of the vehicle
Adaptation:	Adapting to the specific stimulus encountered	Adapting to rotation plus head movement (to generalize to target stimulus)[a]			
Medications:[b]	Scopolamine or promethazine (plus stimulant)	Meclizine or dimenhydrinate			

[a] This is the key to airsickness desensitisation programs worldwide, in combination with education, biofeedback, etc.
[b] Chronic use is not recommended; some side effects incompatible with operational duties; policies differ by agency.

28.7 FACTORS CONTRIBUTING TO SUSCEPTIBILITY

- Occupant's relation to vehicle:
  - Pilots experience less airsickness than other aircrew, partly because of better visual cues and reafferent information.
  - Sea-based studies suggest that being oriented facing the bow (forward) is less sickening than sitting athwart it (sideways).
- Age:
  - Low incidence below age 2.
  - Rises until puberty.
  - Tends to decline during adulthood.
- Motion experience:
  - A critical protective factor.
    - Therefore, adaptation training is a key countermeasure (see Table 28.4).
- Sex:
  - In approximately half the studies comparing sexes, women were more susceptible.
  - Difference is stronger in survey studies than controlled lab experiments.
  - Numerous interpretation confounds exist and difference is not proven.
- Aerobic fitness:
  - Positively correlated with susceptibility.
- Heritability:
  - Likely that differences due to heritability (susceptibility of parents) affect susceptibility more than factors above.
  - Prior to a voyage, ask your parents their susceptibility, because most anti-MS medications are absorbed too slowly to be of sufficient benefit if taken after MS onset.

28.8 MS COUNTERMEASURES

- Summarized in Table 28.4.
  - Best approaches currently are motion adaptation and medications.
  - Experimental display countermeasures (that provide orienting cues) are also in development.

CHAPTER 29

Human systems integration (HSI)

Contents

Key Facts
- Defined as systematic process of identifying, tracking and resolving human-related issues to ensure a balance between the technological and human aspects of a system.
- Aims to ensure that human component is adequately considered in system development.
- HSI is term used in the United States, Canada and Australia; Human Factors Integration is equivalent term used in the United Kingdom.

29.1 WHY DO HSI?

Humans have a significant impact on the operational effectiveness of a system and must be seen as an important component of any system.

29.2 HSI DOMAINS

- HSI identifies and trades-off human-related issues significantly impacting a system.
- Issues are categorized into seven domains (see Figure 29.1).
- Each domain is a checklist of questions to consider and highlights relative risk to overall system performance.
- Domains are related to each other, as decisions in one domain impact others.

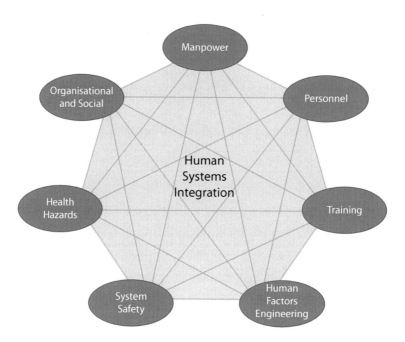

Figure 29.1 Human systems integration domains and interactions.

MANPOWER

- Number of individuals required to operate and maintain, sustain and provide training for a system. Critical questions:
  - Will the right people be available throughout the system life cycle?
  - How will work introduced by the system be allocated between career fields?
  - How will manning numbers, shift size and other factors be balanced to deal with expected workload?

PERSONNEL

- Aptitudes, experiences and other human characteristics necessary to achieve optimum system performance. Critical questions:
  - What physical characteristics, aptitudes and abilities will personnel have?
  - How will personnel be recruited, selected and retained within roles?
  - What previous experience and training would be advantageous or disadvantageous?

TRAINING

- Specification and evaluation of the optimum combination of instructional systems, education and on-the-job training required to develop the knowledge, skills and abilities needed by personnel to operate and maintain systems to the specified level of effectiveness under the full range of operating conditions. Critical questions:
  - What are potential skills gaps?
  - Will automation cause a loss of skill/proficiency?
  - What training methods will be best in teaching personnel to use the new system?
  - How should training be organized and scheduled?

HUMAN FACTORS ENGINEERING

- Comprehensive integration of human characteristics into system definition, including workstation and workspace design and habitability considerations. Critical questions:
  - How will human–machine interfaces be designed to match the cognitive and physical abilities of operators and maintainers?
  - How will decisions be made as to which tasks to automate?
  - What will be the impact of new technology on situation awareness, decision making and communication?
  - Do personnel need to be co-located for effective communication?

SYSTEM SAFETY

- Process of applying human factors expertise to minimise safety risks arising from the system being operated or functioning in a normal or abnormal manner. Critical questions:
  - How will error sources be identified, analysed and mitigated?
  - To what extent could unintentional errors impact safety?
  - What steps are being taken to influence the development and maintenance of safety-related attitudes and behaviours?
  - Does specific consideration need to be given to crashworthiness and protection?
  - How will opportunities for potential misuse that could impact safety be identified?
  - How could abnormal functioning or degraded system status affect safety?

HEALTH HAZARDS

- The process of identifying and addressing conditions inherent in the operation or use of a system that can cause death, injury, illness, disability, or reduce the performance of personnel. Critical questions:
  - Which health and safety standards should be followed?
  - Has the range of environmental issues and risks been considered?
  - What will be done to minimise the risk of personnel exposed to noise, altitude, acceleration, radiation, lasers or toxic material?
  - Could there be risk of injury through use or maintenance of equipment?
  - What activities will be undertaken to ensure the design of appropriate personal protective clothing and equipment?
  - Are personnel required to perform repetitive movements or heavy lifting/load carriage?
  - How will the system be designed to isolate hazards?
  - How will perceptions of risk associated with potential health hazards be managed?

ORGANISATIONAL AND SOCIAL

- The process of applying tools and techniques from organisational psychology, management studies, social science, information science and the system of systems approach to consider the organisational configuration, social environment and ways of working in a system. Critical questions:
  - How will the command structure be supported?
  - How will working with other groups or agencies impact the organization's structure?
  - How will interoperability and shared situation awareness be managed and supported?

- Will the new system or associated ways of working impact on existing cultural, ethical or spiritual norms?
- How will gender differences and evolving social expectations be accommodated?
- How might changes in the mix of military-civilian staff affect the organization?
- How will ways of working be affected by environments that comprise multinational/multiservice interoperability in network enabled capabilities?
- How will issues and risks linked to distributed teamwork be addressed?

29.3 HSI GOALS

The following HSI goals should be pursued to achieve satisfactory outcomes:
- Systematic treatment of human-related considerations through the system life cycle.
- Systematic, rigorous and formal capture, specification and management of human-related requirements necessary to provide the required system capability.
- The adoption of a user-centred design approach.
- The use of established human–systems principles, accepted best practice and suitable methods, tools and techniques and data.
- Design to match the context of use as well as user and organization characteristics.
- Design to meet user needs.
- Involvement of users in system design and evaluation.
- The iteration of design solutions to optimize the solution against human-related requirements and constraints.

29.4 AEROSPACE MEDICINE PRACTITIONER HSI ROLES

- Ensuring early consideration of HSI issues in design and procurement processes.
- Anticipating or diagnosing degraded human performance by screening for gaps at the level of the individual HSI domains.
- Understanding the impact of HSI gaps on health and the potential to aggravate existing medical conditions.
- Integrating HSI domain considerations into aeromedical decision making.
- Developing and updating aeromedical selection and certification standards.
- Participating in the design and/or delivery of training programs.
- Advising organisational leadership on potential human performance challenges and mitigations based on an HSI gap analysis.
- Analysing trade-off benefits and risks of aerospace and occupational aspects of HSI domains.
- Providing human performance consultation as member of an accident/incident investigative team.

30

Selection and training

Contents

> **Key Facts**
> - Pilots undergo continuous selection and training throughout their careers; aerospace medicine supports these processes and by doing so contributes to culture, cost base and safety of organizations in which they work.
> - Aim is to produce pilots who can operate consistently, competently and safely in the flight environment for which they have been chosen, civil or military.
> - It is an iterative career-long process that should be understood by medical professionals involved in the process, as they may be called upon for career defining input.

30.1 HISTORY

- At start of WWI selection process to be a pilot was limited to whether a gentleman could ride a horse; some validity in that the cavalry had to have some coordination and multitask.
- High failure/fatality rate in early training led to an effort to attempt to codify selection processes.
- Simple psychomotor measures such as reaction time, but most emphasis was placed on physiological parameters and simple on-the-job testing; this was not subjected to rigorous validity testing (see Figure 30.1).

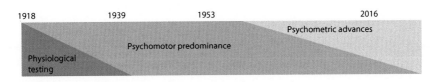

Figure 30.1 The change in pilot selection emphasis.

- Between the World Wars, efforts were made to introduce psychomotor devices; simple hand-eye coordination tasks but remained in use in some form for next 50 years.
- During WWII the requirement for large numbers of pilots to be trained in a short period led to first large-scale trials of selection processes; the Pensacola 1000 Aviator Study assessed the utility of approximately 60 physiological, psychological and psychomotor tests; concluded that latter two had more validity than physiological measures.
- Post–WWII military air forces settled on selection batteries of pencil and paper testing with a small number of psychomotor 'devices'.
- Early civil sector largely relied on ex-military pilots to fill their ranks.
- Selection of aircrew predicated on potential to pass their course becomes more important as training in both civil and military sectors becomes more expensive.
- More recently pilots begin to be selected on more than potential to fly; their fit for the organization and career longevity, promotion to senior roles and the specific skill-set required (e.g. very different for a single seat fighter pilot than airline captain). The old concept of the 'right stuff' is no longer accepted without nuance.

30.2 PRINCIPLES OF SELECTION AND TRAINING

- Tests to be used for pilot selection can be determined only by relating test scores to some later index of skill in the actual job of piloting an aircraft (validation).
- Test must relate to a standard.

RELIABILITY

- Accuracy and consistency of the measurement characteristics of a test is called reliability; when interpreting test scores, they must differentiate the levels of candidate's ability. Common methods of determining reliability are:
  - Test/re-test reliability – same result from the same group over time.
  - Alternate form reliability – several forms of testing the same ability.
  - Observer consistency – higher inter-rater consistency indicates higher reliability.

VALIDITY

- Does the test actually measure what it purports to measure? Commonly assessed by:
  - Face validity – appears to test what it is designed for.
  - Content validity – is test appropriate to the skill under test (e.g. performance of quadratic equations would have little relation to the task of mental dead reckoning)?
  - Predictive validity – what is relationship between a test score and a future measure of task performance? Result should be tracked over time as circumstances in the training pipeline change; new aircraft or roles mean test should evolve.
  - Concurrent validity – measures how well a particular test correlates with previously validated tests.

30.3 SELECTION MODES

- Selection inherent in a pilot's career, from basic training to recruiting a seasoned pilot for a new organization (see Table 30.1).
- Questionnaires – used widely as a precursor to more formal selection procedure; collect basic biographical detail.

Table 30.1 Typical selection procedures

STAGE	TESTING
Advertising	Often unnecessary for ab initio, mostly used to recruit trained pilots.
Basic screen	Often questionnaire biographical data; demographics, education, interests, flying experience. **ICAO Law**: A medical examination, English language proficiency, ability to understand training course (educational level) and human performance guidance.
Advanced screen	**Psychomotor**: Hand-eye coordination, spatial awareness, reaction time, memory and recall ability, 3-D pattern recognition, 2-D data analysis, estimation accuracy. **Psychometric**: Personality 'Big Five'; Extroversion/introversion, tough/tender mindedness, conformity, neuroticism, conscientiousness. Verbal/numerical reasoning, multi-tasking. N.B. Often delivered in one package across 1 or 2 days to avoid exhaustion and mixed with different test modes to repeatedly test the same attribute.
Work sampling	Often conducted in a small aircraft for ab initio or a representative task for trained pilot selection.
Simulation	Much more often used to select trained pilots for civil organisations, higher fidelity; more expense.
Decision	Must be taken in an active manner with review of test procedures inherent in the system to ensure that validity is maintained.

- Interviews – variety used:
  - Free style 'panel of expert' type popular, but research shows they are highly subjective, methodologically weak and poor decision-making tool.
  - Semi-structured interviews capture social and personality traits but difficult to devise and administer.
- Psychomotor tests:
  - Bedrock of aptitude selection from WWII until the sixties; initially mechanical devices but more commonly now computer based.
  - Still part of most initial selection procedures.
- Psychometric testing – Component of most selection procedures since WWII, but has grown in importance as roles of pilots better understood in terms of organisational fit, efficiency and safety.
- Work sampling:
  - Create a typical example of work to be performed; then observe candidate.
  - Common example is military grading in basic training aircraft.
  - Tends to predict success in basic elements of training but is weakly predictive of eventual success.
- Simulation:
  - Used to work sample as above but also to test trained pilots in more complex and stressful scenarios.
  - High cost, therefore not usually used until late in selection process.

30.4 PILOT TRAINING

- Continuous process throughout a pilot's career, line checks with training pilots at least yearly.
- Both ab initio and continuation training can be highly stressful, as threat to future or current career.
- As pilot population ages and flies beyond 55, the medical component becomes a significant source of anxiety.

30.5 LEARNING THEORY

- Most theories agree learning achieved in an experiential fashion; all agree that learning negatively impacted by fatigue, anxiety or poor health.
    - Classical conditioning – The Pavlovian response; humans to some extent learn by associating an action with a stimulus through repetition (e.g. particular action on receiving an emergency warning).
    - Operant conditioning – Reinforcement (reward) depends upon correct response, with negative aspect to not being correct. May risk a negative association with the learning process, rather than the incorrect action.
    - Cognitive theories – Cyclical process of behaviour and cognition resulting in conceptualisation of how new knowledge might be used and experimentation in the mental model and action (see Figure 30.2).

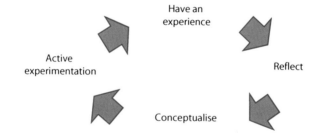

Figure 30.2 Modern learning cycle based on Kolb (1984).

31

The flight deck and cockpit

Contents

Key Facts
- Modern-day cockpits and flight decks are highly complex working environments.
- Application of automation and technology are increasingly replacing traditional crew duties, while individual aircrew tasks shift towards system management.
- Human factors and human systems integration challenges persist and evolve with advancements in human–machine interface, complex multifunction displays and reliance on automation and intelligent systems design.
- Aerospace medicine practitioner must have a functional understanding of the modern-day challenges to pilots and aircrew; regularly flying with crews and observing operations from the flight deck are supremely important.

31.1 ILLUSTRATIVE HISTORICAL PROGRESS AND TRANSFORMATION

WRIGHT BROTHERS FLYER (1903)

- Pilot positioned on wooden beams facing forwards.
- Elevator (front) operated by lifting and lowering wooden beam to control pitch.
- Rear 'T-section' operated by feet which enacted wing warping and allowed aircraft to turn (see Figure 31.1).

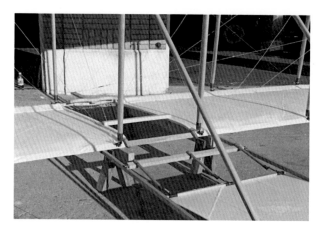

Figure 31.1 Wright Brothers Flyer.

SOPWITH CAMEL (1917)

- Controls comprised of an elevator and aileron operated by a central control column.
- Wire and pulley system connects relevant flying surfaces for control in pitch and roll.
- Rudder controlled with foot pedals; separate system used to steer the tail of aircraft whilst on ground.
- Instrumentation including airspeed, magnetic heading and height incorporated along with elementary engine monitoring by using a tachometer.
- Two machine guns operated using the gang bar synchronised to fire through propeller disc (see Figure 31.2).

DE HAVILLAND CHIPMUNK (1946)

- Basic flying trainer for military recruits in post-WWII era.
- Primary flying instruments arranged in a 3-on-3 configuration.

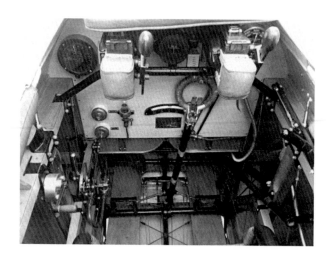

Figure 31.2 Sopwith Camel.

- Engine monitoring instruments surround the 'big six' primary flying instruments; flap select lever on right is used to allow aircraft landing configuration selection (see Figure 31.3).

GROB TUTOR (1999)

- Side-by-side configuration; basic flying trainer for military services.
- 3-on-3 primary flying instruments with turn and slip indicator swapped with altimeter when compared with the Chipmunk.
- May be trimmed in pitch by using the trim wheel (see base of Figure 31.4); GPS has been added to aid navigation.
- View from cockpit is reasonably unobstructed – aids selection of visual attitudes, an important part of basic training flying skill.

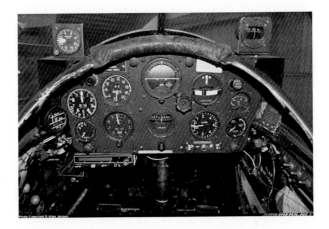

Figure 31.3 De Havilland Chipmunk trainer.

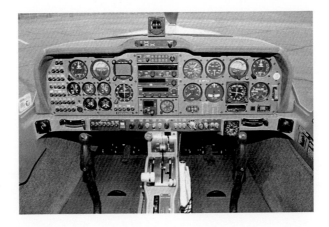

Figure 31.4 Grob Tutor.

SHORTS TUCANO (1986)

- Turbo-prop, tricycle undercarriage, tandem seat aircraft with similar aircraft instrumentation to basic trainer.
- Increased manoeuvrability, time to climb and ability to cruise at 240 knots during low-level navigation.
- Doubling aircraft speed now requires the human brain to process information significantly quicker.
- Focus still aircraft handling with additional skills of instrument flying and 'tail chasing' (follow-my-leader exercise).
- Figure 31.5 highlights ability to motor trim in pitch and yaw (black switch on control column).

BAES HAWK TMK1 (1976)

- Tandem two-seat trainer with a cockpit designed in the early 1970s.
- Used for advanced fast jet training; initially trained pilots to fly the aircraft accurately in day, night, all weather.
- Cockpit is relatively simple and has very few additional features when compared to Tucano (see Figure 31.6).

BAES HAWK TMK2

- Incorporates the need to not only fly but 'fight' the aircraft.
- Tandem seats with full controls available in front and rear; duplication of essential controls with override provided in rear cockpit (e.g. store jettison, landing gear and flaps).
- 'Glass cockpit' avionics suite provides realistic advanced fast jet training platform.
- Three full-colour, multifunction displays similar to those used by modern fighters used to display navigation, weapon and systems information.
- Head-up display (HUD) uses symbols and data comparable current combat aircraft.
- 'Hands-On-Throttle-And-Stick' (HOTAS) controls which are fully representative of front line combat aircraft types.

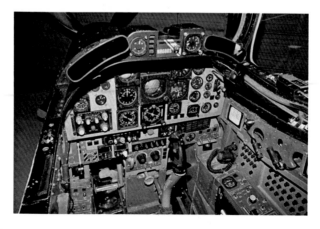

Figure 31.5 Shorts Tucano.

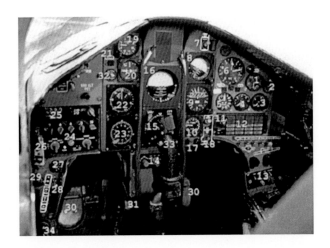

Figure 31.6 BAe Systems Hawk TMk1.

- Twin mission computers hosting simulations of a wide range of sensor and weapon systems as well as a full featured IN/GPS navigation system with moving map display.
- Provides synthetic radar for intercept training and sensor simulation capability to allow realistic electronic warfare (EW) training against surface-to-air missile (SAM) systems (see Figure 31.7).

EUROFIGHTER TYPHOON

- Ability to serve in air-to-air, air-to-ground or multirole capability with large payload.
- Many functions executed by voice command or through HOTAS.
- Combined with an advanced cockpit and helmet equipment assembly (HEA), pilot equipped for all aspects of air operations.

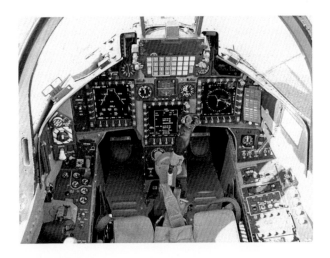

Figure 31.7 BAeS Hawk TMk2.

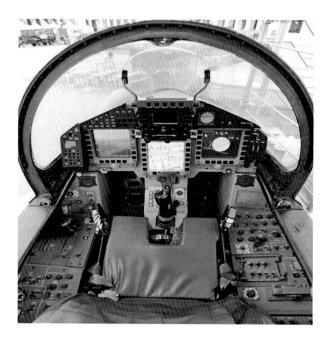

Figure 31.8 Eurofighter Typhoon.

- Wide field of view HUD with ability to display targeting information and assist in defensive manoeuvring.
- Three MFDs allowing different cockpit setups depending on phase of flight to provide right information and right time for rapid decisions.
- Auto-throttle and auto-trim allow the aircraft to be flown easily with focus of pilot on information management within a tactical environment (see Figure 31.8).

31.2 HUMAN FACTORS

- Design improvements and enhancements aid pilots to make the right decision at the right time with high-fidelity situational awareness.
- Realistic and repetitive training important; skills are highly perishable.
- Increased complexity and multiple inputs easily lead to cognitive overload in information management loop.
- Crew resource management highlights the importance of safety, teamwork and synergy.
- Human systems integration addresses the systematic process of identifying, tracking and resolving human-related issues to ensure a balance between the technological and human aspects of a system.

31.3 COCKPIT ERGONOMICS

- Modern-day aircraft cockpits are designed for ease of use and ability to present the pilot with the correct information at the right time.

- Generally engineered to support the 95% of anthropometric population range with static, dynamic, contour and 'eye datum point' considerations.
- Legacy cockpit design often incorporated large amounts of cockpit ironwork which required modified lookout to ensure safe flightpath.
- Ability to target and deliver a weapon in older platforms was highly labour-intensive, with a large number of switch movements and significant cooperation between front and back seat personnel.

CHAPTER 32

Human factors and crew resource management

Contents

32.1 DEFINITIONS

- Accident and incident investigation shows that human error plays a significant contribution in 60–80% of aircraft mishaps.
- All humans make mistakes; human error is unavoidable and inevitable, but in a safety critical environment, consequences may be fatal.
- Human factors (HF) applies the knowledge of human capabilities and limitations to the aviation environment to improve safety and efficiency.
  - HF is a multidisciplinary approach incorporating: psychology, physiology, medicine, sociology, anthropometry, engineering and ergonomics.
- Crew resource management (CRM) is the practical application of HF knowledge using all available resources (team members, other people, information, manuals, procedures, automation) to achieve safe and efficient flight.

32.2 WHY TRAIN HF AND CRM?

- Pilot training traditionally focused on technical and flying proficiency of the individual; assumed that crews made up of well-trained individuals would be able to operate complex systems safely together as a team.

- In the late 1970s/early 1980s, recognised that accidents were occurring primarily due to failures in teamwork, communication, leadership, task management and decision making – topics not traditionally covered in pilot training.
- CRM seeks to address these deficiencies by providing training in HF knowledge and CRM skills to make enduring shifts in attitudes, skills and behaviour in multi-crew operations.
- Proficiency in both technical and CRM skills essential; expertise in one discipline cannot compensate for deficiencies in the other.

32.3 EVOLUTION OF CRM

- CRM training incorporated into ICAO Standards and Recommended Practices (SARPS) in 1980s; mandated requirement for commercial pilots working under most regulatory bodies worldwide, including EASA (Europe) and FAA (USA).
- HF and CRM applicable to single and multi-crew operations; multi-crew cooperation qualification must be attained before operating in a complex multi-crew environment.
- CRM training provides cognitive and interpersonal skills that have evolved through several generations; current focus is on threat and error management (TEM).

32.4 THREAT AND ERROR MANAGEMENT

- TEM accepts that human error is normal and inevitable; shifts focus of training towards error reduction, detection and management (see Figure 32.1).
- CRM provides secondary and tertiary defences by trapping errors that do occur and mitigating the consequences of those that are not trapped.

THREATS

- Occur outside direct influence of the crew.
- Increase operational complexity.
- Require crew attention and management to maintain safety margins.
- Can be environmental (e.g. weather, ATC, terrain, airport factors) or organisational (e.g. operational pressure, aircraft, cabin, documentation and maintenance issues).

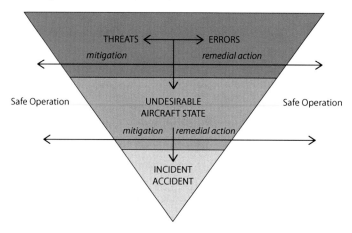

Figure 32.1 Threat and error management principles.

- Can be anticipated, unexpected or latent.
- Mismanaged threats may induce crew errors.

ERRORS

- Flight crew actions or inactions.
- Lead to deviation from intentions/expectations.
- Increase the probability of adverse operational events.

UNDESIRED AIRCRAFT STATE (UDS)

- Aircraft position, speed, altitude or configuration that reduces safety margins.
- Results from incorrectly managed threat or error.
- UDS can be managed effectively to restore safety margins; or flight crew response can induce an additional error, incident or accident.

MANAGEMENT

- CRM skills facilitate crew interventions at each level (threat, error, UDS); by avoiding, reducing, detecting and managing these errors, crew can revert to a safe flight environment prior to an incident/accident occurring.

32.5 CRM TRAINING REQUIREMENTS

AWARENESS/KNOWLEDGE

- Theoretical knowledge delivered via classroom sessions incorporating a variety of participative and interactional teaching methods (see Table 32.1).
- Supported by relevant aviation examples – accident reports, safety reports and data, personal experience and anecdotes.
- Instructor must be credible – Ideally a current line pilot trained in CRM instructional techniques.
- Demonstrated to drive changes in attitude but may not endure or be transferred to flight deck if not supported by training and practice in a flight training device (FTD) or simulator.

TRAINING AND PRACTICE

- Line-Oriented Flight Training (LOFT): Flight simulator exercises designed specifically to provide opportunities to demonstrate CRM skills through interactions with other crew members.
- Scenario design driven by data derived from accident/incident reports, safety reports, fleet and company flight monitoring data, training observations.
- Scenarios should be realistic and relevant, incorporating a number of 'events' with specific targets/objectives designed to elicit interpersonal and cognitive CRM skills in addition to technical expertise.
- Events unfold in real time, so consequences of crew actions and decisions will accrue for the remainder of simulated flight; instructor should allow the scenario to unfold without intervention.
- Sessions followed by an instructor-facilitated debrief, guiding crews to self-critique rather than outlining observed deficiencies.
- LOFT shown to elicit positive and enduring shifts in attitude and behaviour.

Table 32.1 Typical crew resource management training elements

TOPICS	CRM TRAINING ELEMENTS
General principles	HF in aviation, CRM principles & objectives, human performance & limitations, TEM.
Relevant to the individual flight crew member	Personality awareness, human error & reliability, attitudes & behaviours. Self-assessment & self-critique. Stress & stress management. Fatigue & vigilance. Assertiveness, situational awareness. Information acquisition & processing.
Relevant to the flight crew	Automation & automation philosophy. Specific type related differences. Monitoring & intervention.
Relevant to the aircraft crew	Shared situation awareness, shared information acquisition & processing Workload management. Effective communication & coordination inside & outside the flight deck. Leadership, cooperation, synergy, delegation, decision making, actions. Resilience development. Surprise & startle effect. Cultural differences.
Relevant to the operator & organisation	Operator's safety culture & company culture, standard operating procedures (SOPs), organisational factors, factors linked to the type of operations. Effective communication & coordination with other operational personnel & ground services. Case studies.

32.6 CRM ASSESSMENT

- Line Operations Evaluation (LOE) is an assessable form of LOFT.
- Assessing of non-technical skills is challenging; assessment systems must:
  - Be reliable and reproducible.
  - Minimise cultural and organisational differences.
  - Provide feedback to crew collectively and individually.
  - Serve to identify areas for retraining.
- Most widely used method for evaluating CRM is using observable behaviour (behavioural marker) checklists.
- European NOTECH (non-technical skills) system is a generic method for evaluating pilots' CRM/non-technical skills, building on research by Helmreich at the University of Texas.
  - Performance is assessed in four main categories:
    - Situation awareness.
    - Decision making.
    - Cooperation.
    - Leadership and managerial skills.

- Categories further subdivided with behavioural examples provided to illustrate effective and ineffective performance.
  - System validated with a high degree of user acceptability, internal consistency and inter-rater agreement.
- Airlines are free to adapt existing systems or develop their own, but must be acceptable to the regulator.
- Failure cannot be based on non-technical skills alone; there must be a related objective technical consequence where flight safety is actually or potentially compromised.
- Importance of CRM and LOE recognized by EASA Advanced Training and Qualification Program (ATQP) and FAA Advanced Qualification Program (AQP); allow approved operators additional flexibility if incorporating an LOE into pilot training and checking program.

32.7 REINFORCEMENT OF CRM

- HF and CRM should be part of the corporate culture driven from the top of the organization by senior management team.
- Management commitment manifested by:
  - Openness of communication between management and employees.
  - Commitment of resources to training and maintenance.
  - Attitudes and behaviour of critical role models such as training captains.
- Human performance considerations form a critical aspect of any safety management system.
- HF and CRM should be integrated and embedded into every stage of training and can only flourish within a comprehensive framework of standard operating procedures.

32.8 DRAWBACKS OF CRM

- Difficult to assess true impact of CRM.
- Not possible to draw conclusions from accident/incident rates due to variations in training, lack of control group, low accident numbers and incomplete voluntary incident reporting.
- Behavioural changes may be used as a surrogate marker, but behaviour in simulator may not necessarily transfer to flight deck.
- Despite widespread acceptance, small subset of pilots still reject the concept as 'psychobabble' or 'charm school'; paradoxically these individuals are often in greatest need. Others may revert or 'boomerang' back to pre-training attitudes and behaviour.
- CRM cannot be exported; training programs must take into account prevailing national, professional and organisational culture.

32.9 CRM BEYOND THE FLIGHT DECK

- Other groups routinely working with cockpit crew are also essential participants in effective CRM process (e.g. aircraft dispatchers, cabin crews, maintenance personnel and air traffic controllers); joint HF/CRM training now commonplace.

- From commercial aviation roots, CRM has been successfully integrated into military aviation operations, acknowledging the enhanced prioritisation of mission accomplishment.
- CRM programs are being further adapted for use in a number of other safety critical environments such as medicine, nuclear industry, offshore oil industry and fire fighting.

Fatigue and countermeasures

Contents

> **Key Facts**
> - Often considered synonymous with on-the-job sleepiness associated with performance decrement.
> - Function of insufficient sleep, long wakefulness periods, extended time on duty, shift work and/or time zone changes.
> - Physiological reality and not 'just a state of mind'.
> - Cannot overcome fatigue by threats, willpower or incentives.

33.1 FATIGUE IN AVIATION

- Aircrew fatigue associated with involuntary sleep episodes on the flight deck, procedural errors, unstable approaches, attempts to land on the wrong runway, landing without clearances; fatigue identified as co-factor in many crashes and fatalities.
- In the United Kingdom approximately one-third of reports to Confidential Human Factors Incident Reporting Programme blame pilot fatigue for incidents, errors or other flight-related problems.

33.2 FATIGUE FACTORS

- Humans evolved for 7–9 hr of night sleep, to be awake during the day and have a consistent sleep/wake routine.

- Fatigue complicated by sleep–wake patterns that are contrary to biological programming.

HOMEOSTATIC COMPONENT

- Amount and quality of sleep obtained during the last sleep episode.
- Amount of time spent awake since the last sleep episode.

CIRCADIAN COMPONENT

- Alignment between environmental time queues and internal physiological rhythms.
- Synchronization among various internal physiological rhythms.
- Timing of performance relative to the timing of internal rhythms.

SLEEP-INERTIA COMPONENT

- Grogginess associated with short time from wakeup to time of performance.

33.3 MOTHER NATURE'S DESIGN

- Historically, people slept at night and worked during the day; safer with sufficient illumination and easier to sleep without technologically enabled distractions.
- Shift work and jet transportation were non-existent, so circadian disruptions were fewer.
- Homeostatic and circadian components worked in synchrony to keep workplace alertness consistent.
- When both homeostatic and circadian components decline, alertness deteriorates and fatigue increases (see Figure 33.1).
- In the modern work environment, fatigue-related performance decrements are common.

33.4 THE HOMEOSTATIC COMPONENT

- Function of the amount and quality of sleep routinely obtained.
- Average adult needs 7–9 hr of sleep per 24-hr period to feel rested and alert.
- Should be of high quality, progressing through a series of stages without disruptions.
  - Stage 1 – light sleep (*referred to as 'N1' in the newest classification scheme*).
  - Stage 2 – moderate sleep (*'N2'*).
  - Stage 3 – moderately deep sleep (*'N3' includes stages 3 and 4*).
  - Stage 4 – very deep sleep (*also referred to as 'N3'; see note above*).
  - Stage REM – rapid eye movement sleep – when most dreams occur.
- Progression through sleep stages occurs predictably when there is a consistent schedule of wake/sleep.
- Sleep begins in Stage 1 and progresses to Stages 2, 3 and 4, prior to returning back to Stage 2, then to Stage REM.
- Cycle lasts approximately 90 minutes before it begins again.
- During first half of the night, most of the slow-wave sleep occurs.
- During the second half of the night, most of the REM sleep occurs.
- Throughout night, brief transitions to Stage 1 sleep and/or brief awakenings are often observed; a few each night are common for adults and considered normal.

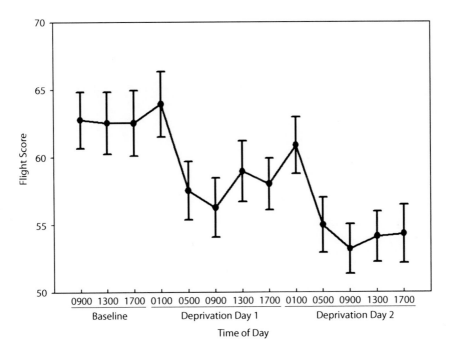

Figure 33.1 Homeostatically based performance decline associated with a build-up of fatigue across three days with no sleep exacerbated by rhythmic circadian influence present on each of the days. Sleep-inertia component not an issue, as no naps permitted immediately prior to performance.

33.5 THE CIRCADIAN COMPONENT

- From the Latin 'circa' meaning about and 'dias' meaning day.
- Somewhat independent from homeostatic component; function of body's internal biological clock.
- Clock kept in synchrony by a combination of internal physiological mechanisms and external environmental cues.
- Many body processes fluctuate on a 24-hr rhythm based on an internal timing mechanism or number of internal clocks which normally work in synchrony unless disrupted by scheduling changes (see Figure 33.2).
- Circadian timing: Body rhythms kept locked to a certain time of day and kept in synchrony by several external cues:
    - Light/sun exposure (primary).
    - Meal times.
    - Work schedules.
    - Social activities.
- Typical circadian pattern (see Figure 33.3): Alertness/sleepiness fairly predictable on a stable schedule of daytime wakefulness and night-time sleep:
    - Opening of the 'sleep gate' – a period of drowsiness that occurs at standard bedtime.
    - Circadian nadir – the point at which sleepiness becomes almost irresistible at 0200 or 0300 in the morning during night-time work.

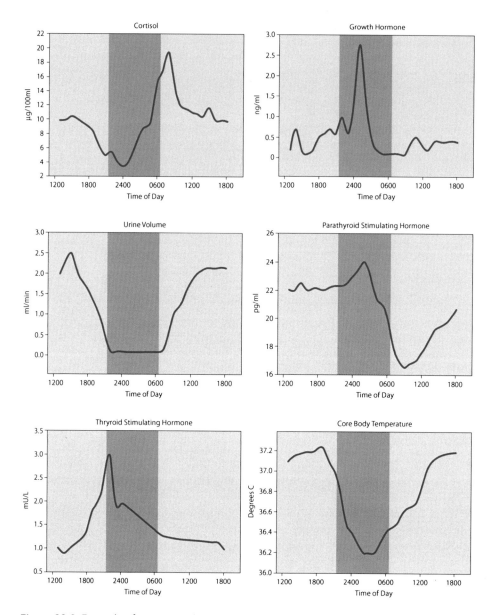

Figure 33.2 Example of processes that evidence circadian rhythms.

- Alertness generally coincides with physiological changes such as body temperature.
- Performance effects sometimes lag behind physiological markers.

33.6 THE SLEEP-INERTIA COMPONENT

- Sleep inertia is degraded vigilance, increased drowsiness and diminished performance that occurs immediately after awakening.

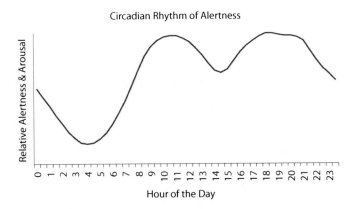

Figure 33.3 Typical circadian rhythm. (Figures from the North American Fatigue Management Program [http://www.nafmp.com/en/].)

- Not usually problematic, as people often have 30 minutes or more between awakening and performance time.
- May be an issue when napping used as an operational fatigue countermeasure; must be weighed against longer-term performance problems without napping.
- Affects mood and cognitive performance.
- Tasks with high cognitive demands or requiring high degree of attention are affected more than simple motor skills.
- Complex decision-making ability may decline by almost 50% within the first 3 minutes after an abrupt night-time awakening.
- Duration:
  - Generally dissipates 15–35 minutes after awakening.
  - Within operational contexts, it is conservative to allow 30 minutes from awakening to the duty time to mitigate effects.
- Factors affecting inertia:
  - Primarily a function of stage of sleep from which awakened.
  - Awakenings from 'deep' or slow-wave sleep (SWS) produce more sleep inertia than from shallower or 'lighter' stages.
  - Worse after awakenings during circadian trough or deep sleep.

33.7 PROBLEMATIC INTERACTIONS AMONG THE THREE COMPONENTS

- Components work in combination favourably under normal schedules to optimize daytime alertness and safeguard night sleep quality.
- Extended duty cycles, shift work and transmeridian travel cause problematic interactions due to the body's inability to adjust to reduced sleep and rapid schedule changes.
- Chronic sleep restriction creates sleep debt that accumulates day to day.
- As sleep/wake schedule is rotated, body's internal clock is disrupted; often becomes desynchronized from work-life demands.

33.8 RECOMMENDATIONS FOR COUNTERING FATIGUE IN AVIATION

- Fatigue-related problems occur due to conflicts between operational scheduling demands and normal physiology.
- Strategies exist to manage fatigue and safeguard performance.
- Inter-individual differences exist in fatigue susceptibility and effectiveness of countermeasures.

OPTIMIZATION OF CREW SCHEDULING

- Implementation of 'human-centred' work routines is crucial for job alertness.
- Assessing proposed crew schedules with modelling (see Figure 33.4) and/or actigraphy permits organizations to identify/avoid schedules at greatest risk for compromised alertness and performance.
- Fatigue metrics can be validated against operational measures from Flight Operations Quality Assurance (FOQA) efforts or pilot self-reports.
- Biomathematical models:
  - Simulate physiological processes that determine fatigue (i.e. performance effectiveness) at any given point in time.
  - Contain homeostatic, circadian and sleep-inertia processes (see Figure 33.5).
  - Have been shown to predict performance effects of different scheduling factors.
  - Validation for specific work environment is desirable.
- Wrist actigraphy:
  - Offers objective sleep/wake information useful to feed models for determination of fatiguing effect of schedules.
  - Actigraphy based on relatively unobtrusive and inexpensive wrist monitors (see Figure 33.6).
  - Wrist monitors contain accelerometer, storage and data-transfer components.
  - Data are processed through automated classification programs to determine sleep/wake patterns of wearer.
  - Information can be uploaded to a biomathematical model to accurately calculate fatigue risk.

IN-FLIGHT COUNTER-FATIGUE STRATEGIES

- The most effective strategies address the homeostatic (sleep) component.
- On-board sleep:
  - Out-of-cockpit bunk sleep is one of the best countermeasures.
  - Crews can estimate times during a flight when increased risk of sleepiness and consider these the best times to schedule in-flight sleep.
- Cockpit naps:
  - One pilot sleeps in the seat while other pilot flies.
  - Extremely beneficial for promoting alertness in the operational context by partially satisfying the homeostatic drive for sleep.
  - 30 minutes of post-nap wakeup time should be allowed for avoiding sleep inertia.

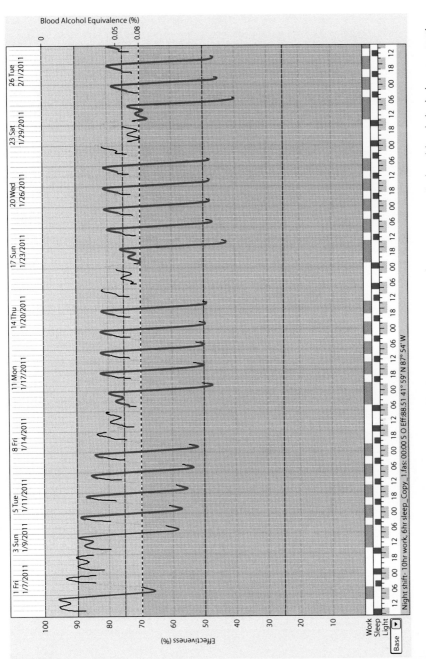

Figure 33.4 Example of Fatigue Avoidance Scheduling Tool (FAST) output, relating performance to equivalent blood alcohol concentration.

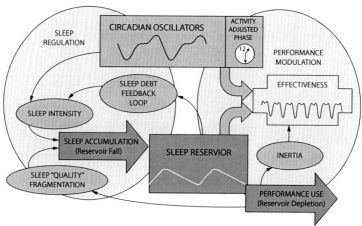

Figure 33.5 Example of a biomathematical model. (From Eddy, D.R., and Hursh, S.R. Fatigue Avoidance Scheduling Tool [FAST] Phase II SBIR final report, Part 1. AFRL-HE-BR-TR-2006-0015.)

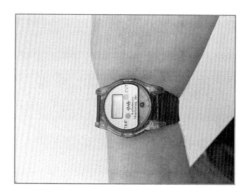

Figure 33.6 Typical wrist activity monitor.

- Controlled rest breaks:
  - Rest break strategy (standing up, walking around, etc.) may be valuable for temporarily combatting fatigue and boredom, especially during lengthy flights.
  - Breaks can improve physical comfort and reduce eyestrain during prolonged, repetitious tasks while also attenuating unintended sleep episodes and subjective sleepiness.
  - Positive benefits are transient (15–20 minutes) but they are noteworthy, particularly within the circadian trough.
- Alertness aids:
  - Caffeine is a widely available valuable pharmacological fatigue countermeasure.
  - Caffeine increases vigilance and improves performance in fatigued individuals; both safe and effective in daily doses of up to 600 mg.

- Caffeine starts working within 30–50 minutes and typically enhances alertness for 4 to 5 hr.
- In some operational contexts, prescription medications are permitted. Dextroamphetamine and/or modafinil reliably improve alertness within 1 hr of ingestion and continue to promote wakefulness for as long as 6–8 hr post-dose (see Figure 33.7).

PREFLIGHT COUNTER-FATIGUE STRATEGIES

- Education: Importance of sleep and proper sleep hygiene, dangers and signs of fatigue, and physiological mechanisms underlying sleepiness:
  - Sleep banking where possible.
  - Operational personnel and schedulers should realize the impact of sleep and circadian rhythms.
  - Focus on maximising the benefits of every available sleep opportunity while minimising circadian disruption.
  - Quality off-duty sleep is the best protection against on-the-job fatigue.

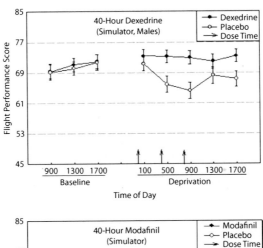

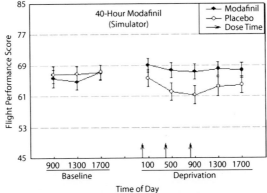

Figure 33.7 Graphs showing how amphetamine and modafinil sustain flight performance after a lengthy period of sustained wakefulness. (From Caldwell, J.A. (2003). Short-term fatigue management: A cross-study analysis of the effects of dextroamphetamine and modafinil in sleep-deprived aviators. AFRL-HE-BR-TR-2003-0059.)

- Sleep hygiene:
  - When possible, stick to same sleep/wake schedule every day.
  - Use sleeping quarters only for sleep and not for work or other activity.
  - Establish a consistent and comforting bedtime routine.
  - Perform aerobic exercise every day, but not within 2 hr of going to sleep.
  - Make sure sleeping quarters are quiet, dark and comfortable.
  - Keep the sleep environment cool (~26°C if you are covered).
  - Move alarm clock out of sight; avoid clock watching.
  - Avoid caffeine in drinks and other forms within 4–6 hr of bedtime.
  - Don't use alcohol as a sleep aid.
  - Avoid sources of nicotine just before bedtime.
  - Avoid computers and smart phones close to bedtime and while in bed.
  - Don't lie in bed awake if sleep doesn't occur within 30 minutes; leave the bedroom and relax quietly until you are sleepy enough to try again.

Sleep-promoting compounds: Helpful for minimising sleep loss and subsequent fatigue; half-life of each compound should be matched to length of available sleep opportunity in order to promote sleep and minimise hangover effects; national military policies vary but the following compounds have been used:

- Temazepam: Useful for maintaining relatively long periods of night-time sleep for day workers or daytime sleep for night workers.
- Zolpidem or zaleplon: Good choices for initiating sleep and/or for shorter sleep periods.
- Eszopiclone: Option for intermediate-length sleep opportunities.

CHAPTER 34

Errors and accidents

Contents

34.1 HUMAN ERROR

- Human error frequently identified as the cause of serious aviation incidents.
- Across definitions of human error, there is a common theme of deviation by one or more human roles; specific description challenging because:
  - Not always possible to determine correct course of action; without knowing correct action it is not possible to specify deviation from it.
  - Definitions of error place strong emphasis on outcome, such that an error may only be identified when it has a negative consequence; however, behaviours frequently deviate from what is expected without a negative outcome.
  - Term 'error' can encompass a broad range of behaviours, including action and inaction, as well as intentional and accidental behaviours.
  - Context in which behaviour occurs is critical, such that the same action could be an error in one situation and correct in another.

34.2 ERROR TYPES

- Early models of human error grouped different types of behaviour based on key characteristics.
- Rasmussen identified three types of human error:
  - Skill-based errors which occur in highly practiced tasks.
  - Rule-based errors which occur in familiar decision-making tasks, such as 'if X, then take action Y'.

- Knowledge-based errors which occur in novel circumstances, where stored knowledge is applied to the situation to select a course of action.
- Reason categorized three types of error:
  - Slips and lapses which refer to failures in executing an action.
  - Mistakes which refer to failures in decision making and judgement.
  - Violations which refer to deliberate deviations from rules and practices.
- Error types can be beneficial to understand nature of errors made and offer some insights into error prevention:
  - However, focus is on actions closest to event of interest.
  - Error is analysed separately from contextual and organisational causes, which limits scope for error prevention.

34.3 ORGANISATIONAL APPROACHES TO ERROR

- Organisational approaches highlight the role of influences outside of the individual performing the action.
- Reason's Swiss Cheese Model is an example of an organisational approach to error (see Figure 34.1).

34.4 HUMAN ERROR ANALYSIS

- Human Error Analysis (HEA), also known as Human Reliability Analysis (HRA), is used to identify the type of errors that can occur when performing a particular task.
- Some techniques also enable the probability of the error to be estimated (producing a Human Error Probability [HEP]).
- Many HEA techniques based on task decomposition:
  - Hierarchical Task Analysis (HTA) identifies actions and decisions required at each stage of a task.

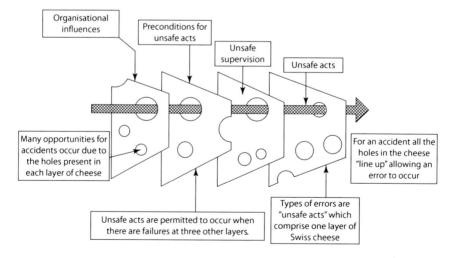

Figure 34.1 Protections in place to reduce the likelihood of an error are conceptualized as slices of Swiss cheese.

- Each action and decision reviewed to identify the potential errors that could occur.
- Examples of such techniques include: Systematic Human Error Reduction and Prediction Approach (SHERPA) and Human Error Template (HET).
- HEA can form part of systems engineering approaches such as Hazard and Operability (HAZOP) assessment, where HF specialist will advise on potential failure modes to be considered in design process.
- Once errors have been identified, probability of an error can be estimated by applying error rates for standardized task types and then adjusting those error rates to reflect attributes of task being performed:
  - Techniques such as Human Error Analysis and Reduction Technique (HEART) and Technique for Human Error Rate Prediction (THERP) provide guidance on process for developing HEP.

BENEFITS OF HEA

- Provides a structured method to identify a wide range of errors.
- Helps understand human error risk in the design process.
- Identifies methods to mitigate errors.

LIMITATIONS OF HEA

- Significant expertise required in human factors and in the system being analysed to apply HEA effectively.
- Can be time-consuming when applied to large and complex systems.
- Less typical error types could be missed.
- Quantification of HEP particularly challenging and often results in a broad range of possible values.

34.5 ERROR PREVENTION

Aim of analysing human error is to implement methods to reduce error risk; typical approaches include:

- **Safety culture**. Safety culture arises from common values, beliefs, attitudes and practices related to safety within an organization.
  - Improvements to safety culture thought to reduce the risk of all error types through positive attitudes to error, safety leadership and open communications.
- **Training**. Training improvements could include:
  - Training on specific tasks where there is a risk of error.
  - Improving overall expertise or system knowledge to support task performance.
- **Procedures**. Putting a procedure in place for correct conduct of a task changes it from a knowledge-based to a rule-based task, which is associated with a lower probability of error.
  - However, when there are a very large number of procedures, it is impossible for users to remember them all, which increases the risk that procedure will be unintentionally violated.

- **System design**. Potential errors can be 'designed out' by use of various safety features.
  - In other cases, design can be used to reduce likelihood of error or to make errors easier to detect and correct.

34.6 AVIATION ACCIDENTS – DEFINITION

- ICAO defines an aviation accident as one which results in a fatality or serious injury, significant damage to the aircraft or the aircraft being missing (see Chapter 35).
- Following an aviation accident, an investigation will be instigated to identify the cause of the accident.
- Investigations undertaken under ICAO Annex 13 are performed with sole aim of preventing further accidents.
- However, investigations may also be undertaken with aim of determining culpability, or to address specific questions regarding the technical or operational aspects of the accident.
- Aviation accident investigation explores the range of issues which could have contributed to the accident; the investigation will identify what, if any, errors occurred during the accident and what caused those errors to occur.

34.7 AVIATION ACCIDENTS – HUMAN ERROR INVESTIGATION TECHNIQUES

- Many techniques available to support the analysis of human error during aviation accidents; these can be grouped into three categories:

CHAIN OF EVENTS MODELS

- These models propose that an error is a result of a series of events which can be traced back from the error through proximal causes to distal factors.
- Based on principle of cause and effect such that error occurs as a result of identifiable contributory factors; by identifying those contributory factors it is possible to determine the root cause or causes of an error.
- Examples of a chain of event model are fault and event trees:
  - In a fault tree, multiple causal factors can be identified for each event and for each causal factor. Each factor in the event tree is linked by either AND or OR relationships, enabling the model to be both explanatory and predictive. Fault tree analysis is widely used in safety engineering, and there are software tools that can support its use.

EPIDEMIOLOGICAL MODELS

- The epidemiological approach accepts that not all factors can be attributed a specific role in contributing to an error.
- Therefore, there are both latent conditions which increase the likelihood of error in general, as well as those specific to the error that occurred.
- Swiss Cheese Model (see Figure 34.1) is an example of an epidemiological model; this was further developed by Weigmann and Shappell into the Human Factors Analysis

and Classification System (HFACS), which provides definitions of specific factors which make up each of the holes in the cheese (see Figure 34.2).

- Accident Route Matrix (ARM) used by UK military is another example of epidemiological model (see Figure 34.3):
    - ARM is grounded in HFACS approach with some adaptations to categories and the introduction of a timeline and a breakdown of accident phases.
    - ARM allows errors to be linked to specific stages of an accident sequence, and the factors which led to those errors to be mapped by both the nature of the factor and time of effect.

SYSTEMIC MODELS

- Systemic models move away from simple cause and effect relationships and re-evaluate apparent errors as failures in control systems.
    - Focus on relationships between components rather than individual system elements.
    - Highlights how elements which are individually effective can come together to cause accidents.
- Example of the systemic approach is the Systems Theoretic Accident Model and Processes (STAMP) developed by Leveson:
    - Safety maintained by a series of control loops, such as tasks performed by a human operator interacting with aircraft systems.
    - Control loop includes multiple interrelated human and technical components working in a closely coupled way.
    - When error occurs, there is some form of disturbance to which control loop does not adapt effectively.

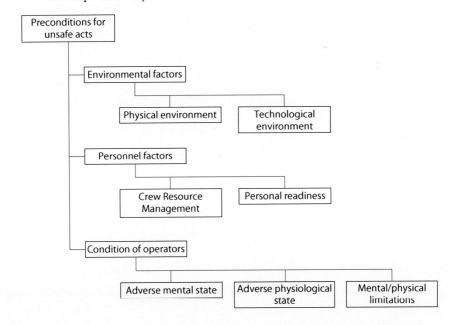

Figure 34.2 Example of categories defined in the Human Factors Analysis and Classification System (HFACS) for one layer of 'Swiss cheese'.

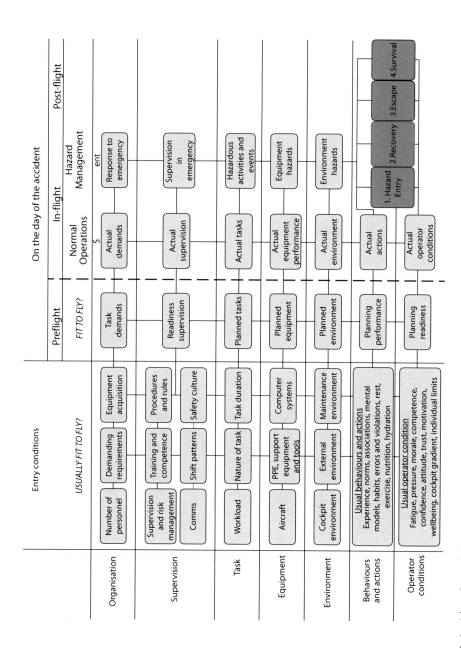

Figure 34.3 Accident Route Matrix.

Accident investigation

Contents

35.1 PRINCIPLES OF AVIATION ACCIDENT INVESTIGATION

- Aircraft accident defined as: 'occurrence which takes place between the time any person boards the aircraft with the intention of flight, until such time that all such persons have disembarked, in which a person is fatally or seriously injured, the aircraft incurs damage or structural failure, or the aircraft is missing or is completely inaccessible'.
- Aims of investigation are to:
  - Determine cause of the accident (to prevent similar accidents recurring).
  - Determine consequences of the accident.
- Approaches to investigation of human error in aircraft accidents are described in Chapter 34.
- Approaches to investigation of aerospace medicine aspects of aircraft accident include:
  - Causes of injuries or fatalities.
  - Specific interactions between victims and aircraft that resulted in injuries or fatalities.
  - If the aircraft had provision for in-flight escape, why did victims fail to escape?
  - Did the in-flight escape system contribute to causes of injuries or fatalities?
  - If fatalities survived deceleration forces of impact, why did they fail to escape from the lethal environment of the wreckage?
  - Did pilot incapacitation or physiological aberrations cause or contribute to the crash?
  - What changes could be made to prevent injuries or fatalities from occurring if an accident were to happen again under similar circumstances?
- Injury pattern can be analysed by relating various combinations of injuries, and certain characteristic patterns, to the sequence of events.
- Analysing injuries can enable dynamic forces involved to be estimated, which together with the investigation of forces of the impacting aircraft (e.g. by measurement of ground contact witness marks) will provide a more detailed picture of the crash event.

- When injury has occurred, investigation must address what could be done to prevent similar injuries in the future:
  - Changes to improve accident survivability may simultaneously introduce other risks that could outweigh any advantage.
  - Any protection system represents a compromise between factors, including system weight, comfort, mobility and occupant anthropometry.
- Aerospace medicine investigators should:
  - Understand requirements within the investigative team.
  - Be aware of organisational policies, manuals and directives of the investigation process.
  - Have knowledge of aircraft flown including design, operational capabilities, technical limitations and life support equipment and systems.

35.2 ON-SITE ACCIDENT INVESTIGATION

- Police and emergency services are likely to be first at scene; their first concern will be saving lives.
- Site safety is paramount and the site should be made free of explosive hazards, fire or excessive heat, smoke or fumes.
  - Crash site can be a biohazard due to presence of biological tissues and fluids.
  - May contain toxic materials, man-made fibre composites, ordnance, fuels, lubricants, flares and compressed gasses.
  - Military fast jet aircraft may also contain ejection seats; should be considered as hazardous explosives and treated with care until made safe.
- All crash sites should be considered as a potential crime scene until proven otherwise:
  - Evidence should be disturbed as little as possible; site's wreckage plot, position of survivors and deceased should be documented.
- Life support systems, aircrew equipment assemblies and survival equipment should be examined to determine their functionality.
- Seating plan is critical; passenger manifest should indicate seating positions, but passengers may have moved seats during flight.
  - Identification of seating positions will assist in injury causation analysis, detection of hazardous aircraft structures and identify improvements to crash survivability.
- Analysis of impact forces and accelerations used to determine injury causation and survivability:
  - Crash considered survivable if impact forces are within limits of human tolerance, occupiable space remains intact and restraints retain the seated occupants.
- Injuries can be caused by whole body acceleration, impact with other components or contents of vehicle, impact with loose objects, body displacement.

ANALYSIS OF AIRCRAFT CRASHWORTHINESS

- Crash survivability and human tolerance to impact can be analysed using: **C**ontainer, **R**estraints, **E**nvironment, **E**nergy absorption and **P**ost-crash factors (CREEP).
  - Container – the occupied space (e.g. cockpit and cabin volume):
    - Container should be a solid structure, or safety cell, which prevents intrusion of outside objects.

- Should resist deformation; restitution (spring-back) can be misleading as it could suggest erroneously that little intrusion of the occupiable space had occurred.
- Restraint – analysis should evaluate forces applied through the restraint system and identify any failings of straps, inertia reel and harness's locking mechanisms.
- Environment – the volume space of the container:
  - During frontal impacts, a seated occupant will flail forwards; if objects located within flail envelope, then contact injuries result.
  - Effects of flail injuries can be limited by adopting a brace position.
  - Brace position will pre-position occupant's body against whatever it was most likely to collide with during the crash; should be designed to take into account magnitude, direction and sequence of crash forces, interior layout, seat and restraint system design and orientation, and size of occupant.
  - Accident investigator should assess the brace position used to determine its efficacy in mitigating injury.
- Energy absorption – should reduce impact energy reaching occupants.
  - Aim is to increase stopping distance and hence time over which impact deceleration occurs.
  - Achieved by crumple zones outside occupiable container which deform in a controlled manner.
  - Energy attenuation can also be incorporated into aircraft seats (stroking seats or energy attenuating foam cushions).
- Post-crash factors – including:
  - Escape from wreckage. Aircraft should have sufficient numbers and appropriately sized aircraft exits; in passenger aircraft, cabin crew should be able to evacuate all passengers through only half the available exits in less than 90 seconds. Helicopters may roll over and ditch; underwater escape training advantageous (see Chapter 22).
  - Post-crash fire survival and smoke inhalation can rapidly incapacitate passengers and crew. Smoke hoods can alleviate risk from poisonous fumes, but passengers should probably spend limited time available escaping rather than putting on smoke hoods.
  - Environmental survival.
  - Provision of medical care.
  - Escape and evasion (military).

35.3 OFF-SITE ACCIDENT INVESTIGATION

The aeromedical investigator should:
- Interview survivors, liaise with treating physicians and attend post-mortem if fatalities have occurred.
- Determine if a medical condition was responsible for, or contributed to, the cause of the crash.
- Identify if any medication (prescribed or over-the-counter) contributed to the accident:
  - May be appropriate for blood/urine analysis for therapeutic substances, alcohol or substances of abuse; before taking such specimens, investigator should ensure that there are no local legal contraindications.

- Analyse the nature, severity and frequency of all injuries sustained:
  - To allow analysis of forces encountered, relate injuries to parameters of aircraft at ejection or impact, including the airspeed, altitude, attitude, angle of roll, pitch and yaw.
- Examine aircrew helmet with respect to retention on the crew's head, evidence of contact with structures, site of impact damage, aerodynamic forces and impact standard:
  - Damage patterns can be replicated using helmet impact test rig to estimate energies sustained during head impact.
- Document whether anthropometric measurements of crew are within aircraft cockpit/cabin space limits:
  - Weight should be within ejection seat, or static seat, limits.
- Examine aircrew equipment and survival equipment:
  - Deficiencies should be rectified, as safety in aviation and aircraft accident investigation is, in part, a matter of learning from what has gone wrong.

CHAPTER

36

Assessing risk and making decisions

Contents

36.1 BACKGROUND

- Assessment of potential clinical risk is the *raison d'etre* of the aeromedical examiner and others involved in aircrew health.
- Determining risk of incapacitation is the usual benchmark, but distraction may be as likely to jeopardize safe flight operations.
- The most common cause of in-flight incapacitation is acute gastrointestinal disease, which is usually mild in nature and self-limiting.
- Conditions that cause acute pain or loss of consciousness (cardiac or neurological) are likely to be immediately incapacitating; loss of mental capacity (including psychoactive substances [alcohol and drugs], organic brain disease and psychiatric illness) may render aircrew unable to safely perform critical flight duties.
- The most common cause of restriction/loss of flying privileges is cardiovascular disease. Cardiovascular risk underpins the 1% rule – the current, if limited, foundation for most 'objective' risk assessment in aviation (see below).
- When assessing risk, it is important to consider not just the underlying medical condition, but the long-term success rates of any intervention (e.g. surgery) and potential aeromedical risks associated with any ongoing pharmacological management.

36.2 THE 1% SAFETY RULE

- In dual pilot flying operations, current threshold for an acceptable level of controlled risk (of death) is usually 1% per annum.
- This is derived using engineering principles to ensure the incidence of a fatal air accident is no greater than 1 per 10^9 hr of flying (see Table 36.1); includes assumptions from simulator studies that 10% of flight time is critical, during which incapacitation would cause an accident (see below).

Table 36.1 Derivation of the 1% rule

Engineering principles
Total failure rate <1 in 10^9 flying hr
• Any single system failure rate must be <10%. • Any sub-system failure rate must be <10%.
Medical equivalence
Pilot flies 10^4 hr per year
• If annual mortality is 1% 1 in $10^{6\,(4+2)}$ • 10% flight time is critical 1 in $10^{7\,(6+1)}$ • 1% deaths results in fatal accident 1 in $10^{9\,(7+2)}$

36.3 LIMITATIONS OF THE 1% SAFETY RULE

● There are several limitations of the 1% rule that mean it should be used as guide to decision making, not a rigorous rule. These include:
  ○ Cardiovascular mortality rates ≠ incapacitation rates.
  ○ Cardiovascular mortality ≠ only death from coronary artery disease.
  ○ Aircrew may be healthier than the 'normal' population.
  ○ Cardiovascular disease is not the only cause of incapacitation.
  ○ Distraction may be fatal.
  ○ The duration of flight may not be 1 hour and % of flight deemed flight critical may not be 10%.
  ○ Does not take into account summative/polymorphic risk.
  ○ Only applies to 'dual-crew' pilot operations.

36.4 PROBABILITY AND CONSEQUENCE OF MEDICAL EVENTS

● Determination of risk requires assessment of likelihood and impact of the event.
● Usually captured in a standard risk matrix (risk along one axis, consequence along the other), with green (i.e. acceptable), amber (i.e. restricted flying) and red (i.e. grounded) boxes set against organization level of risk tolerance (see Figure 36.1).

MEDICAL EVENTS

● Impact of medical event can vary and may:
  ○ Have minimal impact on a flight (e.g. occasional asymptomatic ectopic heart beat) even if relatively frequent.

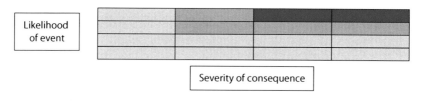

Figure 36.1 Standard form of risk matrix.

- Compromise military mission effectiveness (if symptomatic in a weapons system operator).
- Produce a flight safety hazard (if a single seat pilot).
- Result in a critical flight safety event (if associated with syncope).

AIRCREW ROLE

- To understand the consequence more clearly, the aircrew role must be considered:
  - In many flight operations this may include more than just the pilot.
- Aerospace medicine specialist needs to be clear as to whether the individual is flight, mission or safety critical:
  - Flight critical individual: Includes single, dual or multi-crew pilots.
    - Incapacitation of these individuals jeopardises the flight and if not mitigated will lead to the loss of the aircraft.
    - Acceptable risk will depend on ability/likelihood of additional crew members to take over the safe flight of the aircraft.
  - Mission or safety critical individual: May include navigators, rear-crew, weapons systems operators, flight surgeons/aeromedical staff.
    - Incapacitation will impact the mission (that in itself may be life-compromising).
    - Incapacitation will not jeopardise the immediate flying of the aircraft.

36.5 AEROMEDICAL DISPOSITION

- Single-seat aircrew, especially if flying high-performance aircraft (including helicopters), do not have much leeway with regards to conditions that distract or incapacitate.
- Most multi-crew pilots can expect to return to flying duties if their condition and/or treatment has a 10-year incapacitation risk of less than 10%.
- For non-pilot aircrew a 10-year incapacitation risk may be acceptable, depending on flight/mission or safety criticality of their role.
- For military aircrew, more caution and certain physiological considerations may be required, due to deployment to remote/austere locations and potential operational impact in the event of an adverse clinical episode.

CHAPTER 37

Medication in aircrew

Contents

37.1 DEFINITION

- Medication is any form of medicine that is used to treat or prevent disease. It includes over-the-counter medication, prescribed drugs, herbal medicines and homeopathic remedies.

37.2 TREAT THE PATIENT, THEN THE PILOT

- When treating aircrew, it is crucial that their care is not compromised by prescribing 'pilot-friendly' medication rather than more efficacious drugs which may limit or preclude flying; however, where there is more than one treatment option, one that will impact least on flying should be chosen.

37.3 CONSIDERATIONS WHEN PRESCRIBING

- Few resources available to guide prescribing in aircrew; however, some aviation authorities will give specific guidance for common clinical conditions.
- The following should be considered when prescribing to aircrew:
  - Efficacy. Does it work?
  - Side effects. Can be ignored if minor or transient, and predictable.
  - Observation. Aircrew should be grounded or undertake restricted (multi-crew) flying until medication proven to work without significant side effects; usually 2 to 4 weeks.
  - Dependency. What happens if treatment is suddenly stopped (e.g. lost on stop-over)? Consider rebound or withdrawal symptoms.
  - Frequency. Once daily preferred.
  - Route. Tablets and inhalers preferred. Subcutaneous and intramuscular treatment may be acceptable. Patches fall off and have variable absorption profiles dependent on body and ambient temperature.
  - Storage. Avoid medication that needs to be refrigerated.
  - Supply. Unusual drugs may be difficult to source overseas (e.g. when medication runs out or is lost).

37.4 HERBS AND HOMEOPATHY

- There is compelling evidence for efficacy of many herbal medicines; this is not the case for homeopathic remedies.
- Limited regulation of these treatments, and both raise several aeromedical concerns:
  - Efficacy and side effects. Often limited evidence of efficacy and profiling of side effects, including interactions with other medications.
  - Ingredients. May be undisclosed or inconsistent; some contain high concentrations of alcohol.
  - Concealment. Can be acquired without prescription and taken covertly.

37.5 DEAR DR

- The following mnemonic may be useful when prescribing medication to aircrew:

D	DIAGNOSIS Needs to be confirmed.
E	ETIOLOGY Gives clues to the symptoms that might be present.
A	AEROMEDICAL CONCERNS Focusing on those symptoms which might interfere with flying.
R	REMEDY Treat the patient, then the pilot.
D	DISPOSAL Fitness to fly will depend on the condition, treatment and response.
R	REVIEW Regular review is essential to monitor for symptoms and side effects.

- Below is a working example for a pilot thought to be hypothyroid:

D	Hypothyroidism. Confirmed by demonstrating low TSH.
E	Lack of thyroxine.
A	Slowness of thought, slow reaction times.
R	Thyroxine replacement.
D	Unfit flying until symptomatically well with normal TSH.
R	Initially 6-weekly to reflect time-to-effect of treatment.

CHAPTER

38

International regulation of medical standards

Contents

38.1 FRAMEWORK FOR REGULATORY ACTIVITY IN CIVIL AVIATION

- International Civil Aviation Organization (ICAO) was created to promote safe and orderly development of civil aviation.
- Specialized agency of the United Nations.
- Develops international Standards and Recommended Practices (SARPs).
- SARPs represent consensus view of contracting states and are found in 19 annexes to the 1944 Chicago Convention.
- Chapter 6 of Annex 1 to Convention covers medical aspects of licencing.
- An ICAO 'standard' is mandatory. If state unable or unwilling to comply, they must notify ICAO, thereby 'filing a difference'. Other states may refuse permission for airlines regulated by non-compliant states to overfly or land in their territory – in practice this rarely occurs.
- 'Recommended practices' are desirable but not mandatory.

38.2 FLEXIBILITY AND ACCREDITED MEDICAL CONCLUSION

- SARPs cannot cover every circumstance, and in some places are open to interpretation.
- Special procedure for assessing cases where an ICAO medical standard is not achieved but which may nevertheless permit a certificate to be issued in an individual case.
- Involves obtaining 'accredited medical conclusion' (conclusion reached by one or more medical experts acceptable to the licencing authority for the purposes of the case concerned, in consultation with flight operations or other experts as necessary) and applying 'flexibility'.

- If accredited medical conclusion indicates that an individual applicant's failure to meet medical standard is not likely to jeopardise flight safety, then a fit assessment may be made. In reaching such a conclusion, relevant ability, skill and experience must be considered and the licence endorsed with any necessary limitations required to protect flight safety.
- 'Flexibility' can be applied, and no 'difference' needs to be filed with ICAO, as standards are being followed.
- Can lead to variability in the application of SARPs throughout the world.

38.3 OVERVIEW OF REGULATORY MEDICAL REQUIREMENTS

- Various classes of medical certificate with different medical requirements.
- The ICAO standard for some licence categories are:
  - Class 1 – Airline transport, commercial and multi-crew pilot (aeroplane and helicopter).
  - Class 2 – Private pilot (aeroplane and helicopter), glider and balloon pilot.
  - Class 3 – Air traffic controller.
- Note that US FAA designates Class 1 as airline transport, Class 2 as commercial and multi-crew and Class 3 as private pilot; under 'BasicMed', pilots can fly light aircraft with driving licence equivalent medical standard (no FAA medical certificate).
- Periodicity of examinations and frequency of investigations (e.g. resting electrocardiogram, audiogram) depends on class of certificate and increases with age.
- ICAO does not designate medical examiners to undertake medical examinations but sets out in the SARPs the requirements for such designation.

38.4 REQUIREMENTS FOR MILITARY AIRCREW

- Military aircrew are subject to a variety of additional stressors in and out of the cockpit resulting in separate standards and regulatory systems.
- Personnel must be deployable in as wide a range of military roles as possible.
- Once in service, trained military pilot is a valuable asset, and military often has an occupational mechanism to redeploy a pilot with medical limitations while protecting both individual and employer (e.g. transfer from helicopters to fixed wing aircraft or from solo fast jet to a multi-pilot platform).
- Military medical licencing may be centralised to a medical board (acting as the medical assessors) or delegated to military aeromedical examiners.
- Smaller number of military aircrew means that evidence base for best practice is much slower to accumulate than in civilian operations. Benchmarking against civilian standards and aggregating data between different services and nationalities helps with review and revision of medical standards.
- Most militaries have an assessment protocol that classifies personnel with respect to their medical fitness:
  - For example, UK military Joint Medical Employment Standard is a common grading system to communicate an individual's employability and deployability.
  - This addresses fitness to fly (A), for ground duties (L), maritime duties (M) and to operate in particular climatic zones (E).

38.5 SETTING AND MONITORING INTERNATIONAL MILITARY MEDICAL STANDARDS

- No military equivalent to ICAO.
- To facilitate interoperability, share costs, foster co-operation and further evidence-based practice, allied forces have formed interoperability agreements.
  - Countries in the North Atlantic Treaty Organization (NATO) have a set of standardised agreements (STANAGs).
    - Medical aspects compiled by a joint international aeromedical panel.
    - Mandates minimum medical standards within NATO.
    - Member states free to set higher standards as required (and often do).
  - Five Eyes Air Forces Interoperability Council (AFIC), consisting of Australia, Canada, New Zealand, the United Kingdom and the United States, also has an aerospace medicine working group.

CHAPTER

39

Aircrew medicals

Contents

39.1 INTRODUCTION

- Aircrew undergo comprehensive initial examination prior to flying training and regular periodic medical examinations (on at least an annual basis).
- Purpose of the aircrew medical is medical assessment of an individual's ability to fly safely, and to identify those who are at increased risk of incapacitation during the relevant period of certification subsequent to the examination.
- Medicals are conducted by authorised aviation medical examiners (either civilian or military).
- It is recognised that untargeted testing and physical examination alone is of limited value; the number of abnormalities detected in aircrew medicals is usually very low, but occasionally asymptomatic disease is identified, and it is an opportunity for health promotion.
- Some of the following parameters are taken from EU standards and may vary in non-EU countries.

39.2 AVIATION MEDICAL EXAMINERS

- Aeromedical Examiners (AMEs) are doctors with specialist aviation medicine training.
- Approved by national regulator (or military) to carry out aircrew and Air Traffic Controller (ATCO) medical examinations and to give aviation medicine advice.
- For civilian AMEs, approval type determines which class of certificate (airline transport, commercial, private and/or ATCO) they can assess, based on the training and experience level of the AME.
- International Medical Standards are described in more detail in Chapter 38.

39.3 MEDICAL EXAMINATIONS

- Every doctor has their own routine for performing a medical examination.
- Standard forms usually employed to gather correct information.

COMPONENTS OF TYPICAL AIRCREW MEDICAL

- Height and weight.
- Eye and hair colour.
- Blood pressure.
- Pulse rate and rhythm.
- ENT:
  - Examine ears with an otoscope and look in the mouth and nostrils.
  - Visually inspect the head and neck; assess any restriction to neck movements.
  - Inspect mouth to include teeth, soft palate and tonsillar beds.
  - Inspect the nostrils and assess nasal airways.
  - Assess Eustachian function by any appropriate method (may include simple enquiry).
  - Palpate for thyroid lesions and lymphadenopathy.
- Visual acuity – Uncorrected vision should be recorded for all and correct vision if glasses are worn:
  - Distant visual acuity should be assessed at 5 m or 6 m using an appropriate chart.
  - Intermediate vision should be assessed at 100 cm using an appropriate chart.
  - Near vision should be assessed at a distance between 30 and 50 cm using an appropriate chart.
  - If contact lenses are worn for flying, vision should also be tested using a spare pair of spectacles.
- Ophthalmology:
  - Observe the eyes and surrounding structures.
  - Assess eye movements and check for diplopia.
  - Perform a field assessment by confrontation (or any other method used in routine optometry practice).
  - Assess pupil size and reaction to light and perform fundoscopy.
- Cardiorespiratory:
  - Observe the precordium and look for the jugular venous pulse.
  - Palpate the apex beat and auscultate over the cardiac valves and carotid areas.
  - Observe, percuss and auscultate over the upper, middle and lower segments of the lungs anteriorly and posteriorly.
  - Palpate the peripheral foot pulses and assess for dependant oedema and varicose veins.
  - Where the applicant undertakes regular self-examination, self-reported findings may be accepted; if breast examination is performed, it should be clear that this is with appropriate consent.
- Gastrointestinal:
  - Observe and palpate the abdomen, including liver, spleen, kidneys and hernial orifices.
  - Percussion and auscultation may also be appropriate.
  - Where the applicant undertakes regular testicular self-examination, self-reported findings may be accepted.
  - If there are clinical indications for performing genital or rectal examinations, then it should be clear that this is with appropriate consent.

- Endocrine system:
  - Many signs of endocrine disorders may be detected during examination of other systems; thyroid examination may be included as part of head and neck examination (see above).
- Musculoskeletal:
  - Observe applicant during the process of examination.
  - If they have any difficulty in movement, formally examine the range of movements of any affected joints.
  - Examination of movement of cervical and lumbar spine, and shoulder joints, should be undertaken to ensure adequate range of movement for flying/controlling.
- Neurology:
  - Observe applicant during the process of examination, including gait and posture; formally examine the neurological system if the subject appears to have any difficulty.
  - Assess cognitive function, including memory during history and examination.
  - Elicit upper and lower limb reflexes, including plantar response.
  - Cranial nerve abnormalities may be detected during other parts of the examination; targeted examination indicated if there are concerns.
  - Perform a Romberg's Test.
- Psychiatric:
  - Assess psychiatric history and mental state under the broad headings of appearance/speech/mood/thinking/perception/cognition/insight (see Chapter 64 for more detail).
  - Look out for any signs of alcohol or drug misuse.
- Skin, lymphatics, identifying marks:
  - Document any identifying marks.
  - Look for melanomas, especially on sun-exposed areas.
  - Examination for lymphadenopathy may be included in examination of other systems (e.g. abdomen or head and neck).
- General systemic:
  - Record significant abnormalities that have not been covered elsewhere (e.g. exceptional over or under weight, general examination findings such as clubbing or palmar erythema).
  - Opportunity to offer appropriate health promotion advice (recommended by ICAO).
- Hearing:
  - Perform Spoken Voice Hearing Test in a conversational voice at 2 m; test each ear individually by asking the subject to digitally occlude one ear at a time.
  - If hearing aids are worn, perform test with and without aids.
  - Document presence of hearing aids.
  - If audiometry is performed, it should similarly be undertaken with and without hearing aids:
    - Class 1: requirement becomes increasingly frequent with age.
    - Usually no hearing loss beyond 35 dB at 500, 1000 or 2000 Hz and beyond 50 dB at 300 Hz allowed.
    - Beyond these limits demonstrated proficiency may be used to determine fitness.

- Urinalysis:
  - Test a mid-stream specimen of urine with an appropriate reagent strip.
  - A trace of blood or protein is considered acceptable, but any other abnormality mandates further testing/investigation.
- Haemoglobin:
  - Requirement depends on national civilian or military policy.
  - If abnormal results are repeated once, and if the second reading is normal, then this is acceptable.
  - Usually if haemoglobin level recorded at the medical or from measuring full blood count shows haemoglobin is below 11.5 g/dl in males or 10.5 g/dl in females, then applicant should be assessed as temporarily unfit and further (specialist) assessment is required.
- Cholesterol:
  - Requirement depends on national civilian or military policy.
  - For civilian aircrew, usually required at initial class 1 and the first class 1 examination over age 40.
  - Otherwise on clinical indication.
  - Results should form part of a cardiovascular risk assessment (discuss results with applicant).
- Electrocardiogram (ECG):
  - Requirement depends on national civilian or military policy.
  - Increasing frequency of ECG examination with age; typically 6-monthly for over 50 year olds.

39.4 FREQUENCY OF MEDICALS

- Varies between civilian and military; typically annually becoming 6-monthly for older aircrew:
- The following is taken from the EU civilian requirements:
  - Class 1 (see Section 38.3):
    - Under 40 – annual.
    - Over 40 – 6 monthly for single pilot commercial.
    - Over 60 – 6 monthly all commercial.
  - Class 2 (see Section 38.3):
    - Under 40 – 5-yearly.
    - Over 40 – 2-yearly.
    - Over 50 – annual.

CHAPTER

40

Anthropometry

Contents

Key Facts
- Anthropometry is study of human body size.
- Certain measurements (e.g. sitting height and functional reach) highly important in aviation.
- Measurements need to be repeated for consistency.
- Anthropometry informs aircraft design and selection of crew.

40.1 DEFINITION

- Anthropometry is the study and measurement of the human body and its segments.
- Anthropometry is a key aspect of ergonomics and essential for designers to match equipment, workstations and working environments to human users.
- Anthropometry considers the wide variations in human form to ensure that individuals fit into the environment in which they will be working and can operate all of equipment requiring operation within that workspace.

40.2 WHY IS ANTHROPOMETRY IMPORTANT IN AVIATION?

AIRCRAFT DESIGN

- Aircrew must be able to fully utilise the functions of their aircraft for safe and effective operation; anthropometry permits designers to properly accommodate aircrew, permitting:
  - Adequate space and reach to instruments and controls.

  - Acceptable control movement and seat adjustment.
  - Adequate views of the external scene and instruments inside the cockpit.
- Design should permit this for maximum number of potential crew, within physical and engineering limits of the aircraft, cockpit space, seat and control design, plus their ranges of adjustment.

AIRCREW SELECTION

- Aircrew must be able to conduct all tasks required before, during and after flight safely and effectively.
- Once an aircraft has been designed, aircrew must be selected to ensure that they can achieve:
  - Full preflight and post-flight inspections.
  - Correct lookout.
  - Reach to all controls and avionics.
  - Full ranges of control movements.
  - Egress in an emergency.
  - Correct fit of clothing and survival equipment. For military aircrew this includes helmets, anti-G protection, oxygen systems, life preservers, life rafts, body armour, load carriage.

ANTHROPOMETRIC SURVEYS

- Anthropometric surveys may be conducted on new aircraft to confirm design and acceptable aircrew sizes.
- May also be conducted on population to define population's size (e.g. for future design of clothing, equipment or aircraft).

40.3 WHAT HUMAN CHARACTERISTICS ARE USED IN ANTHROPOMETRY?

- Typical anthropometric measures include:
  - Stature.
  - Buttock–heel length.
  - Buttock–knee length.
  - Functional reach.
  - Shoulder breadth.
- Over 180 potential measurements have been described, including detailed measurements of hands and heads; in general, most users will limit data used to suit required purpose.

40.4 HOW ARE ANTHROPOMETRIC CHARACTERISTICS ASSESSED?

- Anthropometric measures may be either static or dynamic.
  - **Static**. Static (or structural) dimensions taken with subject in a rigid position; easy to measure but do not recognise the flexibility of joints.
  - **Dynamic**. Dynamic (or functional) dimensions take body movement and flexibility in working positions into account; they are harder to achieve.

- Many organisations use a combination of static measures, with functional assessments of individuals to ensure dynamic performance if static anthropometry is borderline.

MANUAL MEASURES

- Manual measures can be taken using:
  - Tape measures.
  - Anthropometric rods.
  - Callipers.
  - Anthropometric rigs, some with electronic measurement and recording.
- Manual measures relatively simple to obtain and simpler equipment is mobile.
- Rigs have advantages in removing some observer errors, but they still need consistent operation and are frequently fixed in location (see Figure 40.1).

AUTOMATIC MEASURES

- 3-D surface anthropometric scanning:
  - In development for a considerable time.
  - Uses either white light or lasers to provide contour as well as body landmark data.
  - Can produce much accurate data, but is expensive and until recently had not found extensive practical application.
  - Now possible to scan and model cockpits and equipment as well as individuals.
  - Along with accurate computer modelling of ranges of movement of the body, it is possible to conduct integration studies and cockpit anthropometric assessments using computer models.
  - In use for scanning of heads to manufacture custom fit helmet liners.

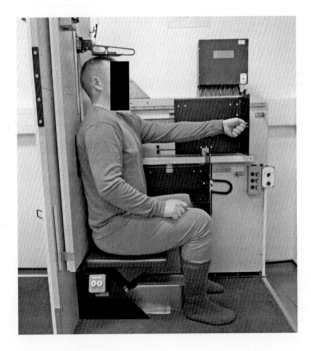

Figure 40.1 A typical anthropometry rig.

- Choice of anthropometric method will be influenced by numerous factors, including purpose, measurements needed, location of subjects and availability of equipment.
- Essential that only appropriate measures are used, that operators are properly trained and method consistently applied to reduce errors.

40.5 WHAT FACTORS INFLUENCE ANTHROPOMETRIC RANGES?

- Anthropometric data for populations are normally obtained by surveys of groups, but results will differ depending on target population factors:
    - Gender. Population data for females will, in general, produce smaller results than data for males, although there is individual overlap.
    - Region. Results for a population will vary with nation and even region within a nation; can be due to factors such as genetics or nutrition.
    - Confounding. If a military aircrew population were sampled to obtain data for a new aircraft design, the results would differ from the general population because military aircrew have already been selected to conform to a set of anthropometric requirements for existing aircraft.
    - Time. In general, populations appear to be getting larger both in physical size but also in weight, so results from surveys in the 21st century may yield larger measurements of the same parameters than surveys conducted in the mid-20th century.

40.6 HOW ARE ANTHROPOMETRIC DATA DESCRIBED?

- Anthropometric data may be used to describe a population, or an individual within a population:
    - Population data can be analysed to assess the central tendency, typically the mean value for each parameter.
    - However, usefulness of mean value is limited in aerospace medicine.
    - Consequently, means are used to derive the percentile range of measurements within which proportions of subject population will be found.
- Designers usually aim to accommodate the 5th to 95th centiles:
    - Means that 10% of the population (5% at each extreme of range) would be excluded.
    - However, no individual has all of their measurements at a specific centile; when considering multiple parameters, even though each one may be designed to accommodate the 5th to 95th centiles, far more than 10% of the population may be excluded.
- Ideally, design would encompass a whole population:
    - Design challenges increase disproportionately when trying to include the 5% at each end of the range.
    - For example, the space and mechanical requirements to increase the ranges of seat and control adjustment may be impossible or cost prohibitive.

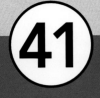
The health of the cabin crew

Contents

- Assessment of the cabin crew is to ensure that the individual is medically, physically and psychologically fit for the role and should consider:
  - Standards of health necessary to carry out the required tasks safely and effectively.
  - Positive and negative impacts of the job on the employee's health and well-being.

41.1 CABIN CREW DUTIES

SECURITY AND SAFETY

- Crew must be alert on the ground prior to boarding, ensuring that all areas of the plane are secure, with no potential threats left on board by previous passengers, maintenance or cleaning staff.
- Must make assessments of the fitness to travel of passengers who may have a health problem that might deteriorate on board.
- Must assess potential impact on the safety and security of the flight posed by intoxicated or abusive passengers.
- Must understand detailed safety instructions and be able to deliver, receive and action these safety instructions in the routine preflight, takeoff, cruise (including possible turbulence) and landing phases of flight, including emergency situations.
- Must be physically able to open emergency doors and render instructions and assistance to passengers in the event of any emergency.
- Require first-aid proficiency and calmness under pressure to attend to medical emergencies.

CUSTOMER SERVICE ROLE

- Must be able to assist passengers throughout the flight with their needs, within the bounds of sensible manual handling guidelines (e.g. handling of refreshment carts, assisting with baggage into or out of overhead lockers, assisting a passenger with reduced mobility).
- Crew require empathy with children and mothers with infants.
- Should display calmness and authority when dealing with physically and verbally abusive (potentially intoxicated) passengers.

41.2 PHYSICAL AND PSYCHOLOGICAL ATTRIBUTES

PHYSICAL

- Size and mobility. Cabin crew must:
  - Be able to manoeuvre freely in the confines of the aircraft environment and tall enough to reach and use overhead lockers:
    - Obesity, too small stature or physical disability may preclude a satisfactory assessment.
- Strength. Cabin crew must:
  - Have sufficient strength to open the doors both during normal flight operations and in an emergency.
  - Have physical strength, stamina, coordination and mobility to enable safe access and egress in an emergency and survival situation (e.g. use of an escape slide, swimming and entry into a life raft).
  - Fitness and aptitude can be reassessed during recurrent training.
- Vision and hearing. Cabin crew must have:
  - An appropriate level of vison and hearing so that emergency signals can be seen, heard and delivered.
  - Safe (rather than normal) colour vision.
  - No evidence of severe myopia; use of corrective spectacles or contact lenses is permitted.

PRE-EXISTING MEDICAL CONDITIONS

- There must be no pre-existing medical or psychological conditions that might cause sudden or subtle incapacitation thereby rendering the cabin crew member unable to carry out their safety critical duties.
- Initial assessment requires the applicant to truthfully declare all previous significant medical history.
- Assessing physician and the applicant need an awareness of the impact of altitude on pre-existing conditions (e.g. hypoxia in chronic respiratory or cardiac conditions, problems caused by gas expansion or auditory tube dysfunction, pneumothorax or inflammatory bowel disease).

SOCIAL AND MENTAL HEALTH

- Crew should not have pre-existing mental health issues which may cause problems in an environment that has potential to be pressured and socially isolating down route far from friends and family; additionally, cabin crew do not often work with the same individuals on a regular basis.

- Need for additional rest and preparation before and after flights due to disruption of circadian balances can affect relationships and psychological well-being.

41.3 POTENTIAL HEALTH RISKS

CABIN ENVIRONMENT

- Hazards of cabin environment include: Hypoxia (see Chapters 9–22), pressure change (see Chapter 7), cosmic radiation (see Chapter 14), motion sickness (see Chapter 28), low humidity.
- Cabin air quality: Adverse health effects due to 'fume' events relating to engine bleed air is a very contentious issue. Cabin air is subject to regular intake of fresh air with removal of stale air and use of high efficiency particulate air (HEPA) filters. There is no substantial evidence for any significant health hazards, and long-term health effects are believed to be very unlikely, but a number of individuals believe they have suffered ill health effects as a result of poor cabin air quality.

DESTINATION

- Potential hazards include:
    - Infectious disease.
    - Malignant melanoma due to frequent sun exposure.
    - Sexually transmitted diseases.
- Disruption of circadian rhythm and fatigue caused by shift work and patterns of working, crossing of time zones; requires management with flight time limitations.

TRAVEL ADVICE

- Cabin crew require aeromedical advice to ensure appropriate vaccinations, malaria prophylaxis; advice on preparing for flights (by ensuring adequate pre-trip rest), lifestyle, personal safety and security.

41.4 MEDICAL ASSESSMENT/CERTIFICATION OF FITNESS

- Assessment of fitness is usually required; format often mandated by regulatory authorities. The outcome may be a medical certificate or report of fitness.
- Basic premise is to document that a satisfactory medical assessment (either by questionnaire or face-to-face) has been carried out, and that the prospective cabin crew member is physically and psychologically fit to carry out their role safely and effectively with little or minimal risk to their own health and well-being.
- Medical examinations or assessments are repeated periodically; usually a requirement for reassessment after a period of unfitness or decreased medical fitness.
- If a crew member becomes pregnant, the majority of airlines will 'ground' the cabin crew member for the duration of the pregnancy once it has been declared.

CHAPTER 42

Air traffic control

Contents

42.1 ROLE OF AIR TRAFFIC CONTROL

- The International Civil Aviation Organization (ICAO) has set out basic requirements for Air Navigation Service Providers (ANSPs) to:
    - Prevent collisions between aircraft.
    - Prevent collisions between aircraft, vehicles and obstructions on the ground manoeuvring area.
    - Expedite and maintain an orderly flow of air traffic.
- Airspace can be:
    - 'Controlled' by an ANSP; where pilots are given detailed instructions where to fly (usually found around airports, centres of population and areas used by commercial aviation); or
    - 'uncontrolled'; where pilots are free to fly according to basic rules.
- Current technology requires ANSPs to use Air Traffic Control Officers (ATCOs) to deliver the service.
- ATCOs prevent collisions by maintaining separation of aircraft in blocks of airspace known as 'sectors' using:
    - Position – known from radar, navigation aids.
    - Route – known from flight plans, flight strips (paper or electronic).
    - Characteristics of aircraft types, weight and performance to instruct pilots via radiotelephony to climb, descend, turn or change speed.

42.2 ATCO WORK ENVIRONMENTS

TOWER OR THE VISUAL CONTROL ROOM (VCR)

- Depending on airport complexity, these may have ATCOs managing:
  - Air arrivals (glide slope to leaving runway).
  - Departures (taxiway onto runway and departure).
  - Ground Movement Controller (taxiing around airport de-conflicting with road vehicles).
  - Release/Delivery (prioritising aircraft from stands).

APPROACH OR TERMINAL RADAR

- Usually control aircraft about 60 miles to 5–6 miles out and altitude 24,000 ft to 6000 ft before handover to tower or VCR for inbound aircraft or area controller for outbound.
- Traffic is complex, as is usually climbing/descending and turning.
- Often co-located at airport tower building.

EN-ROUTE OR AREA CONTROL CENTRES

- Usually in a centre that may be remote from airports.
- Usually controls air traffic above 24,000 ft.
- Sectors are usually larger, as aircraft are on established routings.

OCEANIC CONTROL CENTRES

- Radar coverage is not possible over large expanses of sea.
- ATCOs use procedural control with timed separations and 60-mile horizontal separation.

42.3 OCCUPATIONAL HAZARDS AND REQUIREMENTS

- Interaction between tasks, environment and health should be considered (see Table 42.1).
- Compared with flight crew, better opportunities for mitigating against incapacitation means slightly higher incapacitation risk may be acceptable.

VISION

- Assimilation of information from multiple screens in varying light conditions.
- Near, intermediate and distance vision for Tower ATCOs looking at ground and air movements.

Table 42.1 Interaction between task, work environment and health conditions in air traffic control

SPECIFIC TASKS	WORK ENVIRONMENT	HEALTH CONDITION
Tower	1G/normoxic/normobaric	Vision
Approach	Multi-controller/solo operation	Hearing
En-route	Day/night/shift	Musculoskeletal
	Workplace pressure	Fatigue
		Mental health

- Area and Terminal Control ATCOs require near and intermediate vision for radar consoles.
- Consider effects of presbyopia and correction for the functional tasks of each position.
- Colour dense environment when using visual display units (VDUs) observing airfield lights such that many jurisdictions require normal trichromacy demonstrated by advanced colour vision testing.
- Technological advances may determine 'safe' colour vision levels.

HEARING

- Headsets used for aural transmissions.
- Must have sufficient hearing to discriminate speech from air-air and ground-air communications, which are routed to each ear separately.
- Must retain situation awareness of instructions from within the operations room.
- A functional hearing assessment and specialist review to rule out underlying conditions is required for those who do not meet standards.
- Hearing aids may be allowed provided operational function is not compromised.

MUSCULOSKELETAL/ERGONOMIC

- Workstation has at least two VDUs, keyboard/mouse/touch screen/bench top.
- Task analysis required for posture, neck rotation, standing/sitting for prolonged periods, upper and lower limbs for use of mouse/keyboard/touch screens/foot-pedals.
- Visual hazards/fatigue – glare in towers or low light conditions with reduced contrast sensitivity.

SHIFT WORK AND FATIGUE MANAGEMENT

- Most ATCOs exposed to shift work.
- Regulatory protections may exist.
- Rostering should take account of:
  - Circadian rhythm phase shifts.
  - Individual preference for more time off/longer shifts.
  - Risk management based approach with shorter shifts during high workload periods.
  - Any impact of clockwise or anti-clockwise shift patterns – no clear evidence one is more fatiguing.
- Individual education should emphasise actions to prevent performance drop-off during times of overload and underload that may coincide with the circadian nadir.
  - Responsibility to ensure adequate recovery during rest days, which may conflict with social life.

WORKPLACE PRESSURE

- Not necessarily inherent to the role.
- Potential hazards include:
  - Loss of confidence with controlling ability, particularly during training or post-incident.
  - Adverse personal events.
  - Interpersonal relations with colleagues or managers.
  - Reduced mental agility with ageing.

- Protective factors include:
  - Personal resilience.
  - Strong collegial and personal networks.
  - Organisational resources such as peer support and employee assistance programs.
- Early identification by supervisors and open communication with aeromedical professionals is key to returning or maintaining operational fitness.

42.4 NEW TECHNOLOGIES AND FUTURE WORKSTATIONS

- Route planning integration with ATC systems.
- Data links transmitting instructions direct to aircraft.
- ATCOs monitoring systems rather than making interventions.
- Change from physical rooms to portable systems.

Passenger fitness to fly

Contents

43.1 THE AVIATION ENVIRONMENT

- Patients flying on commercial aircraft face the following challenges:
  - Dry, hypoxic, hypobaric environment of the aircraft at altitude.
  - Busy and complex airport with long distances between check-in and departure; busy queues; halls packed with passengers; security body scanners; stairs to climb onto aircraft; fitting into narrow seat spaces and other small spaces (e.g. aircraft toilets).
  - Ease of manoeuvring wheelchairs in these environments.
- Passengers should be advised to:
  - Wear comfortable and appropriate clothing for the flight and destination.
  - Remain well hydrated and mobilise every couple of hours.
  - Place any regular medication in their hand luggage, together with a prescription and/or letter from the GP certifying their legitimate use to avoid problems at customs with opioids (e.g. codeine phosphate or stimulants such as pseudoephedrine).
  - Ensure there are no important restrictions on medications.
  - Consider how changing time zones may affect when they take/administer their medication (e.g. insulin).
- Cabin crew cannot toilet or feed passengers or administer injections.

43.2 PREFLIGHT ASSESSMENT

- Most passengers are healthy and mobile, fit to fly.
- As a rule, unstable or acute clinical conditions are considered unacceptable, but others may be approved following a preflight assessment.

- Stable conditions may deteriorate during (as well as in between) flights, thus compromising the return; consider asthma, diabetes, epilepsy.
- Post-surgical cases may be affected by the expansion of trapped gas (up to 30%) which may lead to deterioration of a previously stable condition.
- Most major airlines work within similar medical guidelines, usually based on those established by the International Air Transport Association (IATA).
- To avoid rejection on arrival at the airport, delays or diversions due to deterioration of the passenger, an early approach to the airline's medical clearance unit or advisor is essential:
  - Provide a GP's letter and/or complete a MEDIF in advance (see below).

CONDITIONS LIKELY TO BE REJECTED FOR TRAVEL

- Severe anaemia (Hb <7.5 g/dl), sickling crisis (within 10 days), bleeding/clotting disorders.
- Severe otitis media or sinusitis; middle ear surgery (within 10 days).
- Acute or active contagious/communicable disease.
- Congestive cardiac failure or other cyanotic conditions if not fully controlled.
- Uncomplicated myocardial infarction (within 2 weeks of onset) or complicated myocardial infarction (within 6 weeks of onset).
- Angioplasty (3 days if no stenting; 5 days if stenting).
- Severe respiratory disease:
  - Breathless after walking 50 metres on flat ground or on continuous oxygen therapy on ground.
  - Recent pneumothorax (not fully inflated or within 14 days of full inflation).
- Gastrointestinal lesions which may cause haematemesis, melaena or intestinal obstruction.
- Recent surgery:
  - Simple abdominal operations (within 10 days).
  - Thoracic surgery (within 21 days).
  - Invasive eye surgery (excluding LASER); up to 6 weeks if gas in the globe.
  - Introduction of air to body cavities for diagnostic or therapeutic purposes (within 7 days).
  - Following procedures likely to bleed (e.g. tonsillectomy within 1 week).
- Pregnancy (see below).
- Neonates within 48 hr of birth.
- Recent scuba diving (within 24 hr).
- Symptomatic cases of decompression illness (minimum of 72 hr, up to 10 days depending on condition).
- Fractures in plaster will require bi-valving if they have occurred within the previous 48 hr.

CONDITIONS THAT MAY BE ASSESSED FIT IF APPROPRIATELY ESCORTED

- Fractures of the mandible with fixed wiring of the jaw (wire-cutters required).
- Unstable mental illness (suitable medication may be required).
- Uncontrolled seizures (suitable medication must be available).

- Nasogastric or gastrostomy feeding.
- Oozing wounds and conditions requiring frequent change of dressings (wide surface burns); drains or wounds that require aspiration.

43.3 PREGNANCY

- Any woman planning to travel beyond the 29th week of pregnancy must carry a medical certificate/letter signed by an appropriately qualified doctor (or midwife) stating:
  - Confirmation of a singleton or multiple pregnancy.
  - That pregnancy is progressing without complications.
  - Estimated date of delivery.
  - That there are no health problems and no reasons known that would prevent her from flying.
- Limits to flying in pregnancy:
  - Singleton pregnancy – beyond the end of 35th week for journeys of >4 hr; beyond 36th week for journeys of <4 hr.
  - Uncomplicated multiple pregnancy – beyond the 32nd week.

43.4 MEDICAL INFORMATION FORM (MEDIF)

- IATA publishes a standard form for its members.
- Although modified by most companies, the forms are similar and can be found at the airlines' websites.
- MEDIF should be submitted at least 48 hr in advance by a medical attendant who knows the passenger's medical conditions well when:
  - Fitness to travel is in doubt (as proven by recent illness, hospitalisation, injury, surgery or instability).
  - Where special services are required (e.g. oxygen, stretcher or authority to carry accompanying medical equipment such as a ventilator or nebulizer).
- For frequent travellers with stable, chronic medical conditions, the airline may give a FREMEC card to avoid the need for repeat medical clearance.

43.5 OXYGEN REQUIREMENTS

- First-aid bottles are available to provide oxygen in cases of a medical emergency:
  - Note these are in addition to emergency drop-down oxygen supply available in cases of cabin decompression.
- No aircraft oxygen supplies can be used for pre-planned ('scheduled') therapeutic oxygen therapy:
  - For this, the airline must be informed before the flight in order to load sufficient bottles.
  - Patients are not allowed to carry their own, as certain approved aviation standards must be met.
- Portable oxygen concentrators may be used if approved for flight use (e.g. by FAA); may require higher oxygen flow setting than usual ground use; need sufficient batteries.

43.6 DEEP VENOUS THROMBOSIS (DVT)

- Prolonged periods of immobility (stasis) in long-haul flights >6 hr are associated with lower limb DVT but absolute risk is low.
- See Chapter 63 for risk-based prophylaxis strategy.

43.7 MILITARY PASSENGERS

- Passenger is defined as any person not directly concerned with the operation of the aircraft or its systems, or critical for the mission (i.e. supernumerary crew).
- Any medical assessment should additionally consider:
    - Likely highest cabin altitude (fast jet, air dispatch).
    - Rates of ascent/descent.
    - Acceleration forces.
- Passengers may be categorised according to these factors, and this will determine level of medical assessment required, anthropometrical assessment and need for preflight training or briefing.

43.8 ADDITIONAL INFORMATION

For more information on passenger assessment, see websites of:
- Specific airlines.
- Aerospace Medical Association.
- IATA.
- British Thoracic Society.

CHAPTER 44

Travel health and infectious diseases

Contents

44.1 INTRODUCTION

As air travel becomes more accessible worldwide, the potential hazards are increasingly more diverse, and health needs can be more complex. Ideally, all travellers' needs, regardless of their individual health status, should be identified prior to departure to mitigate for these travel health risks.

- Data on true incidence and therefore risk of travel-associated infections is incomplete worldwide.
- However, sufficient country/region-specific information is usually available to guide advice and management.
- Worldwide trends are constantly changing, and therefore up-to-date information should always be used. Recommended websites include:
  - WHO: http://www.who.int/en/
  - PHE: https://www.gov.uk/government/organisations/public-health-england
  - FCO: https://www.gov.uk/foreign-travel-advice
  - CDC: https://wwwnc.cdc.gov/travel/
- Table 44.1 shows potential travel-related infections. Mitigation includes vaccination and behavioural strategies:
  - Faecal-oral prevention includes hand and food hygiene and sanitation.
  - Blood-borne infection prevention includes avoidance of exposure of body fluids to mucous membranes and skin cuts/penetrating injuries, and intercourse barrier protection.
  - Direct contact prevention includes avoidance of exposure to body fluids and hand hygiene. Indirect contact prevention includes hand hygiene and cleaning.
  - Mucous membrane exposure and broken skin prevention includes avoiding exposure sources.
  - Insect (e.g. mosquito) prevention includes bite prevention and vector control.
  - Droplet prevention includes hand hygiene, respiratory and mucous membrane protection.

Table 44.1 International infectious disease risk

DISEASE	GEOGRAPHY	TRANSMISSION	INCUBATION	VACCINE	ADDITIONAL PREVENTION	ACUTE TREATMENT
Viruses						
Hepatitis A	WW	Faecal-oral	15–50 days	Yes	Shellfish can harbour virus. Post-Exposure: Vaccine +/- HNIG.	
Hepatitis B	WW	Blood-borne infection	40–160 days	Yes	Post-Exposure: Vaccine +/- HNIG.	
Hepatitis C	WW	Blood-borne infection	4–26 weeks			
Hepatitis E	WW	Faecal-oral	2–9 weeks		Uncooked pork is significant source. Post-Exposure: HNIG (limited evidence).	
Influenza	WW	Droplet/Indirect contact	0.5–5 days	Yes	Post-Exposure: Viral neuraminidase inhibitors.	Yes
Common Respiratory Viruses	WW	Droplet/Indirect contact	Variable			
Novel Coronavirus MERS	ME	Droplet/Indirect contact	2–14 days		Avoid camel exposure.	
Novel Coronavirus SARS	Far East	Droplet/Indirect contact/Faecal-oral	2–10 days		Variable human to human transmission.	

Afr = Africa; CA = Central America; SA = South America; ME = Middle East; Med = Mediterranean; WW = Worldwide.

(*Continued*)

Table 44.1 (Continued) International infectious disease risk

DISEASE	GEOGRAPHY	TRANSMISSION	INCUBATION	VACCINE	ADDITIONAL PREVENTION	ACUTE TREATMENT
Dengue	Trop & Subtrop	Mosquito	5–8 days		Limited vaccine to population of endemic countries. Possible aircraft transmission if no disinsection.	
Zika	Trop & Subtrop	Mosquito/Blood-borne infection	3–14 days		Usually asymptomatic but risk to unborn child.	
Yellow Fever	Afr, CA/SA	Mosquito	3–6 days	Yes		
Chikungunya	Trop and Subtrop	Mosquito	2–12 days			
Japanese Encephalitis	Asia	Mosquito	5–15 days	Yes		
West Nile Virus	Worldwide	Mosquito	2–14 days			
Sandfly Fever	Med, ME and E Asia	Sandfly	3–6 days			
HIV	WW	Blood-borne infection	2 weeks–3 months*		PrEP. *Seroconversion lag time.	Yes
Hand, foot and mouth	WW	Faecal-oral/Droplet/ Indirect contact	2–5 days			
EBV, CMV	WW	Direct contact	2–6 weeks		High seroprevalence in population.	

Afr = Africa; CA = Central America; SA = South America; ME = Middle East; Med = Mediterranean; WW = Worldwide.

(Continued)

Table 44.1 (Continued) International infectious disease risk

DISEASE	GEOGRAPHY	TRANSMISSION	INCUBATION	VACCINE	ADDITIONAL PREVENTION	ACUTE TREATMENT
Rabies	WW	Bite/Membrane	10 days - 2yrs	Yes	Avoid animal bites. Post-exposure: Vaccine +/- HRIG.	Yes
Polio	Pakistan, Afghanistan Nigeria	Faecal-oral	3–21 days	Yes		
Measles	WW	Droplet/Direct contact	7–18 days	Yes		
Viral Haemorrhagic fevers (e.g. Ebola, Lassa, CCVHF)	Trop and Subtrop	Direct contact/Indirect contact	3–21 days			
Bacteria						
Travellers' Diarrhoea	WW	Faecal-oral	6–72 hr		Antibiotics may be appropriate.	No*
Meningitis	WW	Droplet	2–10 days	Yes	Post-Exposure: Antibiotics for close contacts.	Yes
Typhoid	WW	Faecal-oral	7–21 days	Yes	Chronic carriage can exist.	Yes
Cholera	Asia, Afr, CA	Faecal-oral	0.5–5 days	Yes	Antibiotics may be appropriate for individual treatment.	No*
Legionella	WW	Droplet	2–10 days		Control of sources (e.g. air-conditioning).	Yes
Leptospirosis	WW	Membrane	5–19 days		Control exposure to zoonoses, soil, water.	Yes

Afr = Africa; CA = Central America; ME = Middle East; Med = Mediterranean; WW = Worldwide.   SA = South America;

(Continued)

Table 44.1 (Continued) International infectious disease risk

DISEASE	GEOGRAPHY	TRANSMISSION	INCUBATION	VACCINE	ADDITIONAL PREVENTION	ACUTE TREATMENT
Rickettsiae (e.g. Tick-borne encephalitis, Rocky Mountain Spotted Fever)	WW	Insect	2–28 days		Antibiotic prophylaxis may have a role.	Yes
Tuberculosis	WW	Droplet	Wide	Yes	Vaccine (BCG) for prolonged exposure risk.	Yes
Tetanus	WW	Inoculation	3–21 days	Yes	Wound care. Post-Exposure: Vaccine/Ig/Antibiotics.	Yes
Lyme disease	Northern Temperate	Tick	3–30 days		Prompt removal of ticks reduces transmission.	Yes
Brucellosis	WW	Direct contact/Indirect contact	2–4+ weeks		Control exposure to zoonoses (e.g. unpasteurised milk).	Yes
Protozoa						
Malaria	Trop and Subtrop	Mosquito	6–30+ days		Increased mortality with *P. falciparum*. ABCD approach to control (Awareness, Bite prevention, Chemo-prophylaxis, Detection early).	Yes
African Trypanosomiasis (Sleeping sickness)	Sub-Saharan Afr	Tsetse	2–28 days		Population screen and treat.	Yes

Afr = Africa; CA = Central America; SA = South America; ME = Middle East; Med = Mediterranean; WW = Worldwide.

(*Continued*)

Table 44.1 (Continued) International infectious disease risk

DISEASE	GEOGRAPHY	TRANSMISSION	INCUBATION	VACCINE	ADDITIONAL PREVENTION	ACUTE TREATMENT
American Trypanosomiasis (Chagas)	CA/SA	Membrane, Blood-borne infection	1–4 weeks		Transmission low in travellers.	Yes
Leishmania Cutaneous & Visceral	CA/SA, N Afr, ME & E Asia	Sandfly	2–4 weeks Cutaneous 2–4 months Visceral		Possible aircraft transmission if no disinsection.	Yes
Giardiasis	WW	Faecal-oral	5–25 days			Yes
Amoeba						
Amoebic dysentery	Trop and Subtrop	Faecal-oral	2–6 weeks			Yes
Helminths						
Schistosomiasis – acute	Afr, Asia, Eastern SA	Skin	2–6 weeks		Freshwater avoidance.	Yes
Strongyloidiasis	Tropical	Skin			Sanitation, isolation of faecal matter.	Yes
Mycoses						
Histoplasmosis	Americas, Afr, SE Asia	Inhalation	3–17 days		Avoidance of exposure (e.g. caves, guano).	Yes
Coccidioidomycosis	Americas	Inhalation	7–21 days		Avoidance of exposure (e.g. soil disruption).	Yes

Afr = Africa; CA = Central America; SA = South America; ME = Middle East; Med = Mediterranean; WW = Worldwide.

44.2 CONSULTATION

Travellers should aim to be seen at least 6–8 weeks prior to departure for a risk assessment consultation with a travel medicine specialist where possible, or have suitable information made available.

- Consultations should identify:
  - Planned regions of travel.
  - Duration (including stopovers).
  - Purpose.
  - Modes of transport.
  - Activities planned.
  - Accommodation.
- Education and recommendations for risk management should include preparation for last minute schedule changes as well as awareness of increase in risky behaviour which can happen in travellers.
- Specific health issues to address are:
  - Injury (including road traffic collisions).
  - Pre-existing medical and dental conditions.
  - Infection (e.g. travellers' diarrhoea, malaria and other vector borne infections, skin and soft tissue conditions).
  - Travelling with medication.
  - Vaccinations/antimalarial medication.
  - Safe sex.

44.3 TRAVEL ADVICE

PRE-TRAVEL ADVICE

- Make appointment with primary care physician to address chronic medical conditions and requirements for travel.
- Manage timing of travel to avoid high-risk times/areas.
- Travel with sufficient medication in temperature appropriate storage:
  - Keep copy of any prescription with you and have physician's letter for controlled substances.
  - Some countries have strict drug policies and do not allow certain medications (e.g. codeine).
  - Keep medication in hand luggage.
- Arrange to have required vaccinations and/or start antimalarial medication.
- Consider dental fitness.
- Take appropriate documentation (e.g. health certificates, exemption certificate, copies of passport and insurance, next of kin and emergency contact information).
- Ensure you have sufficient travel insurance.
- First-aid kit.
- Take any necessary action to prevent veno-thromboembolic disease (see Chapter 63).

ADVICE WHEN OVERSEAS

- Take precautions with food and water.
- Beware of heat exhaustion and sun exposure.
- Follow insect bite prevention advice.
- Reduce risk of animal bites and stings.
- Consider good road safety practice.
- Be aware of region-specific safety and security risks.
- Consider effect of jet lag and reduce where possible.
- Minimise effects of motion sickness.
- Take appropriate precautions for sexual health.

ADVICE AFTER TRAVEL

- On returning home, travellers should be encouraged to seek medical attention early if unwell, and they should declare their travel history.
- Fever in a traveller from an area with malaria is a medical emergency.

44.4 RISK ASSESSMENT

There is a higher risk in travellers with:

- **Pregnancy** – Note airline restrictions, availability of healthcare facilities and risk of infections (e.g. Zika)
- **Children** – Increased risk of death from road trauma and drowning, plus increased risk from infectious diseases, bites, stings and poisons.
- **Elderly** – Pre-existing comorbidities, poly-pharmacy and vaccine response may be weaker and delayed.
- **Diabetes** – Increased risk of infection, time changes will affect meal times and insulin dosing and high temperatures increase insulin absorption.
- **Immunosuppressed/compromised (e.g. asplenic, transplant recipients, HIV)** – Increased risk of severity of infections, delayed or muted response to vaccination and live vaccines may be contraindicated.

Aviation public health

Contents

45.1 INTERNATIONAL AVIATION PUBLIC HEALTH

- CAPSCA (Collaborative Arrangement for the Prevention and Management of Public Health Events in Civil Aviation):
  - Partners include World Health Organization (WHO), Centers for Disease Control and Prevention (CDC), International Civil Aviation Organization (ICAO).
  - Key objective of public health protection.
- The International Health Regulations 2005 (IHR):
  - Binding for 194 countries.
  - Aims to prevent, protect against, control and respond to the international spread of disease while avoiding unnecessary interference with international traffic and trade.
  - Aims to reduce the risk of disease spread at international airports, ports and ground crossings.
  - Provides the regulatory health framework under which airlines operate.
  - Requires states to strengthen core surveillance and response capacities within healthcare systems, designated international ports, airports and ground crossings.

45.2 PREVENTING INTERNATIONAL SPREAD OF DISEASE

- Passengers and crew should avoid air travel whilst potentially infectious to others:
  - To avoid international carriage.
  - To reduce risk to fellow passengers (particularly those who may be immunocompromised).

- Infectious periods of some common illnesses once symptoms have developed are up to:
  - Chicken pox: 5 days from onset of rash (traditionally until all lesions crusted).
  - Hepatitis A: 7 days after onset of jaundice.
  - Measles: 4 days from onset of rash.
  - Mumps: 5 days from onset of swelling.
  - Rubella: 4 days from onset of rash.
  - Whooping cough: 5 days after commencing antibiotics or 21 days after onset.
  - Pulmonary TB: 2 weeks antibiotics and sputum negative for Acid Fast Bacilli (AFB).
- Aircraft air-conditioning systems have High-Efficiency Particulate Air (HEPA) filters and airflow predominantly downwards.
- On-board transmission is only likely directly from person to person rather than circulation through the cabin.

45.3 INFECTIOUS DISEASE OUTBREAKS

After identifying a disease threat, evidence-based risk assessment by local public health bodies is required.

AT THE AIRPORT

- Measures to prevent infected persons/carriers boarding aircraft may include:
  - Local communication of public health messages.
  - Administration of questionnaires to travellers.
  - Temperature monitoring.
  - These are the responsibility of the authorities and not the airline.

ON BOARD

- Identification, control and communication of suspected infectious disease cases through:
  - Crew training.
  - Guidelines for suspected infectious or communicable disease include persistent temperature of 38°C (100°F) or more and one or more of the following:
    - Persistent coughing.
    - Impaired breathing.
    - Persistent diarrhoea.
    - Persistent vomiting.
    - Skin rash.
    - Abnormal bleeding.
    - Confusion.
  - Reduction of risk of on-board transmission by:
    - Isolation or segregation as far as practicable.
    - Designation of a single toilet for the affected passenger.
    - Use of a 'universal precaution kit'.
    - Cleaning and removal of contaminated fluids (e.g. using spill clean-up kit).
  - Collection of adjacent passenger details using the WHO Passenger Locator Form.
  - Notification to public health bodies at destination via Air Traffic Control.

AT DESTINATION

- Medical care for the individual.
- Passenger screening via questionnaire and/or temperature monitoring.
- Aircraft cleaning using appropriate disinfectants, bearing in mind compatibility with aircraft components.
- Where appropriate, contact tracing (limited to two rows in front and behind index case unless highly infectious) by local public health bodies using:
  - Information from passenger locator form.
  - Airline data (disclosure likely to be subject to local data privacy laws).
  - Targeted local publicity.
- For TB, contact tracing only if:
  - Flight was within previous 3 months.
  - Passenger was likely to have been infectious at the time of travel.
  - Total flight duration >8 hr.
- Limited to two rows in front and behind index case.

45.4 PREVENTION OF SPREAD OF INSECT VECTORS

- In accordance with IHR (2005), countries may require aircraft disinsection in order to prevent import of insect vectors (principally mosquitoes) which may be locally viable:
  - 1 hr preflight using permethrin (25:75 cis trans).
  - Pre-departure (doors closed) or top of descent using D-phenothrin.
  - Residual disinsection using permethrin (25:75 cis trans) emulsifiable concentrate at (not exceeding) 2-monthly intervals.

45.5 FOOD SAFETY

Food poisoning outbreaks on board aircraft are uncommon but can be serious if they occur. Measures to prevent outbreaks include:

- Avoiding high-risk foods on the menu.
- High standards of food preparation and storage:
  - At airport kitchens (or at subcontractors' facilities).
  - In transportation vehicles which carry the food from the ground source to the aircraft.
  - On the aircraft.
- Monitoring temperature during storage and after reheating.
- Crew training in hygiene, food preparation and service.
- Exclusion of anyone involved in the food chain, including cabin crew, from the workplace following diarrhoea and/or vomiting until symptom free for 48 hr and on no treatment.

CHAPTER 46

Planning for aeromedical evacuation

Contents

46.1 ORGANISATION

NATO definitions of aeromedical evacuation (AE) used widely by militaries:

- MEDEVAC – Medically supervised patient movement to/between medical facilities.
- CASEVAC – *Not* medically supervised.

PRINCIPLES

- Must offer advantage to patient.
- Weigh against maintenance of ground-based care and risks of AE.
- Carefully plan and risk assess.
- Consider *whole* patient journey, not just aircraft portion.
- Maintain (at least) current level of clinical care.
- Good aeromedical risk assessment throughout.
- Communication/clinician-clinician handover.
- Reassess until completion.

FORMS

- Forward: Point of wounding to first medical facility.
  - Strategies: 'Scoop and run' (minimal medical intervention before travel) vs. 'Stay and play' (high level of intervention before/during flight).
  - Balance: Speed of delivery vs. life-saving care ability.
- Tactical: Between medical facilities within military theatre of operations.
- Strategic: Move away from military theatre of operations.

CATEGORISATION

- Priority: Urgency of patient movement (e.g. as soon as possible, within 24–48 hr, within 7 days); must separate clinical from military operational priorities.
- Classification:
  - Psychiatric. Severity, restricted numbers, patient restraint (for aircraft safety), or wait for treatment.
  - Stretcher-bound. Size of stretcher, access to aircraft (tail ramp/high bodied – air-bridge/K-loader/catering truck), access to stretcher (door, turn, aisle), availability of emergency decompression oxygen, total number of stretcher patients.
  - Stretcher-available. Or flat-bed seat - offers mobility.
  - Sitting.
  - Unescorted. May need mobility assistance, baggage handling.
- Dependency. In-flight clinical requirements (e.g. critical care, IV fluids).

46.2 CAPABILITIES

FORWARD AE

- Limit catastrophic haemorrhage:
  - Combat application tourniquets.
  - Israeli First Field Dressing.
- Provide early intervention:
  - High-quality pre-hospital care.
  - Golden hour, platinum 10 minutes.
- Provide rapid evacuation.
- Correct hypovolaemia, acidosis, hypothermia (most critical factors):
  - Intravenous and intraosseous access.
  - Infusion systems.
  - Blood product replacement (blood, plasma, clotting factors).
  - Blood warming system.
  - Survival blanket.
  - Patient heating system.

TACTICAL/STRATEGIC AE

- Nurse/paramedic-led.
- Augmentation with clinical specialists.
- Critical care in the air.
- Extracorporeal membrane oxygenation.
- Infectious disease transfer teams.

46.3 PLANNING CONSIDERATIONS

- Medical information quality:
  - Language translation.
  - Consider escort pre-positioning.
- Aircraft capability:
  - Type – military transport, commercial scheduled/charter, civilian air ambulance.
  - Available space.
  - Availability and type of stretchers and stanchions.
  - Clearance of electromedical equipment:
    - Effect of aircraft and pressurisation on equipment.
    - Effect of equipment on aircraft – transmitting devices, power cables affecting aircraft defensive aids.
    - Equipment lighting, including NVG compatibility, equipment alarms – patient safety.
  - Cabin altitude restrictions:
    - Unrestricted.
    - Some restriction (e.g. 2000 ft).
    - Ground level transfer.
  - Routing and mission duration, likely diversions and delays.
  - Weather.
  - Airfield suitability for aircraft type.
  - Oxygen arrangements – aircraft, cylinder, Liquid Oxygen (LOX) or concentrator; flow rate and volume required.
  - Power requirements – plug in (converters), battery.
  - Cost and alternative options.
- Aeromedical crew:
  - Training.
  - Aircraft type knowledge.
  - Responsibilities.
  - Medical competency – sufficient to deal with anticipated risks.
  - Escort numbers sufficient for medical care needs and emergency egress.
  - Importation of drugs.
  - Aeromedical crew duty/rest rules.
  - Travel health preparation:
    - Malaria prevention.
    - Immunisations.
    - Occupational health/fitness for role.
    - Passport and visa.
- Patient and aeromedical crew logistics:
  - Transport to/from aircraft.
  - Medical escorting and equipment required from bed-bed.
  - Destination hospital admission status confirmation.
- Aeromedical risk assessment:
  - Anticipate/mitigate medical and operational risks.
  - Tasking appropriately trained medical personnel.

- Aeromedical equipment:
  - Sufficient for task and patient deterioration.
  - Redundancy.
- Airline medical clearance – MEDIF (define oxygen and mobility requirements). Engage airline medical department early (see Chapter 43).

46.4 GENERAL MEDICAL CONSIDERATIONS

- Gas expansion with altitude.
- Hypobaric hypoxia.
- Vibration.
- Temperature control.
- Noise.
- Air sickness.
- Turbulence.
- Anxiety/fear of flying.
- Medication and time zone changes.
- Fatigue.
- G-forces.
- Isolation.

46.5 SPECIFIC CLINICAL CONSIDERATIONS

- Fitness to fly (see Chapter 43).
- See IATA Medical Manual, AsMA, BTS and BCS guidelines.
- Consider oxygenation and ventilation.
- Gas expansion in cavities (skull, abdomen, etc).
- Haemoglobin:
  - Acute vs. chronic anaemia.
  - Acidosis, Bohr effect.
- Recent surgery or trauma:
  - Pneumocephalus.
  - Trapped gas, recent bowel anastomoses.
  - Eye surgery: persistence of gas.
- Swelling and compartment syndrome (bivalve plaster casts).
- Wire cutters if required (discuss security with airline).
- Pregnancy.
- Infectious disease and isolation.
- Deep vein thrombosis risk: see Chapter 63.

46.6 BASIC AEROMEDICAL RISK ASSESSMENT

- Pulse.
- Respiratory rate.
- Blood pressure.
- Temperature.
- Haemoglobin.

- Oxygen saturation.
- Patient can clear ears (perform Valsalva).
- Pain relief adequate including step-up.
- Prepare patient before transfer to minimise in-flight issues.

46.7 QUALITY CARE AND GOVERNANCE

- Recording of preflight risk assessment and decision making.
- Access to further aeromedical specialist opinion.
- In-flight, handover records.
- Record-keeping quality.
- Organisational learning:
  - Clinical governance.
  - Clinical case review.
- Specified standards:
  - Commission on Accreditation of Medical Transport Systems (CAMTS).
  - European Aeromedical Institute (EURAMI).

46.8 SOURCES OF FURTHER INFORMATION

- Medical Manual 10th Edition. International Air Transportation Association. https://www.iata.org/publications/Documents/medical-manual.pdf.
- Aviation Health Unit. UK Civil Aviation Authority. www.caa.co.uk.
- Air Travel Recommendations. British Thoracic Society. www.brit-thoracic.org.uk.
- Fitness to fly for passengers with cardiovascular disease. British Cardiovascular Society. www.bcs.com.
- Dangerous Goods Regulations. International Air Transportation Association. www.iata.org.
- International Health Regulations (IHR). World Health Organisation. www.who.int.
- Tuberculosis and Air Travel. World Health Organization. www.who.int.
- Medical Guidelines for Airline Travel. Aerospace Medical Association. www.asma.org.
- Oxford Specialist Handbook of Retrieval Medicine, ISBN 9780198722168.
- Commission on Accreditation of Medical Transport Systems (CAMTS). www.camts.org.
- European Aeromedical Institute (EURAMI). eurami.org.
- North Atlantic Treaty Organisation (NATO) AMedPs.
- Air and Space Interoperability Council agreements.

Clinical considerations in prolonged aeromedical transfer

Contents

> **Key Facts**
> - Aeromedical evacuation of clinically volatile critical patients is challenging.
> - Both medical and physiological considerations must be countered.
> - Physician should address patient and aircraft factors.
> - Tissue oxygen delivery must be optimized through the manipulation of FiO_2, haemoglobin level and cabin altitude restriction.

47.1 BACKGROUND

- Life-threatening medical or traumatic injuries must be addressed prior to transport of critically ill patients.
- Thorough patient preparation required to minimise secondary insult associated with aeromedical evacuation (AE) with its potential for excess morbidity and mortality.

47.2 MEDICAL CONSIDERATIONS

- Equipment: Equipment preparation prior to evacuation (e.g., monitor/defibrillator, IV pumps, ventilator, portable suction):
  - All equipment should be regularly inspected by biomedical engineering.
  - Batteries should be fully charged; spare set of batteries available.
- Medication: Medications needed during flight should be anticipated and carried. Typical medications:
  - Analgesia (morphine/hydromorphone/fentanyl).
  - Sedatives (lorazepam, midazolam, propofol).
  - Anti-emetics (ondansetron, metoclopramide).
  - Cardiac medications (diltiazem, metoprolol, amiodarone).
  - Emergency medications (epinephrine, norepinephrine, D-50, diphenhydramine).

- IV fluids (lactated Ringers, normal saline, ½ normal saline with 40 meq KCL/litre).
- Packed red blood cells and fresh frozen plasma (trauma patients).
- Peripheral IV access (preferably two lines) and central lines placed prior to flight (with chest x-ray or ultrasound confirmation).
- A 2-day supply of medications is good practice (avoids shortages should aircraft divert to remote location).
- Be aware of time zone changes on dose regime.
- Intubation: For intubated patients:
  - Obtain preflight arterial blood gases; ensure endotracheal tube is secure.
  - Following trauma, neck tenderness/neurologic deficits cannot be assessed; C-collar should stay in place even if C-spine CT is negative (since ligamentous injury/neurologic deficits cannot be excluded).
- Capnography: Mechanically ventilated patients should have end-tidal CO_2 monitoring with an easily visible wave form.
  - Permits immediate detection of ventilator circuit disconnections and ventilator failures.
  - Identifies potentially deleterious trends in CO_2, prompting timely arterial blood gas determinations or ventilator adjustments.
  - Waveform is easier to detect than an alarm on a noisy aircraft (see Figure 47.1).
- Oxygen: Each mechanically ventilated patient should have their own dedicated oxygen supply (portable liquid oxygen if possible) in case aircraft-based oxygen fails.
- Environment: Heat and moisturizer exchangers should be employed where possible to protect against decreased humidity at altitude.
- Aspiration: To protect against aspiration and to gravity-assist ventilation, ensure head of the bed elevation to 30 degrees, unless contraindicated.
- Chest tube care: After chest tube placement for pneumothorax or haemopneumothorax, it is crucial that the chest tube is not clamped or kinked during transport, otherwise a tension pneumothorax could ensue.
  - For haemopneumothorax, clots that could block the tube should be extricated prior to flight and normal drainage of blood/serosanguinous fluid should be confirmed.
  - Large clot obstructing a chest tube can also result in a tension pneumothorax.
- Blood loss: Ongoing haemorrhage prior to flight must be corrected either with surgery or with tourniquet or occlusive dressings:

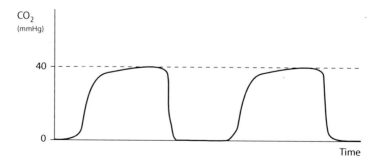

Figure 47.1 Typical normal end-tidal CO_2 (capnograph) display.

- Check haemoglobin/haematocrit (H/H) prior to flight. Various guidance exists for lowest acceptable H/H; no widely agreed limit; a very low H/H (e.g. 6 g/dl and 18%) would not provide optimal tissue oxygen delivery at altitude, suggesting transport be delayed.
- Should an H/H be unavailable, simplified mathematical estimate of blood loss based on current ATLS recommendations for a 70-kg patient is shown in Table 47.1.
- Numerous potential reasons for tachycardia and/or hypotension (i.e. sepsis, cardiogenic shock); in a trauma patient with a low H/H, serious consideration should be given to delaying transport.
- Without H/H, heart rates suggesting 30–40% blood loss should prompt transport delays.
- If higher level of care needed, blood and fresh frozen plasma should be transfused in-flight; platelets have a higher potential for infection – preferentially administered prior to flight in clean hospital environment.
- **Pelvic fractures**: Stabilization of pelvis is required either with a Velcro band/sheet or external fixation (definitive treatment), optimizing pelvic venous injury haemostasis.

Table 47.1 Blood loss estimate based on ATLS recommendations

BLOOD LOSS PERCENTAGE	BLOOD LOSS (ml)	HEART RATE	BLOOD PRESSURE
10%	500 ml	110 s	
20%	1000 ml	120 s	
30%	1500 ml	130 s	hypotension
40%	2000 ml	140 s	hypotension

47.3 PHYSIOLOGICAL CONSIDERATIONS

- Acceleration/deceleration:
    - Forces associated with takeoff, landing and in-flight manoeuvres can produce rises in intracranial pressure, especially in supine patients.
    - Elevated intracranial pressure reduces cerebral perfusion pressure, resulting in relative brain hypoxia; traumatic brain injuries susceptible to secondary insults from hyperglycaemia and hypoxia.
    - Head-first loading should counter the takeoff acceleration; long, slow landings should mitigate the landing deceleration.
    - Restraint required in accordance with litter/aircraft guidelines to prevent unwanted movement during takeoff, landing, turbulence.
- Decreased humidity:
    - Humidified oxygen advised for long duration use to prevent mucosal drying/nosebleeds.
    - Insensible fluid loss should be countered with increased IV fluid rate.
- Vibration:
    - Extremity fractures should be stabilized/splinted prior to transport.
    - Splints must be well padded (especially bony prominences).

- All casts should be bi-valved (i.e. split into two parts similar to a clamshell) since degree of tissue oedema at altitude is unpredictable.
- Neurovascular checks should be performed before and after splinting/casting as well as during flight to avoid numbness/neuropathy/compartment syndrome.
- Air splints present a constant clinical threat as internal pressure rises with altitude (Boyle's law); if used, air must be released from splint at altitude and added on descent.
- Anticipate an increase in pain, particularly with orthopaedic injuries, and dose pain medicaments accordingly.

- Thermal instability (hypothermia/hyperthermia):
  - Temperatures may vary widely within the aircraft depending on season and specific aircraft.
  - Extremes will increase patient metabolic rate and oxygen demand/consumption.
  - Temperature monitoring extremely important; an external temperature probe or Foley catheter (if patient is intubated) should be readily available.
  - With decreased temperature at altitude, space blankets preferred, as lightweight heat-reflective thin sheets add very little weight to the equipment load.

- Noise:
  - Operating aircraft is loud; noise levels often exceed 85 dB.
  - Hearing protection (e.g. ear foamies) should be routinely considered for patients.

- Hypobaric hypoxia:
  - General principles explained in Chapter 9.
  - Imperative that patients are adequately oxygenated on the ground prior to flight, as oxygen requirements only increase with altitude.
  - Based on Air Travel and American Thoracic Society Guidelines, estimated P_AO_2 at normal cabin altitude can be determined by multiplying $0.7 \times P_AO_2$ at sea level. For example, P_AO_2 of 60 mmHg at sea level would be 42 mmHg at 8000 feet. While at altitude, a P_AO_2 of at least 60 mmHg should be sustained.
  - The 30–60//60–90 rule:
    – P_AO_2 of 30 mmHg corresponds to an oxygen saturation of 60%.
    – P_AO_2 of 60 mmHg corresponds to an oxygen saturation of 90%.
  - For non-intubated patients, there are commonly used tables to determine oxygen requirements for maintaining ground equivalent FiO_2 at altitude (see Table 47.2).
  - Patients requiring FiO_2 >70% and/or PEEP >14 prior to an AE flight are extremely difficult to oxygenate at altitude; delay of transport should be considered until patient's pulmonary status has moderated.
  - Congestive heart failure, acute lung injury or acute respiratory distress syndrome demand particular attention as provision of adequate oxygenation is often challenging.
  - A cabin altitude restriction should be considered for patients with high oxygen requirements (see below).

- Pressure change:
  - The IV lines should be free of air bubbles, as will expand at altitude and lock up IV pumps.
  - Chest x-rays should be obtained prior to flight in an intubated patient.

Table 47.2 Clinical oxygen requirements to maintain sea level equivalency

Oxygen Requirements to Maintain Sea Level Equivalency*

Altitude (Ft)	Atmospheric Pressure (mmHg)	Oxygen 21% (mmHg)	0.21	0.25	0.30	0.35	0.40	0.45	0.50	0.55	0.60	0.65	0.70	0.75	0.80	0.85	0.90	0.95	1.00
10000	522	110	32	38	45	53	60	68	75	83	90	98							
9000	543	114	30	36	43	50	58	65	72	79	86	93							
8000	565	119	29	34	41	48	55	62	69	76	83	89	96						
7000	587	123	28	33	40	46	53	59	66	73	79	86	92	99					
6000	609	128	27	32	38	44	51	57	63	70	76	82	89	95	101				
5000	633	133	26	30	37	43	49	55	61	67	73	79	85	91	97				
4000	656	138	25	29	35	41	47	53	59	64	70	76	82	88	94	100			
3000	681	143	24	28	34	39	45	51	56	62	67	73	79	84	90	96			
2000	707	148	23	27	32	38	43	49	54	59	65	70	76	81	86	92	97		
1000	733	154	22	26	31	36	42	47	52	57	62	68	73	78	83	88	94	99	
0 (PiO₂)	760	160	150	178	214	250	285	321	357	392	428	463	499	535	570	606	642	677	760
FiO₂			0.21	0.25	0.30	0.35	0.40	0.45	0.50	0.55	0.60	0.65	0.70	0.75	0.80	0.85	0.90	0.95	1.00

O2 Source: RA | Nasal Cannula (1–6 L/min) | Simple Mask (5–8 L/min) | Partial Rebreathing Mask (7–15 L/min) | Non-Rebreathing Mask (7–15 L/min) | Partial Rebreathing Mask with Bag (7–15 L/min)

Pertinent Formula:

$$PiO_2 = FiO_2 \times (P_{sea\ level} - P_{H_2O})$$

$$Required\ FiO_2 = [FiO_2 \times (P_{sea\ level} - 47\ mmHg)]/(P_{altitude} - 47\ mmHg)$$

- Pneumothorax on the ground can easily become a tension pneumothorax at altitude; insertion of a chest tube at altitude is fraught with hazard and should be studiously avoided.
  - Confirmation of correct endotracheal tube (ETT) placement is essential; ETT is generally inserted to $3\times$ ETT size (e.g. 8.0 mm tube should be aligned with lips/teeth at 24 cm).
  - ETT cuff pressure should be monitored on the ground, on ascent, at altitude, and on landing (normal $= 20-30$ cm H_2O, as measured with a manometer).
    - Air removed from cuff on ascent and added on descent.
    - Overinflation can lead to tracheal necrosis/stenosis and/or cuff rupture.
    - Underinflation can lead to cuff leak with consequent inadequate oxygenation/ventilation and/or aspiration.
  - For patients with abdominal surgery and ileus, orogastric/nasogastric tubes can prevent air expansion at altitude, avoiding the potential for abdominal compartment syndrome and aspiration.
    - Gastric decompression is important for patients post-splenectomy as gastric over-distention has been known to disrupt ligatures on the short gastric arteries with resultant haemorrhage.
    - Cabin altitude restriction should be considered for patients with trapped gas.
  - Possible role of hypobaria with inflammatory upregulation, evolved bubbles and ischemia-reperfusion cascade.
- Also consider:
  - Motion sickness.
  - Fear of flying.
  - Fatigue.
  - Isolation.

47.4 TISSUE OXYGEN DELIVERY

- Tissue oxygen delivery (DO_2) often used in intensive care.
- Concept also valuable in AE, particularly in relation to hypobaric hypoxia.
- Tissue oxygen delivery described by:
  - Alveolar gas equation (see Chapter 9).
  - Arterial blood oxygen content equation.

$$C_aO_2\left(ml\,O_2\,/\,dL\right) = \left(1.34\times Hb\times SaO_2\right) + \left(0.0031\times P_AO_2\right)$$

  - Tissue oxygen delivery equation.

$$DO_2 = \left(CaO_2\times CO\right)/\,wt$$

  - Oxyhaemoglobin-dissociation curve (see Chapter 10).
- Tissue oxygen delivery can be improved by FiO_2, haemoglobin level and cabin altitude restriction (CAR):
  - FiO_2 can be raised with supplemental oxygen.
  - Haemoglobin level can be raised with transfusions.

- Traditional indications for the CAR have been limited to trapped gas, severe pulmonary disease and decompression illness:
  - Most commonly prescribed cabin altitude restriction is 5000 feet followed by 6000 and 4000 feet.
  - Reduced cabin altitude is often accompanied by lower cruising altitude; may result in more fuel consumption, greater cost and longer flights, but these may not be operationally relevant.
  - Recent research suggests that a CAR is considered to raise tissue oxygen delivery. Morbidity in CAR patients appears to be decreased (e.g. reduced number of post-flight procedures and complications) – clinical groups that may benefit include those with traumatic brain injury.
- Tissue oxygen delivery can be calculated for individual patient or inserted into a spreadsheet graphic user interface (in development).

CHAPTER 48

Hypertension

Contents

48.1 BACKGROUND

- Hypertension (HTN) affects over 1 billion individuals globally.
- Usually defined as blood pressure (BP) ≥140/90 mmHg.
- May be elevated by stress and anxiety:
  - 'White coat' hypertension is a well-recognised phenomenon not thought to convey additional cardiovascular risk.
  - 'White coat' hypertension should not be assumed – risk of missing true hypertension.

48.2 DIAGNOSIS

- Diurnal variability, environmental factors, recent exercise, consumption of caffeine or alcohol can affect blood pressure readings.
- Ambulatory blood pressure monitoring (ABPM) is reliable and cost-effective; it should be used to confirm diagnosis in aircrew with BP readings of >140/90 mmHg.
- When making diagnosis of HTN with a 24-hr ABPM:
  - Average blood pressure of ≥135/85 mmHg confirms stage 1 HTN.
  - ≥150/95 mmHg confirms stage 2 HTN.
  - These values correlate with >140/90 mmHg and >160/100 mmHg in the office setting.

- Aircrew with stage 2 HTN should be grounded until appropriately treated.
- Stage 3 (severe) HTN is defined as a BP >180/110 and should be referred for same-day specialist opinion.
- Assessment of average and range of BP readings should be made; lack of a nocturnal dip carries a significant and additional cardiovascular risk.

48.3 GLOBAL CARDIOVASCULAR RISK ASSESSMENT

- Aircrew with HTN should have overall cardiovascular risk assessment using a validated risk-score calculator (JBS3, Q-risk, New Zealand Coronary Event Risk Chart, etc.).
- HTN is often one manifestation of multiple interrelated cardiovascular risk factors (e.g. raised lipid or glucose levels, increasing body mass index):
  - Whole system approach is required.
  - Weight loss and exercise program may prevent the need for pharmacological intervention, even in a healthy population such as aircrew.
- Clinical examination should include:
  - Assessment of end-organ damage.
  - Checking of peripheral pulses (exclude radio-radio or radio-femoral delay in coarctation).
  - Fundoscopy.
  - Cardiac and renal auscultation.
- Further investigations should include:
  - Urine dipstick to check for haematuria, proteinuria; spot albumin to creatinine ratio (ACR).
  - 12-lead electrocardiogram (ECG).
  - Fasting blood screen for electrolytes, glucose, lipids and renal function.
- Evidence of left ventricular hypertrophy (LVH) on 12-lead ECG:
  - Common in aircrew as an incidental finding.
  - Further cardiovascular assessment with echocardiography required in aircrew with HTN to assess for concentric LVH or left atrial dilatation (which suggest long-standing hypertension and increased cardiovascular risk).
- Younger patients (<40 years old) or severe/resistant cases:
  - Give special attention to exclude secondary causes of HTN.
  - Onward referral for specialist evaluation and management recommended.

48.4 AEROMEDICAL CONCERNS

- HTN associated with increased risk for myocardial infarction, heart failure, atrial fibrillation, chronic kidney disease, cognitive decline and premature death.
- Major risk factor for ischaemic and haemorrhagic stroke and coronary artery diseases:
  - Every 10 mmHg rise above normal (130/80 mmHg) thought to contribute an additional 30% to coronary mortality risk.
- Increased likelihood of arrhythmia, especially atrial fibrillation (AF), also a major concern:
  - AF twice as likely in patients without nocturnal dip.

48.5 MANAGEMENT – GENERAL MEASURES

- Aircrew with HTN must be treated as having a significant, but usually modifiable, cardiovascular risk factor.
- Simple lifestyle changes have been demonstrated to be effective:
  - Smoking cessation.
  - Minimising alcohol intake.
  - Reduced salt (sodium chloride) intake.
  - Weight loss.
  - Increased exercise.
- Optimal level of blood pressure control remains controversial:
  - Average BP of <140/90 mmHg is deemed essential.
  - Many would regard <130/80 mmHg as more optimal.

48.6 MANAGEMENT – PHARMACOLOGICAL MEASURES

- Caution is advised when selecting the most appropriate pharmacologic agents to treat HTN in aircrew.
- Alpha-blockers, loop diuretics, adrenergic blocking agents and other centrally acting agents (e.g. methyl-dopa) should be avoided due to risk of unpredictable postural and central effects.
- Usually preferable to initiate multiple agents at sub-maximal doses than to use a single agent at the top of the therapeutic range (where side effects more prevalent).
- All aircrew should be grounded for a short period to exclude idiosyncratic reactions to new drugs (usually 2 weeks in civilian flying and 28 days for military aircrew) at the initiation of a new agent and following a change in dose regimen; also allows assessment of adequate blood pressure control prior to resumption of flying duties.
- Most classes of modern antihypertensive agents are deemed compatible with continued flying.

THIAZIDE DIURETICS

- Long history of use in aircrew.
- Lack of evidence for the use of bendroflumethiazide 2.5 mg, so if this class of agent is introduced, either indapamide or chlorthalidone is now recommended.

ANGIOTENSIN CONVERTING ENZYME (ACE) INHIBITORS AND ANGIOTENSIN RECEPTOR BLOCKING (ARB) AGENTS

- Considered acceptable and are positively indicated in patients with diabetes mellitus.
  - ARB may be preferred to ACE inhibitors due to the incidence of a bradykinin-related irritating dry cough associated with the latter.
  - Both classes acceptable for unrestricted flying duties, even in high-performance aircraft, with no detrimental effect on Gz tolerance.

CALCIUM CHANNEL BLOCKERS (CCB)

- Usually well tolerated.
- Especially useful in aircrew with diabetes or hyperlipidaemia, as exert no effect on these metabolic pathways (do not require routine screening of renal or liver function).
  - Dihydropyridine CCB (such as amlodipine) are acceptable in aircrew, both civil and military.
  - Phenylalkylamine agents (such as verapamil) and benzothiazepine agents (such as diltiazem) have both negative inotropic and chronotropic effects and should be used with caution in aircrew; restricted to aircrew of non-high-performance aircraft only.

BETA-BLOCKERS

- No longer recommended as first-line agents in hypertension.
- Poorly tolerated by younger individuals who often feel profoundly lethargic on this medication.
- Cardio-selective beta-blockers remain acceptable agents for civilian pilots; however, military aircrew are restricted to non-high-performance aircraft and multi-crew environments.

48.7 RESISTANT HYPERTENSION

- If persistently hypertensive despite three agents, a diagnosis of resistant hypertension should be considered:
  - Non-compliance should be considered.
  - All causes of secondary hypertension should be actively excluded.
- At this point beta-blockers can be considered in aircrew, with the alternatives such as alpha-blockers usually incompatible with the retention of an aircrew license.

48.8 AEROMEDICAL DISPOSITION

- Pilots with severe hypertension (BP $\geq$160/100 mmHg) should be grounded, promptly investigated and treated.
- For aircrew with lesser degrees of hypertension, a full subjective assessment of overall cardiovascular risk is required.
- Most aircrew will be able to continue flying (with a multi-crew limitation) whilst under investigation.

48.9 ONGOING REVIEW

- Regular review required once commenced on therapy or lifestyle interventions:
  - Check eGFR and electrolytes of all patients commenced on ACE inhibitors or ARB to ensure renal impairment is not precipitated in those with renal artery stenosis.
  - For all other aircrew, review of electrolytes, glucose and lipids is recommended 4 to 6 weeks after starting treatment.
  - Many individuals require multiple pharmacological agents to control their hypertension; up to half of patients fail to achieve target blood pressure despite pharmacological intervention.

- Repeat clinic and ABPM measurements required to confirm adequate control.
- Some evidence suggests use of regular ABPM may allow adequate control at lower doses when compared to traditional clinic-based recordings.
- Most civilian aircrew can return to unrestricted flying duties following successful treatment and stable blood pressure control:
    - Unless 10-year cardiovascular risk exceeds 10% – then may be restricted to multi-crew operations.
- For military aircrew, more caution is required:
    - Certain physiological limitations may be required depending on the prescribed pharmacological therapy.
    - Aircrew must be normotensive for a minimum of 4 weeks prior to resumption of military flying.
    - Treatment with beta-blockers or rate slowing calcium channel blockers will restrict aircrew to lower Gz environments (max + 2.5 Gz); treatment with beta-blockers is also only permitted in multi-crew environments due to concerns with regards to subtle cognitive and motor retardation.

CHAPTER 49

Atherosclerosis

Contents

49.1 BACKGROUND

- Most coronary artery presentations in aircrew result from atherosclerosis.
- Atherosclerosis is a progressive process, starting as early as the second decade.
- Other rare coronary artery conditions include:
  - Coronary artery spasm (Prinzmetal angina).
  - Coronary artery dissection.
  - Aberrant coronary anatomy.

EFFECT OF STENOSIS

- Enlargement of atherosclerotic plaques over time may obstruct coronary blood flow and impair ability to meet myocardial oxygen demand when increased (e.g. with exercise).
- Failure to meet myocardial demand usually occurs when plaque (stenosis) occludes at least 70% of the arterial lumen, at which point symptoms may develop (angina). Even mild hypobaric hypoxia may be enough to exacerbate this in aircrew.
- At <70% stenosis, coronaries dilate to try to maintain blood flow:
  - However, the effect of this is limited, and so any stenosis of ≥50% is deemed significant in aircrew.
- Plaques may become calcified, but non-calcified ('soft') plaque is particularly vulnerable to rupture and ulceration:
  - This leads to thrombus formation potentially occluding the vessel, leading to an acute coronary syndrome (ACS).

- ACS includes unstable angina (UA), and myocardial infarction – with or without ST elevation (STEMI and NSTEMI, respectively).

49.2 CORONARY ARTERY DISEASE (CAD)

- Fortunately, the majority of aircrew do not present with overt ischaemic heart disease (IHD) but are picked up secondary to minor abnormalities on routine ECG screening.
- Abnormalities on the ECG may precede clinical manifestations of CAD:
  - T wave inversion, ST segment flattening or depression or new bundle branch block on aircrew ECG usually requires further investigation.
  - Usual investigations are exercise tolerance test (ETT), 24-hr Holter ECG and echocardiogram.
- Additional investigations may be required, including:
  - Anatomical assessment of the coronary vasculature (coronary artery calcium score [CACS], CT or invasive coronary angiography [CTCA/ICA]).
  - Myocardial perfusion scan such as nuclear myocardial perfusion scintigraphy (MPS), perfusion cardiac MRI scan (pCMR) or stress echocardiogram.
- The level of investigation will be stipulated by the relevant licencing agency.

MILD CAD

- Mild CAD is a common finding in asymptomatic adults and confers a future risk of cardiovascular events.
- Evidence from aircrew populations suggests the risk of death for stenosis <30% is approximately 0.2% per annum, rising to 0.5% per annum for stenosis between 30 and 50%. This compares to a risk of 0.1% p.a. in those with normal angiography.

MODERATE TO SEVERE CAD

- Data suggest a 15–20% 10-year risk of death for asymptomatic patients with moderate CAD (50–70% stenosis).
- This exceeds the 1% rule for multi-crew operations and is incompatible with flying privileges.

49.3 ISCHAEMIC HEART DISEASE (IHD)

- IHD occurs when CAD is sufficiently advanced to result in associated ischaemia.
- May be picked up in asymptomatic aircrew following a myocardial perfusion scan, or in symptomatic aircrew with anginal chest pain:
  - Stable angina (by definition) is brought on by exercise.
  - Unstable angina may occur at rest.
- IHD is a bar to flying (whether symptomatic or not), with or without medication and requires investigation.
- Following successful coronary revascularisation, aircrew may be able to resume flying duties, usually in a limited capacity, after comprehensive assessment.

ACUTE CORONARY SYNDROMES

- Acute coronary syndromes include UA, NSTEMI and STEMI.
- All are associated with adverse outcomes and require immediate assessment and treatment.

- Distraction due to ischaemic pain, and incapacitation due to malignant arrhythmias are major sources of concern in aircrew.
- Management for aircrew should be as for non-aircrew.
- Invasive coronary angiography is to be expected, and revascularisation is also likely.

49.4 REVASCULARIZATION

SCOPE

- To regain flying privileges, aircrew must be completely revascularised.
- Aircrew may, therefore, require intervention on diseased vessels beyond those deemed to be clinically significant.
- Revascularisation may be with percutaneous coronary intervention and stenting (PCI) or with coronary artery bypass grafting (CABG) according to standard clinical practice.

METHODS

- With PCI, drug eluting stents and bare metal stents are both acceptable in aircrew. Balloon angioplasty alone (i.e. without placement of a stent) is not acceptable due to the high rate of re-stenosis.
- For aircrew undergoing CABG, arterial and venous grafts are considered acceptable, although better longer-term patency has been demonstrated with arterial grafts. In military aircrew, full arterial revascularisation may be required in order to regain flying privileges.

FOLLOW-UP

- Regardless of the method of revascularisation, regular follow-up is mandatory for aircrew to maintain a licence.
- This must include assessment and aggressive management of risk factors, such as obesity, smoking, diabetes and lipid profile.
- Periodic assessment for recurrent ischaemia may be required by licencing agencies.

49.5 AEROMEDICAL RISK ASSESSMENT IN CAD

- CAD in aircrew carries the potential for distraction and/or incapacitation due to angina, infarction and arrhythmia.
  - Hypobaric hypoxia and exposure to Gz increase myocardial oxygen demand and may unmask occult CAD.
  - For these reasons, any stenosis of >50% in one of the main coronary arteries (or 30% in the left main stem) is significant in aircrew.
- When CAD is suspected, aircrew should be grounded until thoroughly investigated and assessed by a cardiologist with aviation medicine experience.
- Complete revascularisation is required for individuals with significant stenosis.
- Evaluation following ACS and/or revascularisation should include assessment of:
  - Ventricular function, including consideration of presence of myocardial scar.
  - Symptoms (off anti-anginal medication).
  - Ischaemia.
  - Arrhythmia.
  - Risk factor modification.

- Treatment for risk factors must be with acceptable therapies.
- If assessment of these factors is satisfactory, aircrew *may* be able to return to commercial or military flying in a limited capacity; non-commercial aircrew *may* be able to return to unrestricted flying.

50

Congenital heart disease

Contents

50.1 BACKGROUND

Adult congenital heart disease (ACHD) is uncommon in aircrew; however, with advances in childhood surgery and adult care, an increasing number of individuals with ACHD seek advice with regards to flying, both in the civilian and military sectors.

- Simple ACHD, especially if repaired in childhood, may be acceptable in aircrew:
  - Conditions that require sustained cardiovascular follow-up, have residual physiological consequence or increase the risk of developing incompatible conditions may preclude individuals from successfully applying to fly.
  - In the military, additional considerations, such as the risk of endocarditis to either native cardiac defects or surgical interventions, may also affect the assessment of suitability for both aircrew candidates and existing aircrew.

50.2 RISK ASSESSMENT IN AIRCREW

- The aeromedical significance of ACHD will be determined by the potential physiological consequences of the underlying pathology in the aviation environment.
- Any abnormality that increases the risk of arrhythmia also of concern.
- Side effects of common pharmacological agents such as those that reduce Gz tolerance need to be considered.
  - Anticoagulation remains a disqualifying condition for some commercial pilots.
- Return to flying sometimes possible in a limited occupational role on non-high-performance airframes.

50.3 SPECIFIC CONDITIONS

- All aircrew with a suspected diagnosis of ACHD require extensive investigation and usually require restriction or grounding whilst these are undertaken.
- Investigation is often extensive and time-consuming, and aircrew should be counselled accordingly.
- For detail of cardiovascular investigations, refer to Chapter 54.

CORONARY ARTERY ANOMALIES

- Anomalous coronary anatomy is present in around 1% in the general population; may be identified following an abnormal 12-lead or exercise ECG.
- May occur in isolation but significantly more prevalent in individuals with other congenital heart disease.
- Most aberrant coronary anatomy is clinically insignificant with little or no physiological effect on myocardial perfusion.
- Most anomalous coronary variants compatible with unrestricted flying duties.
    - Rarely aircrew have clinically important anomalous anatomy that may impair coronary blood flow on exercise.
    - Clinical implications are related to the exact origin and course of the affected coronary artery and the clinical presentation.

CONGENITAL VALVE DISEASE

- See Chapter 51.

PATENT DUCTUS ARTERIOSUS (PDA)

- PDA is usually recognised early in life and closed pharmacologically with surgical ligation or a percutaneous closure device:
    - If closed in childhood, with appropriate follow-up, a closed PDA is usually compatible with unrestricted flying.
    - If a percutaneous device closure has been used, then this may preclude applicants from military flying.
- If small and untreated, rarely PDA may present in adulthood.
    - PDA associated with an increased risk of endocarditis and may result in pulmonary hypertension.
    - Pulmonary hypertension may manifest in aircrew as palpitations, secondary to right atrial dilation, dyspnoea on exertion, or hypoxia.
    - Pulmonary hypertension is a bar to initial flying certification and usually associated with restriction of flying privileges, or grounding, if diagnosed in existing aircrew.

PATENT FORAMEN OVALE (PFO)

- PFO present in 25–33% of the population.
- Often an incidental finding in asymptomatic aircrew undergoing echocardiography for investigation of other suspected cardiac disease.
- Unless associated with an embolic event or decompression sickness (DCS) it should be regarded as a normal variant.

- In individuals with confirmed cerebrovascular accidents (CVA), management usually involves anticoagulation and/or device closure.
- Following any event, either CVA or DCS, aircrew should be grounded, investigated and treated.
    - Return to limited aircrew duties is often possible, depending on type of aircraft operated and the aircrew role performed.

ATRIAL SEPTAL DEFECTS (ASD)

- ASD may occur in isolation or as part of a wider constellation of ACHD.
- If isolated, ASD may be asymptomatic in childhood and may be detected incidentally, in aircrew, with an ejection systolic murmur.
- Unless closed early in adulthood, all ASD are associated with atrial arrhythmias, particularly atrial flutter and atrial fibrillation (AF).
- If presenting late they are usually not compatible with unrestricted flying.
- Risk of paroxysmal embolization that may be exacerbated by positive pressure breathing in certain aircrew roles.
- Nearly all ASD are now detected and closed in childhood, either with percutaneous closure devices or surgically.
    - Small residual shunts do not usually require further intervention clinically but require further assessment in aircrew, especially if positive pressure breathing may be undertaken.
    - Long-term data to support aeromedical disposition following ASD closure are lacking, and there remains a small increased risk of endocarditis and arrhythmia, meaning aircrew are usually restricted.

VENTRICULAR SEPTAL DEFECT (VSD)

- Isolated VSD accounts for about a third of simple ACHD.
- Small VSD may cause a palpable thrill and loud pan systolic murmur.
- VSD associated with an increased risk of endocarditis.
- Small VSD:
    - In civilian commercial flying, applicants with small VSD may be considered for unrestricted aircrew roles
    - If found incidentally in trained aircrew, restrictions are usually not required.
- Large VSD:
    - Usually associated with significant haemodynamic manifestations, such as pulmonary hypertension unless closed either surgically or percutaneously.
    - Repair is associated with a long-term increase in incidence of arrhythmias and aortic regurgitation.
    - For these reasons, professional aircrew applicants are likely to be unsuccessful.

Valvular heart disease

Contents

51.1 BACKGROUND

- The incidence of acquired valvular heart disease (VHD) has fallen with the reduction in rheumatic heart disease but does still occur in aircrew.
- Congenital valve disease is common and is often asymptomatic until later in life. Due to periodic medical examinations, asymptomatic aircrew with VHD may be detected secondary to ECG changes, or murmurs, on clinical examination.
- In the military, additional considerations such as the risk of endocarditis to either native cardiac defects or surgical interventions may also affect the assessment of suitability for both aircrew candidates and existing aircrew.

51.2 RISK ASSESSMENT IN AIRCREW

- Assessment of VHD is like that of ACHD (see Chapter 50), both for native disease and following intervention.
  - All aircrew with a suspected diagnosis of VHD require extensive investigation and usually require restriction or grounding whilst these are undertaken.
  - For detail of cardiovascular investigations, see Chapter 54.
- Simple VHD, especially if mild, may be acceptable in aircrew; however, conditions that restrict cardiac output also restrict the compensatory physiological response to sustained acceleration.
- Stenotic VHD is usually problematic if more than mild, whereas regurgitant valve lesions are less problematic until moderate in severity.
- Due to the significant economic investment in aircrew applicants, individuals identified as having VHD on selection may not be successful if applying to fly professionally.
  - It is possible to return to flying after a diagnosis of VHD, however, often in a limited occupational role and on non-high-performance airframes.

51.3 CONGENITAL VALVE DISEASE

BICUSPID AORTIC VALVE DISEASE

- Bicuspid aortic valve (BAV) disease is the most common form of ACHD.
- Prevalence of 1–3%.
- Usually asymptomatic in childhood and often found incidentally in aircrew undergoing a periodic medical examination.
- BAV disease is associated with dilatation of the ascending aorta and aortic coarctation, and both should be actively excluded in aircrew.
  - Surgery may be required if the ascending aorta is >4.5 cm in diameter.
  - Usual treatments such as β-blockers, with their significant impact on Gz tolerance, may result in restriction or grounding of certain aircrew.
  - Disease progression is highly variable, and the risks associated with high Gz forces are unknown.
- As with all valve disease, there is an increased associated risk of endocarditis.
- Mild stenosis and moderate regurgitation are likely to lead to flying restrictions.

PULMONARY STENOSIS

- Pulmonary stenosis (PS) may occur in isolation or as part of a wider constellation of congenital heart defects (CHD):
  - Intervention for severe PS usually carried out in childhood and is generally incompatible with aircrew licencing, as is sub- and supra-valvular PS.
- Progression of mild PS is not uncommon:
  - Aircrew may remain asymptomatic, even with significant disease, with a systolic murmur often the clinical finding that highlights the condition.
  - Associated risk of atrial arrhythmia and additional endocarditis risk.
- Fitness to (continue) to fly is dependent on disease severity, and after exclusion of additional CHD, decisions based on the same criteria as acquired disease.
- Pulmonary valve replacement is usually incompatible with ongoing flying due to the associated complication rate being approximately 5% per annum.

51.4 ACQUIRED VALVE DISEASE

AORTIC VALVE DISEASE

- Valve degeneration may involve leaflet thickening and/or calcification. This may lead to stenosis, regurgitation or a combination of both (mixed disease), although one form usually predominates.
- Aortic valve disease is often part of a wider aortopathy and dilatation of the aortic root and ascending thoracic aorta should be excluded in all aircrew.
- Regurgitant disease is associated with inflammatory conditions such as inflammatory bowel disease, rheumatoid arthritis and ankylosing spondylitis, as well as connective tissue disorders.
  - Isolated, mild to moderate regurgitant disease is usually compatible with unrestricted flying, but requires regular follow-up (usually annually) to monitor for disease progression, including volume overload and arrhythmia.

- Aortic stenosis is less well tolerated in the aviation environment:
  - Aircrew identified with suspected aortic stenosis should be grounded until investigated.
  - Mild disease may be asymptomatic and aircrew with mean gradients on transthoracic echocardiography of <20 mmHg are usually able to fly without restriction.
  - Depending on aircrew role and airframe operated, restriction, including potential withdrawal of flying privileges, is often required.
- The aortic valve is usually not amenable to repair, and the choice of surgical procedure and prosthetic material used in valve replacement surgery are often critical in the determination of licence renewal:
  - Following surgery and post-operative follow-up, additional investigations are required, and most aircrew will be restricted in their roles (i.e. unfit high Gz, unfit pressure breathing, unfit solo).
  - The AME should always liaise with the pilot's cardiothoracic surgeon prior to any proposed surgery and the pilot, surgeon and AME should be cognisant of the ramifications of various courses of action, and the need for certain clinical investigations to determine suitability to return to flying after surgery.

MITRAL VALVE DISEASE

- Mitral valve disease is uncommon in aircrew:
  - Congenital stenosis is usually detected in childhood.
  - Acquired mitral stenosis is rare with the decline in rheumatic heart disease.
  - Regurgitant disease is usually seen secondary to mitral valve leaflet prolapse, but can also be associated with ischaemic heart disease.
- Mild mitral valve disease with no evidence of left atrial dilation (<4 cm) is usually compatible with unrestricted flying.
  - Left atrial enlargement is associated with atrial fibrillation, which is unpredictable and has significant ramifications in aircrew (see Chapter 53).
- Mitral prolapse is usually detected following the auscultation of a loud late systolic murmur, but may also present with palpitations.
  - Echocardiography and arrhythmia assessment are mandatory, and mitral valve prolapse requires regular follow-up (usually annually) to monitor for disease progression, including volume overload and arrhythmia.
  - If aircrew are aged over 40, consideration should be given to assessing the coronary arteries with CT coronary angiography (Chapter 54).

CHAPTER 52

Heart muscle disease

Contents

52.1 BACKGROUND

- Heart muscle disease (HMD) includes many disorders, but this block will focus on cardiomyopathies and myocarditis.
- HMD is detected surprisingly commonly, usually secondary to ECG change identified during aircrew medical examinations.
- Cardiomyopathies are often detected in asymptomatic aircrew; however, individuals may present with palpations, dyspnoea or with reduced exercise tolerance.
- Cardiomyopathies may be secondary to hypertension or ischaemic heart disease but in the young are often familial or genetic in origin.
- HMD should be considered in aircrew with family history of sudden cardiac death (SCD), implantable cardiac defibrillator (ICD) implantation or cardiac transplantation.

52.2 RISK ASSESSMENT IN AIRCREW WITH HMD

- HMD may be associated with increased risk of distraction and incapacitation in aircrew, even in mild disease.
  - Investigation is often extensive and usually involves advanced imaging with cardiac MRI (CMR) and genetic testing.
  - Investigation of coronary artery disease may also be required in older aircrew.
  - All aircrew with a suspected diagnosis of HMD require further specialist investigation and usually require restriction or grounding whilst these are undertaken. For details of cardiovascular investigations, refer to Chapter 54.
- Mild disease may be compatible with continued flying in existing aircrew if the ejection fraction is >50% and there is no evidence of rhythm disturbances.
  - However, given the increased risk of arrhythmia and SCD, return to flying will often be restricted to low-performance aircraft and multiple crew roles.

- Pharmacological treatment, ICD implantation and ultimately cardiac transplantation may all be required.
- A diagnosis of HMD will likely adversely affect the assessment of suitability for aircrew candidates.

52.3 CARDIOMYOPATHY

DILATED CARDIOMYOPATHY (DCM)

- DCM is a progressive disease that is characterized by ventricular chamber enlargement and contractile dysfunction.
  - It can affect both ventricles.
  - DCM may be caused by viral infection, immune dysregulation, toxic, metabolic, inherited and tachycardia-induced conditions (such as severe ventricular ectopy).
- DCM is the third most common cause of heart failure and the most frequent reason for heart transplantation.
  - Disease progression in DCM is variable, from stable asymptomatic to rapidly progressive disease, despite treatment with ACE inhibitors and β-blockers.
- DCM is associated with electrical instability and SCD.
- Both the underlying condition and treatment options require restrictions and often withdrawal of flying privileges.
- Determination of HMD, such as dilated cardiomyopathy (DCM), can be challenging in young, very fit individuals:
  - They often have low normal ejection fraction (EF) with high stroke volumes that may mimic pathologic findings.
  - If there are no pathognomonic signs such as late gadolinium enhancement (LGE) on cardiac MRI (CMR), or confirmed genetic mutations, then ongoing follow-up may be required to determine progression, and individuals may need to be restricted for several years prior to return to full flying duties.

HYPERTROPHIC CARDIOMYOPATHY (HCM)

- HCM is defined as myocardial hypertrophy (>1.5 cm), most commonly affecting the interventricular septum but with variable distribution, following exclusion of hypertension, infiltrative disease and aortic stenosis.
- HCM is associated with many identified gene defects, and detection of these can, in some circumstances, allow more detailed prognostication. The lack of an identified gene defect does not exclude the diagnosis of HCM.
- HCM is the most common cause of SCD in athletes and often leads to restrictive cardiac physiology and valve dysfunction, both of which may impede cardiac output, with significant ramifications for aircrew.
- The distribution of hypertrophy is significant, as is the presence or absence of LV outflow tract obstruction (LVOTO):
  - Apical HCM has a better prognosis and may be compatible with limited flying duties; treatment is usually with β-blockers.
  - Traditional septal HCM without LVOTO may affect both ventricles; there is a spectrum of disease severity, and if hypertrophy is <2.5 cm, restricted aircrew duties may be permitted.

- Septal thickness >2.5 cm, LVOTO (either at rest or on exercise) and any symptoms of dizziness or syncope, in conjunction with any degree of HCM, are a bar to flying.
- Treatment with an ICD, septal ablation or surgical myectomy are all incompatible with flying privileges.

INFILTRATIVE CARDIOMYOPATHY

- Infiltrative (sometimes called restricted) cardiomyopathies include those associated with amyloidosis, hemochromatosis, sarcoidosis and Fabry's disease.
- All are associated with impaired cardiac function, myocardial hypertrophy and restrictive filling.
- All are related to systemic disease, with risk assessment of all affected systems required when considering aircrew disposition.
- Cardiac involvement is usually incompatible with flying duties.

ATHLETE'S HEART

- Athlete's heart (or athletic heart [AH]) is not, as one might assume, a benign condition.
- It represents a probable maladaptive response to intense athletic exercise (usually >1 hr a day) and results in LV hypertrophy and conduction disturbances.
- Differentiation of AH from HCM can be challenging but can often be distinguished by assessing the diastolic filling parameters on echocardiography.
- Whilst AH has a better prognosis than HCM, it is associated with atrial fibrillation, atrioventricular conduction defect and concern regarding ventricular arrhythmia.
- The diagnosis of athletic heart may lead to restriction of flying privileges.

52.4 MYOCARDITIS AND PERICARDITIS

- Inflammation secondary to viral infection may affect the pericardium, myocardium or both.
- The incidence of both reduce with age.
- ECG findings are often typical in pericarditis, with saddle-shaped concave ST elevation and troponin release indicating myocardial involvement.
- Acute pericarditis:
  - May be acutely incapacitating secondary to severe pain.
  - Is usually a self-limiting condition and amenable to treatment with NSAIDS.
  - Can be treated with colchicine if recurrence occurs; this is most likely within 12 months of the initial attack.
  - Can take 3–6 weeks to resolve and aircrew should desist from flying for this period and if ECG changes have resolved.
  - Aircrew should return to restricted (dual-crew) operation for 6 months and echocardiography and assessment of inflammatory markers should be considered.
- Myocarditis and myo-pericarditis:
  - Can both cause acute chest pain and be confused with ischaemic heart disease.
  - Investigation with CMR is often required, with classical LGE changes often confirming the diagnosis.

- Exclusion of coronary disease in older aircrew is often required.
- Aircrew should be grounded for 6 months following an episode of myocarditis.
- Echocardiography, exercise testing and a 24-hr Holter should be performed and be acceptable (excluding DCM and arrhythmias) prior to return to flying duties.

CHAPTER

53

Arrhythmias and electrophysiology

Contents

53.1 BACKGROUND

- Cardiac arrhythmia is a major cause of restriction of flying duties.
- Exposure to sustained acceleration is arrhythmogenic and +Gz acceleration may lead to cardiac dysrhythmias:
  - These are usually benign.
  - +Gz acceleration may precipitate 2nd/3rd degree block, AF, SVT and VT.
  - In aircrew with pre-existing susceptibility, sustained acceleration may provoke and aggravate episodes of severe arrhythmias that may have significant flight safety implications.
- Arrhythmias in aircrew are of concern as they may cause incapacitation secondary to pre-syncope or syncope, or symptoms such as palpitations or dizziness that may impair the safe operation of an aircraft simply by distraction.
- Assessment is complicated when trying to discriminate between benign and potentially significant rhythm abnormalities in pilots, many of whom are young and fit, have a resultant high vagal tone and where underlying cardiac disease has a low prevalence.
- Arrhythmia and conduction disturbances in aircrew may be caused by underlying structural heart disease, endocrine or other organic disorders. Therefore, when investigating arrhythmias in aircrew, thorough cardiac and general (internal) medical assessment is mandatory.
- For aircrew with confirmed arrhythmia, assessment of both the abnormal conduction abnormality and anti-arrhythmic therapy (which may have relevant side effects) is critical as both may have flight safety implications.
- Increasingly many aircrew are recommended, or have undergone, catheter ablation or device implantation and both short- and long-term outcome data must be considered when determining aircrew licencing.

53.2 APPROACH TO SCREENING IN AIRCREW

- Aircrew periodic medical examination should include a thorough medical history, including family history, alcohol and caffeine intake, a physical examination and 12-lead ECG.
  - Symptoms such as palpitations (regular or irregular), dizziness, syncope or pre-syncope should lead to suspicion of an arrhythmic aetiology.
- ECG findings in young individuals with high vagal tone that do not require additional follow-up and are acceptable for unrestricted flying:
  - Partial right bundle branch block (pRBBB).
  - 1st-degree heart block (up to 250 ms).
  - Mild Wenckebach (2nd degree heart block – Mobitz Type 1).
  - Single PVC.
- ECG findings in aircrew that require further investigation:
  - T wave inversion.
  - ST segment flattening or depression.
  - New complete bundle branch block.
  - Multiple ectopic beats.
  - Atrial tachycardia.
  - Delta waves (in Wolff-Parkinson-White).
  - Brugada phenotypes.

SECOND LEVEL INVESTIGATION

- Further investigation should include Holter monitoring (24 hr to 7 day), echocardiography and exercise ECG.
  - When undertaking Holter assessment, the longer the registration period, the more likely it is to reveal abnormal results.
  - In certain scenarios, in-flight Holter monitoring may be appropriate.
  - If episodic, telemetric ECG monitoring and/or external/implantable loop recorders may be appropriate.
- Laboratory investigations should include a blood count, electrolytes and thyroid hormone assessment.
- Other investigations may be required (e.g. urinary catecholamines).

SPECIALIST INVESTIGATIONS

- In some instances, specialist pharmacological testing (e.g. adenosine/ajmaline in an accessory pathway) may be indicated.
- In a minority of cases, invasive electrophysiological (EP) testing may be required.
  - If this reveals a target for ablation, it is often performed concurrently.
- In certain arrhythmias, genetic testing may be indicated.
- In aircrew flying in high-performance aircraft, centrifuge testing, to assess the response of arrhythmias to sustained acceleration, may be useful.
- If underlying structural of coronary artery disease is suspected, stress echocardiography, cardiovascular CT, cardiac MRI or invasive coronary angiography may be indicated (see Chapter 54).

53.3 SYNCOPE

BACKGROUND

- Syncope is a transient, self-limiting loss of consciousness with relatively rapid onset and spontaneous, complete recovery after a short time period.
  - Pre-syncope or 'near syncope' occurs when there are symptoms of a cerebral hypo-perfusion without a loss of consciousness.
  - The aetiology is diverse and may be caused by disturbances in homeostasis or neuronal-mediated reflexes, cardiovascular disease or arrhythmias, neurologic or psychiatric conditions, medications and a variety of metabolic disorders.
- A single episode of loss of consciousness, if associated with a clear precipitant (e.g. venepuncture or prolonged standing), and likely vasovagal in origin, should not lead to aircrew being restricted in their flying duties.
- Recurrent syncope is common, with almost a third of individuals having >1 episode. In aircrew, thorough investigation is mandated, and in some cases, tilt table and an implantable loop recorder (ILR) may be required.

AEROMEDICAL CONCERNS

- In an aviation context, a syncopal attack may lead to sudden incapacitation and loss of aircraft control whilst pre-syncope that causes distraction or incapacitation may also be potentially catastrophic.

- Therefore, loss or disturbances of consciousness, orthostatic or symptomatic hypotension, or recurrent vasodepressor syncope are all disqualifying for flying duties, if recurrent.
- If a clear precipitant is identified and the risk of recurrence is low and/or the underlying condition or triggering factor can adequately be controlled, return to restricted flying duties may be possible after a period of observation.

53.4 SINUS NODE DYSFUNCTION

- Sinus bradycardia and sinus arrhythmia are common findings in active people; they often normalize during exercise and are usually asymptomatic. In isolation they are compatible with unrestricted flying duties.
- In contrast, aircrew with syncope or pre-syncope caused by sinus bradycardia, sinus arrest or sino-atrial block should be grounded.

53.5 ATRIOVENTRICULAR CONDUCTION DISTURBANCE

- 1st-degree AV block in asymptomatic aircrew:
  - Can be regarded as a normal variant up to 250 ms.
  - Is common in young athletes.
  - If the PR interval exceeds 300 ms or is a new finding in aircrew >40 years of age, further investigation is recommended.
  - Most aircrew can remain flying.
- Mobitz type I (Wenkebach) is common and in most cases is an incidental finding in asymptomatic individuals.
  - Further examination is usually not required, and aircrew can fly unrestricted.
- Mobitz type II is rarely seen in aircrew and carries a risk of progression towards third degree (complete) AV block:
  - Aircrew with Mobitz type II and complete AV block must be investigated for underlying structural heart disease and are unfit for flying because of the risk of sudden cardiac death, syncope and bradycardia-related haemodynamic symptoms.
  - In most cases pacemaker therapy is indicated.
- Individuals with implanted pacemakers are primarily unfit for flying:
  - Restricted flying, with a second qualified pilot, may be acceptable if individuals are not pacemaker-dependent, have bipolar lead systems and have regular pacemaker follow-up.

53.6 RIGHT BUNDLE BRANCH BLOCK (RBBB)

- Incomplete RBBB is a very common finding in aircrew and seen in 2–3% of routine aircrew ECG; it can be regarded as a normal variant, and further investigation is not required.
- Complete RBBB should be investigated with an echocardiogram, an exercise ECG and Holter monitoring:
  - If an underlying disease can be excluded, aircrew may be assessed as fit, and flying restriction and follow-up is usually not necessary.
  - In aircrew aged >40 years, coronary artery assessment may also be considered.

53.7 LEFT BUNDLE BRANCH BLOCK (LBBB)

- LBBB is commonly associated with underlying structural heart disease.
  - Isolated LBBB in young people has a good prognosis; however, it can be a marker of coronary artery disease, hypertension, valve disease and cardiomyopathy, and therefore requires investigation in all aircrew.
- Aircrew with LBBB are unfit for flying until thorough cardiological evaluation has been completed:
  - If underlying heart disease can be excluded, return to unrestricted flying duties may be acceptable.
  - Many civil and military licencing authorities mandate an observation period and close follow-up with further (often annual) investigation.

53.8 ATRIAL ECTOPY

- Atrial ectopy (or premature atrial contractions [PAC]) is usually benign and does not require further investigation, or restrictions, for aircrew, as long as not associated with haemodynamic symptoms.
- If associated with symptoms or numerous, underlying heart disease should be excluded.
  - At higher PAC burden, there is concern regarding the development of atrial fibrillation (AF).
  - Therefore, aircrew with more than 5% PACs in a Holter registration should undergo further investigation and regular follow-up with echocardiogram, Holter and exercise ECG, and may be restricted in their flying duties.

53.9 VENTRICULAR ECTOPY (VE)/PREMATURE VENTRICULAR COMPLEXES (PVC)

- VE/PVCs are a common finding in aircrew.
- Single PVC on a 12-lead ECG is acceptable.
- Holter monitoring and additional investigation (exercise ECG and echocardiography) may be required if more than one single PVC or more complex forms are present.
- The ectopy burden on the 24-hr Holter determines the requirement for further specialist work-up.
  - If the VE burden is less than 2%, with less than 10 couplets and no evidence of sustained VT or complex ectopy, no further testing is usually required.
  - If the VE burden exceeds 2%, or complex forms are prevalent, further investigation may be required to exclude cardiomyopathy.
- In aircrew with higher ectopy burden (>2–5%), yearly follow-up with exercise ECG, echocardiography and Holter is recommended for the early detection of tachycardia-related cardiomyopathy. Most aircrew can continue to fly in an unrestricted capacity.
- In those with a VE burden >7.5%, many licencing authorities would restrict aircrew to multi-crew and low-performance aircraft.
  - However, there is no consensus on an upper limit of ectopy that requires disqualification, although if >10% and not suppressed by exercise, many licencing authorities would consider further restrictions.

53.10 SUPRAVENTRICULAR TACHYCARDIA

BACKGROUND

- Supraventricular tachycardia (SVT) consists of:
  - AV nodal re-entrant tachycardia (AVNRT).
  - AV re-entrant tachycardia (AVRT).
  - Atrial tachycardia.
- Requires extensive investigation in aircrew to exclude an underlying aetiology.
  - Information about alcohol or caffeine intake is important, because these agents may be provocative.

AEROMEDICAL CONCERNS

- Tachycardia usually starts suddenly and is usually symptomatic, with distracting symptoms, or haemodynamic symptoms being of significant concern in an aircrew population.
- SVT are initially disqualifying for aircrew and often require prolonged and intensive investigation and management.

MANAGEMENT

- Anti-arrhythmic drug therapy for SVT is unreliable and often associated with side effects that are incompatible with flying duties.
  - As a result, the therapy of choice for symptomatic SVT is often invasive EP testing and catheter ablation.
  - For most SVT, ablation has a success rate of >90%.
  - Depending on the aircraft type and role of aircrew, many can return to previous flying duties; however, with a 5–10% recurrence rate, those who fly high-performance aircraft, or on single seat platforms, may be restricted, even after clinically successful ablation.

53.11 ASYMPTOMATIC PRE-EXCITATION

- Wolfe-Parkinson-White (WPW) pattern on ECG is seen in up to 1% of healthy subjects.
- In contrast to WPW pattern, WPW syndrome requires evidence of tachyarrhythmia for appropriate diagnosis:
  - Only a very small proportion of those with WPW ECG (<2%) have arrhythmia.
- All aircrew with WPW pattern should initially be made unfit for flying and risk stratified:
  - Holter monitoring and Exercise ECG is usually sufficient, but an EP study may be required for single seat aircrew.
  - If the delta wave disappears during exercise, this is reassuring, and the situation can be deemed benign; however, if the delta wave does not disappear, an EP study is recommended.
- Aircrew with WPW syndrome require ablation if they wish to continue flying.
  - This is deemed curative in almost 100% of cases and has a very low risk of complications.

53.12 ATRIAL FIBRILLATION

BACKGROUND

- Atrial fibrillation (AF) is the most common type of cardiac arrhythmia seen in aircrew.
- It may be associated with valvular heart disease, CAD, cardiomyopathies, hypertension or thyroid disease.
  - Other potential causative factors include alcohol excess, smoking, excess caffeine intake, excessive physical activity, fatigue, exhaustion, sepsis, gastrointestinal and respiratory disease or drugs.
- Idiopathic AF (without an underlying aetiology):
  - May rarely occur as a single episode of arrhythmia.
  - Is often paroxysmal (PAF) (≤7 days), but may be persistent (>7 days).
  - In most cases, AF encountered in aircrew is paroxysmal, idiopathic and converts either spontaneously or by medical intervention within 24 hr.
  - A single idiopathic episode occasionally has a clearly identifiable cause, such as acute alcohol excess (so-called 'holiday heart syndrome').
- The investigation and management of AF in aircrew requires a comprehensive and integrated approach, as it may have a cardiac or non-cardiac aetiology; the underlying disease guides treatment.

AEROMEDICAL CONCERNS

- In aircrew, the risk of palpitations, dizziness, shortness of breath, pre-syncope, syncope, exercise intolerance and haemodynamic instability are all of concern.
  - The loss of atrial contribution to cardiac output, loss of atrioventricular synchrony and the rapid ventricular response during an episode may impair cardiac performance, especially during exertion, and can be acutely distracting or incapacitating.
- Aircrew diagnosed with AF are initially to be made unfit for flying.
  - Investigation into underlying causes (with echocardiography, Holter monitoring, exercise ECG and laboratory investigations) is required.

MANAGEMENT

- AF should be managed in accordance with international guidelines.
  - Potential side effects of medication used to restore or maintain sinus rhythm or to control ventricular rate make AF a difficult condition to manage in aircrew.
  - Most anti-arrhythmic drugs are incompatible with unrestricted flying.
  - β-blockers are often used for rate control, but the negative chronotropic effects and blunted blood pressure response on these agents significantly impairs +Gz tolerance and are not recommended in aircrew.
- AF catheter ablation is increasingly recommended as a first-line intervention in aircrew:
  - In PAF, success rates of more than 80% can be achieved. However, the long-term success rate in patients with persistent atrial fibrillation is only 40–60% after a single ablation.

- Within the post ablation observation period, the first 3 months are referred to as the 'blanking period', where procedure-related arrhythmias may occur, and an additional observation time of at least three months is necessary; follow-up investigations to determine the success of the procedure should not be undertaken in this 6-month period.
- For two months following ablation, aircrew should be on oral anticoagulation, regardless of thromboembolic risk scores, because ablation lesions are potentially thrombogenic.
- In both PAF and persistent AF, recurrences may occur years after ablation therapy, and as a result many licencing authorities do not allow a return to single seat flying operations or high-performance flying.
- A return to unrestricted flying is usually only possible after a single episode of atrial fibrillation without underlying disease.
    - In all other cases, restricted flying may be possible after a minimum observation period of 6 months, with extensive investigation to confirm stable sinus rhythm.

53.13 ATRIAL FLUTTER

AEROMEDICAL CONCERNS

- Atrial flutter may coexist with AF or occur in isolation.
- In most cases, atrial flutter is caused by similar underlying pathology to those causing AF with similar aeromedical concerns.
- An additional concern in atrial flutter is the potential for 1:1 AV conduction resulting in extreme tachycardia and acute incapacitation.
- Aircrew with atrial flutter should be grounded and require thorough cardiac and non-cardiac evaluation.

MANAGEMENT

- Anti-arrhythmic medication is only moderately effective and not appropriate for aircrew.
- Catheter ablation is usually the first-line therapy and has success rates of more than 90%. AF recurrence can occur years after the ablation, as can AF.
- Due to the arrhythmogenic +Gz environment, single seat and flying high-performance aircraft is not generally recommended following flutter ablation.
- In selected cases, consideration of a diagnostic EP study to reconfirm bidirectional isthmus block would be recommended if considering a more lenient approach.

53.14 NON-SUSTAINED AND SUSTAINED VENTRICULAR TACHYCARDIAS

BACKGROUND

- Non-sustained ventricular tachycardia (NSVT) usually defined as VT with a duration of less than 30 seconds.
- It may be idiopathic or secondary to conditions such as structural, coronary or heart muscle disease, or ion channelopathies.

AEROMEDICAL CONCERNS

- NSVT for nearly 30 seconds would potentially be catastrophic in an aviation context.
- As a result, the threshold for defining significant VT in aviation cardiology is stricter than civilian guidelines.
    - A cut-off of 11 beats of VT and no more than 4 runs of NSVT in a standard stage IV Bruce Protocol is often used.
- Aeromedical concerns include the presence of haemodynamic symptoms such as pre-syncope or syncope and chest pain, and the risk of acute incapacitation or sudden cardiac death and distraction in the critical phases of flight.
- Aircrew with significant underlying structural or cardiac disease or symptoms are unfit for flying.

MANAGEMENT

- Usual treatment options for symptomatic NSVT, such as β-blockers and calcium channel blockers, are incompatible with many flying roles.
- In aircrew, both RVOT and LVOT VT are usually amenable to ablation and should be considered as a first-line therapy.
    - After successful catheter ablation and a period of observation, return to flying duties may be considered.
- Individuals with primary or secondary ventricular fibrillation are permanently unfit for flying.

53.15 INHERITED ARRHYTHMOGENIC CONDITIONS (CHANNELOPATHIES)

- Aircrew with inherited arrhythmogenic disorders, including long QT syndrome (LQTS) or Brugada syndrome (BrS), are usually unfit for flying.
- Channelopathies are rare, but LQTS and BrS cases predominate in the aviation medicine literature.
- Risk stratification should be performed in specialist centres using international guidelines and can be very challenging.
    - Crucial factors include medical and family history and genetic testing.
    - High-risk patients usually need ICD implantation and are permanently unfit for flying.
    - However, after careful risk stratification; restricted flying might be possible in asymptomatic, lower risk individuals on a case-by-case basis.

BRUGADA SYNDROME (BrS)

- There are three recognized BrS morphology types.
- Type I:
    - Associated with the highest risk of arrhythmia and sudden cardiac death.
    - Symptomatic patients are unfit for flying and are usually treated with an ICD.
    - In asymptomatic aircrew, aircrew with spontaneous type 1 BrS ECG should be grounded.
- Type II and Type III may be compatible with restricted flying duties.

LONG QT SYNDROME (LQTS)

- LQTS can be diagnosed in the absence of a secondary cause for QT prolongation and/or in the presence of:
  - An unequivocally pathogenic mutation in one of the LQTS genes.
  - The presence of a QT interval corrected for heart rate (using Bazett's formula) of (QTc) ≥500 ms in repeated 12-lead ECGs.
- Risk in asymptomatic patients depends on types of genetic mutation.
  - Patients with a QTc >500 ms can be regarded as high risk, and those with a QTc >600 ms as very high risk.
  - For aircrew, a QTc of 470 ms, for asymptomatic individuals, is often used as the cut-off for restrictions to flying.

CHAPTER 54

Cardiac investigations

Contents

54.1 BACKGROUND

- Aircrew who are found to have potential cardiovascular disease are usually required to undergo comprehensive cardiovascular assessment.
- First-line investigations, usually conducted at periodic medical examinations (PME), include:
  - 12-lead ECG.
  - Blood pressure assessment.
  - Investigations of lipid profile.
- If abnormal, referral for second level investigations may be required, often in conjunction with a clinical assessment by an aviation trained specialist; these investigations will depend on the suspected underlying diagnosis but may include echocardiography, exercise ECG/ tolerance testing, 24-hr blood pressure and/or extended ECG (Holter) monitoring.
- Further specialist investigations, such as anatomic imaging with cardiovascular CT (including CT coronary angiography) or cardiovascular MRI; physiological assessment with nuclear, exercise/stress echocardiography, perfusion MRI, or functional flow reserve (FFR) on CT or invasive angiography; or specialist electrophysiological (EP) investigations (loop recorder, ajmaline/adenosine challenge, etc.) may also be required in certain circumstances.

54.2 ELECTROCARDIOGRAPH (ECG)

- The 12-lead ECG is used to highlight underlying cardiovascular disease in aircrew.
- It is cheap and easy to perform.

- It is a good investigation to highlight rhythm abnormalities and may identify those with underlying structural heart disease.
- It is less sensitive for the detection of coronary artery disease.

Aircrew ECG findings that are seen in young individuals with high vagal tone, that do not require additional follow-up, and are acceptable for unrestricted flying, include partial right bundle branch block, 1st-degree heart block (up to 250 ms), mild Wenckebach (2nd degree heart block – Mobitz Type 1) and single premature ventricular complexes (PVC) – see Chapter 53.

Aircrew ECG findings requiring further investigation include T wave inversion, ST segment flattening or depression, new bundle branch block, multiple ectopic beats, atrial tachycardia, delta waves (in Wolff-Parkinson-White) and Brugada phenotypes – see Chapter 53.

54.3 SECOND-LINE INVESTIGATIONS

TRANSTHORACIC ECHOCARDIOGRAPHY (TTE)

- Myocardial functional assessment with TTE should include both global assessment of left ventricular function and regional wall motion assessment.
- To be acceptable, the ejection fraction should be >50% and there should be no evidence of regional wall motion abnormality (RWMA).
- Valvular assessment should include full visualisation of all four valves and include accurate quantification of any stenotic or regurgitant lesions.
- There should be no evidence of additional structural cardiac disease.
- Mild to moderate regurgitation may be acceptable, but even mild stenotic valve disease may be a bar to flying in certain circumstances.

EXERCISE ECG/EXERCISE TOLERANCE TEST (ExECG/ETT)

ExECG/ETT may be performed in a number of scenarios, including assessment of suspected CAD, arrhythmia and global cardiovascular fitness.

- Aircrew must achieve 9 minutes of the Bruce protocol on the treadmill to be diagnostic.
  - This is the minimum standard for enhanced cardiovascular screening in military aircrew to determine a suitable physiological reserve for flying.
- Aircrew should be encouraged to continue until symptomatic (i.e. fatigued, breathless or chest pain).
  - To be deemed acceptable, there should be no ECG changes (ST changes, T wave inversion, bundle branch block, arrhythmia, etc.) and the patient should be free from angina symptoms.
- The main limitation of ETT is its lack of sensitivity and specificity for the detection of significant CAD and results in a high number of false positive tests in aircrew with a low pre-test probability of significant CAD.
  - Positive tests may determine the need for angiography (either CT or invasive) or functional testing depending on the clinical scenario.
- If the ExECG is performed as part of an assessment following coronary intervention, the ETT must be performed off all anti-anginal medication (including beta-blockers even if for treatment of BP, etc.).

- Suppression of arrhythmias on exercise is usually a reassuring finding; the unmasking of others may suggest underlying CAD.
  - In aircrew with extreme resting bradycardia or heart block, appropriate physiological response to exercise can be used to exclude pathologic conduction defects.

EXTENDED HOLTER ECG

- 24-hr Holter monitoring may be required in patients with palpitation or in those with abnormal 12-lead ECG findings.
- Aircrew should be free of significant arrhythmia during all usual activities performed when the tape is fitted.
- Assessment of both underlying rhythm and burden of arrhythmias such as ectopy are important in determining the suitability of aircrew in return to flying duties.
- In individuals with less common symptoms or in whom a greater degree of certainty of potential arrhythmia identification/burden is required, extended Holter assessment (up to 7 days) is possible.
- In those with rare but potentially concerning symptoms, a 2–4 week patient activated recorder (such as King of Hearts or RTest4) can be used, or a subcutaneous reveal device if longer duration assessment is required.

54.4 SPECIALIST CORONARY ANATOMY INVESTIGATIONS

CT CORONARY ANGIOGRAPHY AND CORONARY ARTERY CALCIUM SCORING

Coronary artery calcium scoring (CACS) may be used as a surrogate marker for coronary atheroma. It is often undertaken as part of a full CT coronary angiogram (CTCA) examination.

- Zero is the only normal coronary calcium score.
- Coronary calcium is thought to represent approximately one-fifth of coronary atheroma.
- Low coronary calcium scores (1–10) are often compatible with unrestricted flying but may require further assessment with either an ETT or CTCA to determine suitability.
- Higher coronary calcium scores may preclude single seat flying.
  - The US Air Force threshold for non-waiverable disease is >10.
  - The UK civilian cut-off for further functional investigation for aircrew (MPS, pCMR or DSE) is a CACS >100.

CTCA provides a comprehensive non-invasive assessment of the coronary vasculature with a near 100% negative predictive value. It may be used as a second-line test in patients with low to intermediate pre-test probability of significant CAD with a positive or an equivocal ExECG/ETT.

- Using modern CT scanners, the radiation dose for CTCA in aircrew is often less than 1 mSv.
- The spatial resolution of CTCA is less good than invasive angiography, so calculation as to the exact degree of stenosis should not be performed on CTCA.
- If the CACS is previously known to be >400, CTCA is not recommended in aircrew.

INVASIVE CORONARY ANGIOGRAPHY (ICA)

- Invasive coronary angiography is still regarded by many as the gold standard for anatomical assessment of the coronary arteries.
- If other non-invasive tests are abnormal, it may be warranted in the assessment of aircrew.
- The risk of death from ICA is approximately 1/1,000; however, vascular damage (both coronary dissection and arterial access damage) may be significantly higher.
- It is therefore often difficult to justify ICA investigation for pure occupational assessment and should be discussed fully with aircrew to ensure appropriate consent is undertaken.

54.5 SPECIALIST MYOCARDIAL PERFUSION IMAGING

- Myocardial perfusion scintigraphy (MPS) has been the gold standard myocardial perfusion test for many years.
- Limited by its radiation dose, especially in younger aircrew and those who require serial follow-up.
- Perfusion cardiac MRI (pCMR) and exercise or dobutamine stress echocardiography (Ex echo/DSE) are suitable alternatives to MPS and do not involve ionizing radiation.
- Regional wall motion abnormalities and assessment of hibernating myocardium can be assessed using appropriate protocols.

Regardless of the type of perfusion imaging undertaken, there must be no evidence of reversible ischaemia to be acceptable. For cases with suspicion of reversible ischaemia or silent infarction (as determined by fixed perfusion defects), further anatomical or functional correlates are required to fully risk assess the patient.

CARDIAC MRI (CMR)

- CMR does not involve ionizing radiation, but is contraindicated in patients with metallic implants.
- It is the gold standard for the assessment of suspected cardiomyopathy and allows complete visualisation of the right heart.
- In patients with prior IHD, it is able to accurately delineate areas of partial and full thickness infarction using late gadolinium enhancement (LGE).
- It is also able to distinguish myocarditis from myocardial infarction.
- CMR can be used to determine the prognosis of several cardiovascular pathologies, including LGE and oedema assessment with CMR to determine the potential for arrhythmogenesis, the extent of infarction and severity/prognosis of cardiomyopathy.

CHAPTER 55

Respiratory disease

Contents

55.1 PASSENGER FITNESS TO FLY ASSESSMENT

BACKGROUND

- In passengers with lung disease, the following assessment is recommended:
  - History and examination with particular reference to cardiorespiratory disease, dyspnoea and previous flying experience.
  - Spirometric tests.
  - Measurement of O_2 saturation by pulse oximetry. Blood gas values are preferred if hypercapnia is known or suspected.

HYPOXIC CHALLENGE TEST

- In those with resting oximetry between 92 and 95% at sea level, hypoxic challenge testing can be performed.
- The hypoxic challenge test consists of breathing 15% fraction of inspired oxygen (FI_{O2}) for 20 minutes with blood gas measurements being taken directly after.
  - PA_{O2} > 6.6 kPa (>50 mmHg): oxygen not required.
  - PA_{O2} < 6.6 kPa (<50 mmHg): in-flight oxygen (2 l/min).

- Often, the PA_{O_2} will be measured on 2 litres O_2 in order to ascertain whether a satisfactory improvement has occurred.

SUPPLEMENTARY OXYGEN

- If the person's resting oximetry at sea level is less than 92%, then supplementary oxygen will be required. If the person is on supplementary oxygen at sea level, then the flow rate will have to be increased during flight.
- Patients are usually unable to use their own oxygen cylinders on the flight unless agreed in advance by the airline, and any oxygen that is required will have to be booked well in advance with the airline.
- Oxygen usually can be provided only in flow rates of 2 l/min or 4 l/min via nasal cannulae and often in a breath-activated manner; therefore, if higher concentrations are required, the patient's fitness to fly should be put in doubt.
- In an extreme emergency, higher flow rates are possible but may require a medical escort.
- Portable oxygen concentrators are increasingly allowed on commercial flights:
  - There are a number that have been tested for air worthiness and it is important to check with the airline as to allowed devices, as the list is currently increasing.
  - Note should be made to carry sufficient batteries for the whole flight, and chargers for recharging for the return flight.
  - Power supply for concentrators may be available on some airlines and cabins with sufficient prior knowledge.
- Other general considerations for passengers with lung disease should include:
  - Travelling within the airport and on to the aircraft due to potential long distances in modern airports between check-in and gates.
  - A letter from a doctor may be required if carrying controlled medications, needles, syringes or any trial drugs that are not specifically labelled.
- National guidance and recommendations may be available for air travellers.

55.2 AIRWAY DISEASES (ASTHMA & CHRONIC OBSTRUCTIVE PULMONARY DISEASE)

PASSENGERS

- Theoretical risk is of bronchospasm secondary to bronchial mucosal water loss due to relatively low cabin humidity.
- No studies, however, have shown an increased physiological risk for airway disease passengers in flight.
- Passengers should carry preventive and relieving inhalers in their hand luggage.
- Portable nebulizers may be used at the discretion of cabin crew.
- Some airlines can provide nebulizers for in-flight use, and patients should check with the carrier when booking.
- It is important to stress that spacers are as effective as a nebulizer.
- Patients with frequent attacks or recurrent infections should discuss with their doctor to consider a rescue pack of prednisolone and antibiotics.

AIRCREW AND ATCOs

- For pilots and ATCOs, the risks to aviation include:
  - Sudden incapacitation.
  - Subtle incapacitation.
  - Susceptibility to aircraft fumes or smoke.
  - Hypoxaemia.
- A pilot or ATCO with asthma or a history of asthma may be assessed as fit depending on the severity of their disease and the stability; features of a pilot or ATCO's history that may prevent issuance of a medical certificate include:
  - Severe asthma likely to reduce operational efficiency.
  - Brittle asthmatics.
  - Repeated courses of oral steroids.
  - Poor control on inhaled corticosteroids.
  - Hospital/emergency room attendance.
  - Frequent exacerbations.
  - Those requiring unacceptable medication such as oral steroids or steroid sparing agents.
- Standard spirometry, and in some cases bronchial reactivity tests, will be required.
- Inhaled β2 agonists, inhaled corticosteroids, long-acting β2 agonists, leukotriene receptor antagonists and inhaled cromoglicate are likely to be acceptable.
- For pilots with COPD, only minor impairment is likely to be acceptable.

55.3 SARCOIDOSIS

- For passengers, an assessment of their resting oxygen state is required and a hypoxic challenge test may be performed, and the results interpreted as per the previously stated recommendations.
- Pilots and ATCOs with active sarcoidosis should be assessed as unfit.
  - Before returning to duty, investigation should be undertaken to look for systemic, particularly cardiac, involvement.
  - If the disease is shown to be limited to hilar lymphadenopathy and is inactive and no medication is required, then the pilots and ATCOs may be assessed as fit.
  - Pilots and ATCOs with cardiac sarcoid should be assessed as unfit.

55.4 PNEUMOTHORAX

PASSENGERS AND PATIENTS

- A patient with a current closed pneumothorax should not travel on commercial flights. The patient may be able to fly 1 week after a definitive surgical intervention and resolution of the pneumothorax.
- A patient who has not had surgery must have had a CXR confirming resolution, and at least one week must have elapsed following resolution before travel.
- Following traumatic pneumothorax, a patient is fit to travel 2 weeks after resolution on CXR.

- Following a spontaneous pneumothorax, pilots and ATCOs should not fly or control.
- Restricted flying may be permitted around 2 months after a full recovery from a single spontaneous pneumothorax, but unrestricted flying may require a year after full recovery and without a recurrence.
- Where a recurrent pneumothorax has occurred, a return to flying may be permitted following surgical intervention with a satisfactory recovery.
- Flying will not usually be permitted following a recurrent spontaneous pneumothorax that has not been surgically treated.
- A fit assessment following full recovery from a traumatic pneumothorax as a result of an accident or injury may be acceptable once full absorption of the pneumothorax is demonstrated.
- Acceptable surgical treatment includes thoracotomy, oversewing of apical blebs, parietal pleurectomy and video-assisted thoracic surgery (VATS) pleurectomy.
- Recertification can be undertaken 6 weeks after a VATS pleurectomy. For other procedures, recertification may require a longer grounding period.

55.5 OBSTRUCTIVE SLEEP APNOEA

PASSENGERS

- The condition is usually diagnosed by symptoms and confirmed through sleep studies.
- Passengers may require a letter from their doctor outlining the medical diagnosis and stating that the continuous positive airways pressure (CPAP) machine should travel in the cabin as extra hand luggage.
- Long-haul flight passengers should consider using their CPAP machine.
- The majority of patients will not require CPAP during short flights.
- Battery-powered CPAP machines can be used during the flight but must be switched off before landing.
- Patients should avoid drinking alcohol before and during the flight.
- Patients with significant OSA should use CPAP when visiting high-altitude destinations.

AIRCREW AND ATCOs

- Pilots and ATCOs are likely to be assessed as unfit following diagnosis.
- They should have their OSA sufficiently managed before they continue to exercise their licence privileges.
- If CPAP is used, then a minimum period of use per night and number of nights to be used per week may need to be stipulated.
- It should be used during the sleep period just prior to flight.
- There should be a period of stable use of CPAP prior to a return to duties.
- Cardiovascular risk should also be considered.

55.6 PULMONARY TUBERCULOSIS

- Patients with infectious TB must not travel by public air transportation until they have had a minimum of 14 days treatment and are non-infectious (three smear-negative sputum examinations on separate days).

- Pilots and ATCOs will not be able to exercise the privileges of their licences with active disease.

55.7 PULMONARY THROMBOEMBOLIC DISEASE

PASSENGERS

- All patients with recent pulmonary thromboembolic disease should seek specialist assessment before flying.
- Those with previous pulmonary thromboembolic disease when flying should avoid alcohol- and caffeine-containing drinks, take only short periods of sleep unless they can attain their normal sleeping position and avoid the use of sleeping pills.
- Graduating compression stockings are recommended for those patients not on anticoagulant treatment.
- Patients with recurrent pulmonary thromboembolic disease should use prophylactic subcutaneous low-molecular-weight heparin or DOAC, especially if the flight is greater than 8 hr.

AIRCREW AND ATCOs

- For pilots and ATCOs, screening should have been undertaken for underlying causes, including coagulation abnormalities.
- Those permitted to take warfarin will be required to maintain their INR within a tight target range.
- They should demonstrate stability for a number of months with regular ongoing testing. This may include preflight home testing.
- In all cases of pulmonary embolism, undertake follow-up reviews with a specialist physician.
- Medical certification is possible provided that there is a full recovery and the total incapacitation risk of the medication, the pulmonary thromboembolic disease and any other underlying conditions is acceptable.

CHAPTER 56

Gastroenterology

Contents

56.1 GI PHYSIOLOGY IN THE AVIATION ENVIRONMENT

- GI physiology is affected by:
    - Altitude (change in gas volume leading to increased flatus).
    - Hypoxia and sustained acceleration (decreased gastric emptying and acid secretion).
    - Vibration (increased urge to defecate).
- In normal subjects, these changes usually of little clinical relevance but may affect those with chronic GI conditions.

56.2 AVIATION GASTROENTEROLOGY

- Globally, the most common cause of in-flight incapacitation is acute GI disease; however, this is usually mild in nature and self-limiting.
- Most gastroenterological (GI) disease has no long-term implications for aircrew.
- Many common GI conditions remain compatible with both flying duties, either unrestricted or with some limitations, dependent on risk of relapse and consequence.
- Chronic GI complaints, such as inflammatory bowel disease (IBD), have a relapsing nature and can be unpredictable; specialist advice usually required, but with increasing medical advances, aircrew can often continue to undertake (limited) flight duties.

56.3 GASTRO-OESOPHAGEAL REFLUX AND PEPTIC ULCER DISEASE (GORD/PUD)

- Gastro-oesophageal reflex disease (GORD):
  - Is common.
  - May be affected by the aircrew environment (but no evidence that sustained acceleration or pressure breathing affects symptoms).
  - Is usually easily managed in aircrew with standard lifestyle advice and proton pump inhibitors (PPI), which are safe in aircrew and do not require restrictions.
- Peptic ulcer disease (PUD):
  - Has fallen significantly in prevalence in the era of *H. pylori* eradication therapy and PPI treatment.
  - Endoscopy is mandated in aircrew with symptoms of concern.
  - Aircrew should be fully treated and grounded until the ulcer has healed and this has been confirmed by repeat endoscopy (both gastric and duodenal).
  - Ongoing restrictions may be required (for a limited period) in some cases (such as perforation), depending on aircrew role and likelihood of relapse.

56.4 COELIAC DISEASE

- This gluten enteropathy often presents with diarrhoea, weight loss, anaemia and non-specific abdominal pain.
- Confirmatory diagnosis:
  - Requires both tissue trans-glutaminase (TTG) antibody detection and if positive, subsequent duodenal biopsy.
  - Not all patients are TTG positive, and duodenal biopsy should be considered in individuals if clinical suspicion is high.
  - Biopsy results give useful information about the severity of disease (which is variable).
- Following diagnosis, strict adherence to a gluten-free diet is important due to the longer-term risk of small bowel lymphoma and renal failure.
- Aircrew with systemic manifestations (anaemia, folate deficiency) should be grounded and only return to flying on satisfactory correction of these abnormalities.
- Those with symptoms alone may return to flying when established on a gluten-free diet; this may not be possible in a military operational environment.

56.5 INFLAMMATORY BOWEL DISEASE (IBD)

- Crohn's disease and ulcerative colitis (UC) are remitting/relapsing conditions that have a significant burden on lifestyle and predominantly are diagnosed in younger people (10–40 years).
- Symptoms may include abdominal pain, fatigue, diarrhoea and rectal bleeding.
- Response to medical therapy is highly individual, with high relapse rates, and this makes risk assessment in aircrew challenging.
- It is likely that a period of many months will be required after apparent remission is achieved before a return to flying is permitted due to the risk of relapse.

ULCERATIVE COLITIS

- UC affects the colon, from the rectum, and extends proximally.
- It may present with acute colitis, occasionally requiring surgical resection, but most disease can be managed pharmacologically.
- Diagnosis is confirmed by mucosal inflammation on biopsy, but there is a broad differential, including Crohn's disease and infective colitis.
- If UC of mild to moderate severity, treatment is usually with oral/topical 5-aminosalicylic acid (5-ASA), whilst for more severe disease, steroid treatment or azathioprine may be required. Increasingly patients are treated with anti-TNF monoclonal antibodies (Mab).
- On diagnosis, aircrew with UC:
  - Should be grounded until in remission on maintenance therapy.
  - Those with mild disease, treated and stable on oral/topical 5-aminosalicylic acid (5-ASA), may be able to return to unrestricted flying duties.
  - Those maintained on anti-TNF monoclonal antibodies (Mab), steroids or azathioprine may be able to return to restricted flying duties.
  - However, those with more extensive and relapsing disease are unlikely to be able to return to flying duties.

CROHN'S DISEASE

- Crohn's is a multisystem disorder that may affect any part of the GI tract but most commonly affects the distal ileum. It is associated with anaemia, arthritis, uveitis, dermatological manifestations and sclerosing cholangitis.
- In the GI tract, Crohn's is frequently associated with fistulae, abscess formation, intestinal strictures and perianal disease.
- The clinical manifestations of Crohn's and high recurrence rates result in permanent grounding for most aircrew.
  - A return to restricted aircrew duties may be possible in those few cases with long-term remission confirmed by endoscopy.

56.6 GALLSTONE DISEASE AND PANCREATITIS

- Gallstone disease:
  - Is usually an incidental finding.
  - Is of concern in aircrew if associated with biliary colic, which may be acutely incapacitating.
  - Even if asymptomatic, the chance finding of multiple gallstones may require restrictions for aircrew.
  - Aircrew with colic and multiple small gallstones should be grounded until a cholecystectomy is performed and radiological confirmation of a clear bile duct confirmed.
- Acute pancreatitis:
  - Is a life-threatening condition that causes incapacitating abdominal pain.
  - Has diverse aetiology but most commonly associated with alcohol and gallstones.

- Gallstone pancreatitis requires a cholecystectomy in aircrew but unrestricted flying is often possible thereafter.
- Other causes of pancreatitis usually require flying restrictions and recurrent pancreatitis is usually incompatible with flying duties.

56.7 LIVER DISORDERS

- Aeromedical concern with regards to liver disease is usually related to the severity of symptoms.
  - Aircrew with raised ALT/AST should be investigated, and this includes liver ultrasound, blood tests to include viral, autoimmune and inherited liver disease and an alcohol questionnaire.
- Vital hepatitis:
  - The majority of acute viral hepatitis will not result in long-term flying restrictions but may require temporary downgrading during the acute illness.
  - Chronic viral hepatitis is of more concern, as it may be related to cirrhosis and hepatocellular carcinoma and is associated with acute exacerbations.
  - Antiviral therapy, such as interferon, requires close monitoring due to side effects, and aircrew are often restricted for a period of time following their initiation.
- Autoimmune and inherited liver diseases are uncommon in aircrew, and flying restrictions are often required for patients requiring treatment.
- Venesection (e.g. for haemochromatosis) is compatible with unrestricted flying duties, but aircrew should be grounded for 48 hr afterwards.
- Liver transplantation: Depending on the underlying causes, it may be possible to consider commercial pilots and ATCOs who have undergone liver transplantation for medical certification after careful consideration of the underlying causes, progress post-operatively, medication, monitoring for the various forms of transplant rejection and long-term complications such as post-transplant lymphoproliferative disease.

CHAPTER 57

Metabolic and endocrine disorders

Contents

57.1 BACKGROUND

- The endocrine system is involved in all aspects of an aviator's performance in the cockpit. Manifestations of its disruption range from sudden incapacitation to subtle performance degradation of flight status over many years.
- Evaluation of normal function is readily performed with history, physical examination and access to fundamental tests with skill in their interpretation.
- Early recognition of disruption is paramount, and restoration of normal function can be readily achieved in virtually all cases.

57.2 DIABETES AND GLYCAEMIC DYSREGULATION

GLYCAEMIC DYSREGULATION

- Any disruption in normal accepted levels of plasma glucose can be called glycaemic dysregulation:

- Early recognition of glycaemic dysregulation and correct classification by type and cause are important for the management of the disease, as well as mitigating short- and long-term effects.
- Any condition, drug or disease state affecting the normal function of the pancreas, liver, kidneys, peripheral tissues or glucose receptors can result in glycaemic dysregulation with hyper- or hypoglycaemia.
- The acute effects of hypoglycaemia are a significant concern in the aviation environment.
- Evaluation of the aviator with glycaemic dysregulation must include recognition of symptoms from hyperglycaemia and (treatment related) hypoglycaemia, and surveillance for both short- and long-term complications of disease and treatment (e.g. cardiovascular, renal, neurological and ophthalmological).

DIABETES MELLITUS

- Most common form of hyperglycaemia.
- Best demonstrated by an elevated fasting glucose level or haemoglobin A1C concentration.
- Diabetes treatment:
    - Dependent on correct classification of type (Type 1 or Type 2) and severity.
    - Usually consists of the use of diet, oral medications, injectable insulin or its analogues, or other synergistic agents.
    - Acceptable medications include those that do not cause hypoglycaemia such as metformin.
    - Newer drugs such as glinides, glitazones and gliptins may require multi-crew limitations.
    - Drugs such as sulphonureas, that may cause hypoglycaemia, may be incompatible with certain flying roles.
    - In some countries, regulators have developed protocols that enable the medical certification of pilots who require insulin therapy; this can involve pre- and in-flight testing of blood sugar.
    - Protocols are dependent on control of blood glucose within tight limits and assessing the risk of hypo- and hyperglycaemia.

57.3 THYROID

- Restoration of normal levels of thyroid hormone is easily accomplished in the clinical setting.
- Pilots and controllers likely to be assessed as unfit when diagnosed and reassessed when euthyroid and on stable doses of medication (where it is required).

HYPERTHYROIDISM

- Typically manifests with palpitations, feeling hot, night sweats, anxiety, visual disturbances, insomnia and weight loss. The thyroid may feel enlarged.
- Treatment rests on determination of whether the cause is autoimmune or inflammatory:
    - For autoimmune causes, treatment is with anti-thyroid drugs and perhaps beta-blockade during the acute high-level phase.
- Causes include:
    - Graves' disease (autoimmune stimulation of the thyroid).

- Toxic nodular goitre.
- Solitary toxic thyroid nodule.
- Thyroiditis (infection or inflammation of the thyroid, usually temporary).
- Treatment usually lasts for 18 months, after which there is a 60% chance of resolution.
  - For repeat presentation, definitive treatment with radioactive iodine or surgery is recommended.
- Return to unrestricted duties sometimes possible when euthyroid (restricted duties if taking thyroid suppressants); lifelong monitoring required.

HYPOTHYROIDISM

- Causes include autoimmune thyroid disease (Hashimoto's thyroiditis), radioactive iodine or surgery, medicines (e.g. lithium) or secondary to hypopituitarism (rare).
- Typically manifests with fatigue, feeling cold, hypersomnia, low mood, dry skin and hair, weight gain.
- Treatment is replacement with thyroxine (either T4, T3 or combination); monitoring of levels and TSH to tailor dose to normal range, with return to flying/controlling when euthyroid; indefinite monitoring required.

57.4 PARATHYROID

- Parathyroid hormone regulates calcium, which is vital for most controlling systems in physiology:
  - Calcium levels determined by dietary intake, vitamin D status.
  - Fine control conducted by parathyroid hormone release from the parathyroids.
- Pilots and controllers are likely to be assessed as unfit at diagnosis of parathyroid disorder.
- Aeromedical certification depends on underlying causes and success of management; good cooperation between endocrinologist and aviation physician essential.

HYPERPARATHYROIDISM

- Symptoms are due to hypercalcaemia (renal stones/colic, hypertension, peptic ulcer disease, depression, abdominal pain).
- Diagnosis confirmed by having a high corrected calcium in the presence of measurable or high parathyroid hormone levels:
  - This excludes other common causes of hypercalcaemia (malignancy).
- Treatment is indicated if calcium levels rise to certain thresholds.
- Localisation with MIBI or ultrasound scan of potential parathyroid adenoma is conducted followed by surgical removal.

HYPOPARATHYROIDISM

- Due either to lack of parathyroid activity or secondary to thyroid surgery or neck radiation.
- Symptoms are due to critically low calcium levels and include muscles spasm, cramps and weakness.
- The most important sign is for cramps and tetany, particularly in response to blood pressure; assessment with a sphygmomanometer that precipitates muscle contraction when inflated.

- Diagnosis is made with a low parathyroid hormone in the presence of a low calcium.
- Treatment is with vitamin D replacement.

57.5 PITUITARY DISORDERS

- Conditions of the pituitary gland can be acute and catastrophic or asymptomatic, or subtle and asymptomatic; could present as 'jet lag' or fatigue in aviators, or as sudden collapse.
    - Incidental benign masses of the pituitary are found in approximately 10% of the general population.
- Pilots and controllers are likely to be assessed as unfit at diagnosis.
- Aeromedical certification depends on underlying causes and success of management; military flying may not be possible.

PITUITARY TUMOURS

- Pituitary tumours can cause three types of problems:
    - Hyper-secretion (too much of any of the pituitary hormones).
    - Hypo-secretion (too little secretion of the hormone, usually caused by a large pituitary tumour which interferes with the other normal pituitary).
    - Mass effect due to pituitary tumour pressing on neighbouring brain structures within the close confines of the cranium.
- Occasionally pituitary adenomas can infarct, producing a syndrome called apoplexy, where there is a sudden headache, visual disturbance and loss of pituitary function.
- Microprolactinoma may cause suppression of the production of testosterone in a male aviator and chronic symptoms of depression, fatigue and impaired physical performance.
- Other masses may cause under- or overproduction of hormone by direct or indirect effect.
- The pituitary, although protected both within its own bony pituitary fossa and set within the cranium, is also susceptible to damage from major head trauma.
- If pituitary surgery has been undertaken to remove pituitary tumours, hypopituitarism may develop and will be treated by individual hormone replacement of all of the pituitary axis.

TREATMENT

- Treatment may involve either observation, medication to control or restore normal endocrine function, surgery or radiation therapy.
- Replacement therapy for hypopituitarism may be acceptable in the civil setting but unlikely in military service due to reliability of medication supply and impact of intercurrent illness.
- Acromegaly causing gross physical changes unlikely to be fit even after successful trans-sphenoidal microdissection; specialist endocrinological and ophthalmic review required.
- Hyperprolactinaemia treated by surgery or long-term medication (except bromocriptine) may be compatible with return to civil flying.

57.6 GONADAL DISORDERS

- Disorders of gonadal function are common.
- Physical and cognitive effects on the male aviator can affect performance in the cockpit.
- Imaging is directed by the pattern established by biochemical testing; central causes require imaging of the brain and pituitary, whereas primary testicular failure requires imaging of the scrotum.
- The deficiency of testosterone in the male aviator is subtle at first but can cause depression, impaired concentration and impaired physical performance if unrecognized.
- Restoration of sex hormone concentration depends on gender:
  - In the male patient, age, risk factors and the desire for fertility determine the approach to therapy.
  - The deficiency of oestrogen and progesterone will cause symptoms that are commonly recognized as menopause in the female aviator and unlikely to affect performance in the cockpit.

57.7 ADRENAL

- The adrenal glands mainly produce aldosterone, cortisol, epinephrine, norepinephrine and dehydroepiandrosterone.
- Conditions causing an over- or underproduction of these hormones lead to a spectrum of clinical presentations ranging from secondary hypertension, psychological disturbance, weight loss/gain, diabetes, bone mineral density disorders, haemodynamic collapse.

CUSHING'S SYNDROME

- Cushing's syndrome is caused by an overproduction of cortisol:
  - Can either be due to an adenoma in the cortex of the adrenal glands or by overstimulation from an ACTH-secreting pituitary tumour.
- Treatment is with excision of either the adrenal or pituitary adenoma.
- Occasionally bilateral adrenal removal is necessary to treat pituitary lesions that are unable to be removed; radiotherapy also used to reduce pituitary ACTH output if surgery unsuccessful.
- Excessive use of steroids for medical purposes can also lead to a syndrome of cortisol excess, but such treatment is usually disqualifying for flying or controlling.
- Aeromedical disposition highly individualised depending on lesion and treatment.

ADRENAL INSUFFICIENCY

- Adrenal insufficiency occurs when the adrenal glands do not make enough hydrocortisone and aldosterone.
- Causes include Addison's disease (an autoimmune destruction of the adrenal glands) and malignancy, usually due to infiltration of the adrenal gland.
- Treatment is with replacement of adrenal hormones:
  - Hydrocortisone used to replace cortisol within the body, requiring approximately 20–30 mg a day in divided doses to mimic the diurnal variation, with high levels in the morning and less at night.

- Aldosterone is replaced with long-acting fluorinated compound fludrocortisone that is a very potent mineralocorticoid.
- Return to civilian multi-crew flying may be considered on stable maintenance therapy; military flying unlikely to be acceptable.

PHAEOCHROMOCYTOMA

- Phaeochromocytoma is a rare neuroendocrine tumour of the adrenal medulla and can produce high levels of adrenaline and noradrenaline, which produce volatile and high blood pressure.
- If tumour completely removed, blood pressure control satisfactory, and no significant end-organ damage, then return to civilian multi-crew licence may be possible on case-by-case basis.

57.8 OBESITY

- Obesity is epidemic, and its adverse effects on overall health are important.
- Hypertension, cardiovascular disease, obstructive sleep apnoea, diabetes and orthopaedic problems all have potential significant aeromedical concerns and should be investigated.
- Medical and surgical options for therapy have dramatically risen in the past decade, each with their own short- and long-term complications.

CHAPTER

58

Malignant disease

Contents

58.1 INTRODUCTION

- Cancers in pilot and ATCO populations are representative of the types seen among the general population of working age.
- Most professional licence holders are male; five most common malignancies in aircrew are:
  - Prostate.
  - Colorectal.
  - Lymphoid.
  - Melanoma.
  - Testicular.
- Studies of malignancy in pilots have yet to establish a conclusive occupational link.
  - Reports of increased skin melanoma rates may be due to sun-related behaviour rather than cosmic radiation exposure (see Chapter 14).
- Pilot or ATCO should not exercise privileges of licence whilst undergoing treatment for malignant disease.
- Once remission achieved and full recovery from treatment, obtain specialist reports to include histological diagnosis, stage and grade of tumour, results of blood and radiological tests, treatment used with start and end dates, planned follow-up and prognosis.
- Certificatory assessment should consider both physical and mental state (in relation to the psychological effects of a cancer diagnosis) following treatment and risk of incapacitation secondary to local or distant metastatic recurrence.
- Primary and secondary brain tumours are permanently disqualifying for certification due to unacceptably high risk of incapacitating effects.
- Palliative treatment precludes certification.

58.2 GENERAL CONSIDERATIONS FOR FITNESS

- Surgery: Earliest time to recertification will vary according to the procedure.
- Radiotherapy: General side effects include fatigue, nausea; localised side effects include skin erythema, diarrhoea, cystitis.
  - Cranial irradiation may cause neurotoxicity and cognitive deficits.
  - Small vessel coronary disease may be a late effect for radiotherapy directed at the chest.
- Chemotherapy: Several months are likely to be required before considering a fit assessment after chemotherapy, subject to haematological indices being within normal range and stable. Assessment of incapacitation risk should consider the immediate and possibly delayed side effects.
- Adjuvant hormone therapy: Adjuvant steroid treatment precludes a fit assessment as it may cause euphoria and subtle cognitive changes when given in large doses (also used to treat active tumour).
  - Some therapies used for breast or prostate cancer may be acceptable.
- Tumour markers: Where available, can be a useful prognostic factor and surveillance tool for early detection of recurrence.

58.3 CERTIFICATION AFTER TREATMENT

- Usually only considered after primary treatment, if it has been undertaken with curative intent and there is no residual evidence of tumour.
- Exceptions include some chronic lymphoid malignancies and early prostate cancer where no active treatment may be indicated.

FACTORS TO CONSIDER

There are three main factors to consider when assessing an individual's risk of recurrence of malignant disease in any one year (after primary treatment only), which can be used to assess incapacitation risk as shown in Figure 58.1.

- *Risk of recurrence* – Can be estimated from disease-free survival curves but may need to use overall survival data if these are not available. Usually expressed as a percentage per annum following completion of treatment.
- *Site of recurrence* – Consider those sites most likely to cause incapacitation. Expressed as a percentage likelihood that recurrence will be at a specific site.
- *Tissue weighting* – (According to the propensity of metastasis to result in incapacitating symptoms) – 100% for brain, 20% for bone marrow, 5% for other body sites. The possibility of subtle incapacitation should be considered as many types of recurrence could result in a degradation of performance.

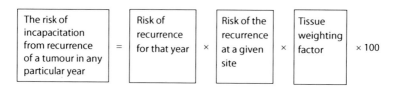

Figure 58.1 Assessment of incapacitation risk from malignant disease.

Example

If a tumour has a risk of recurrence of 5% in year 1 after completion of primary treatment and 3% of recurrences are cerebral (tissue weighting of 100%), the risk of incapacitation in year 1 for this person is 0.05 × 0.03 × 1.00 × 100 = 0.15%.

58.4 COLORECTAL CANCER

- Early recertification generally possible:
  - Risk of incapacitation from recurrence is low.
  - Clinical follow-up surveillance is well established and distant spread rarely presents with symptoms.
- Most common relapse site is liver, then local spread, pulmonary metastases and other abdominal.
- Cancer of the rectum or recto-sigmoid junction tends to have a slightly worse prognosis than cancer of the colon.
- Carcinoembryonic antigen (CEA) levels may be a useful marker of recurrence.

58.5 HODGKIN'S LYMPHOMA

- Very low risk of sudden incapacitation as presentation of relapse.
- As most cases are treated with anthracyclines, professional aircrew and controllers should undertake cardiological evaluation before certification.
- Long-term follow-up is required, as the risk of a second malignancy following chemotherapy may be raised.
- Consideration should be given to the likelihood of central nervous system relapse.
- Certification assessment: known prognostic factors at presentation, such as age, stage, lactate dehydrogenase level, number of extra-nodal sites involved and performance status, related to mobility impairment, are considered on a case-by-case basis.

58.6 MELANOMA

- Prognosis of a primary malignant melanoma depends on the vertical thickness of the excised lesion and whether there is lymph-node involvement or more distant spread.
- Certification is possible only if there has been complete excision of the primary lesion with regular clinical examination for signs of local recurrence and regional and distant metastases.

58.7 GERM-CELL TUMOURS OF TESTICLES

- Two main types: Seminoma and non-seminomatous germ-cell tumours (NSGCTs).
- A staging system based on disease site of origin, histology, tumour size and level of serum tumour markers has been developed by the International Germ Cell Cancer Collaborative Group.
- The prognosis is related to metastatic spread to secondary sites and the level of serum tumour markers, alpha-fetoprotein, human chorionic gonadotrophin and lactate dehydrogenase at presentation
- Central nervous system metastases are rare.

- Even with metastatic disease, the prognosis in testicular cancer is good compared with that of other tumours; unrestricted or multi-crew certificate possible 2–3 years after treatment in many cases.

58.8 BREAST

- The most significant indicators of prognosis are tumour grade, stage as indicated by histological lymph-node involvement and tumour size.
  - The Nottingham Prognostic Index can help predict outcome in individuals.
- In moderate to very poor prognostic groups, the concern is the risk of a sudden incapacitation from covert metastatic disease.
- The most common sites involved are liver, lungs and bone, but also consider cerebral metastases.
- Return to unrestricted flying possible in those with good prognosis (e.g. as assessed by Nottingham Prognostic Index).

58.9 PROSTATE

- Conservative management or active surveillance is acceptable for early disease localised to the prostate.
  - Regular clinical reviews and prostate-specific antigen (PSA) monitoring is essential.
- Main prognostic factors for recurrent prostatic disease are:
  - Pre-treatment PSA levels.
  - Stage.
  - Gleason score.
- Aircrew may remain on unrestricted duty unless disease extends beyond the prostatic capsule, the PSA trend is rising and/or the Gleason score is 8–10.
- Certification is possible after treatment, providing PSA is suppressed on hormonal therapy, and there is no nodal/bony spread:
  - Bony metastases to the vertebra and other skeletal sites can result in pathological fractures and spinal cord compression, plus symptoms of bone pain and hypercalcaemia.

CHAPTER

59

Renal disease and aviation

Contents

59.1 INTRODUCTION

- Chronic kidney disease is common.
- Most renal disease is asymptomatic, but conditions may cause distracting or incapacitating symptoms.
- No identified renal physiological detriment secondary to hypoxia or hypobaria.
- Sustained +Gz acceleration may exert some transient effects:
  - Reduced renal perfusion during +Gz causes reduced glomerular filtration rate (GFR) and increased plasma renin.
  - Reduced central blood volume causes reduced atrial natriuretic peptide (ANP) and increased antidiuretic hormone (ADH).
  - Transient proteinuria has been reported.
  - Evidence for haematuria after +Gz exposure not convincing, although pilots found to have haematuria on routine urine dip after G exposure should have repeat sample.

59.2 THE EFFECTS OF KIDNEY DISEASE ON THE AVIATOR

Kidney disease may cause distraction or incapacitation through the following.

RENAL COLIC

- Rapid and unpredictable onset with severe pain.
- Frequently caused by ureteric obstruction secondary to calculi.
- Transitional cell carcinoma, thrombus or external compression by lymph nodes, tumour or retroperitoneal fibrosis may also produce symptoms.

DECLINING RENAL FUNCTION

- Largely asymptomatic until GFR drops below 20–30 ml/min/1.73 m^2.
- Lethargy, pruritus, dyspnoea, anaemia, acidosis or fluid overload may develop.
- The clinical state of uraemia may cause subtle to severe cognitive impairment or even seizures.
- Platelet dysfunction, gastritis and pericarditis may result in GI haemorrhage and cardiac tamponade.
- Electrolyte abnormalities cause dysrhythmias.

INCREASED CARDIOVASCULAR DISEASE

- Occurs with even mild renal impairment.
- Atherosclerosis is compounded by hypertension, dyslipidaemia, vascular calcification, insulin resistance and uraemia.
- This occurs with reducing GFR or increasing proteinuria and is compounded when both are present.

NEPHROTIC SYNDROME

- Can be idiopathic or caused by systemic illness, drugs, infection.
- Specific diagnoses are made on biopsy of renal tissue, with minimal change, IgA, FSGS and membranous amongst the most common, aside from diabetic nephropathy.
- With increasing nephrosis, venous and arterial thromboembolism rates are increased.

ASSOCIATED CONDITIONS

- Diabetes mellitus is the most common cause of renal impairment.
- Other systemic diseases such as systemic lupus erythematosus, multiple myeloma and connective tissue diseases are also associated with renal disease.

MEDICATIONS

- Diuretics, ACE inhibitors, ARBs, steroids and immunosuppression are often used in the treatment of renal disease or its effects.
- Side effects, compatibility with flying and relevant restrictions must be considered.

59.3 ASSESSMENT OF KIDNEY DISEASE

Comprehensive history and clinical examination are crucial. Investigations include:

- Blood pressure: all-cause renal disease increases blood pressure, and uncontrolled hypertension potentiates renal impairment.
- Urine analysis: not within 24 hr of menstruation, high G exposure or arduous exercise, to reduce false positives.
- Urine microscopy and culture: urine dip sensitive enough for RBC, but white cells, casts or organisms are diagnostically important.
- Quantification of proteinuria: 24-hr collection is no longer necessary.
    - Protein to Creatinine Ratio (PCR) and Albumin to Creatinine Ratio (ACR) require only spot testing on a single sample.
    - From an aeromedical perspective, proteinuria >0.5 g/day (PCR >50 mg/ml, ACR >30 mg/ml) is significant and will require referral; proteinuria exceeding 1 g/day (PCR >100 mg/ml, ACR >70 mg/ml) usually warrants grounding pending further review.
- Renal function: eGFR incorporates gender, ethnicity and serum creatinine and is validated in adults with stable renal function.
    - Caution! Athletic individuals with high muscle mass may have an increased serum creatinine, and consequently reduced serum GFR, despite normal renal function, because serum creatinine is primarily derived from skeletal muscle.
- Imaging: modalities include:
    - Ultrasound (USS), including Doppler for renal blood flow, can assess the size and number of kidneys, scars, stones, obstruction and hydronephrosis.
    - Abdominal x-ray (AXR) for monitoring renal stone disease.
    - CT is the gold standard for the detection, location and measurement of all stones (including radiolucent, uric acid stones).
    - Radionuclide scans can be used to assess split function and urine flow.

59.4 HAEMATURIA AND PROTEINURIA

- Transient haematuria or proteinuria (on urine dip) not frequently pathological, especially in the young, whereas persistent abnormalities require investigation.
- Aircrew with visible haematuria should always be grounded and referred for urological assessment for exclusion of calculi or malignancy.
- Aircrew over the age of 40 with Non-Visible Haematuria (NVH) require urology referral to exclude malignancy and cystoscopy, in addition to radiological imaging.
    - If asymptomatic with normal BP and renal function, and no calcification on USS/AXR, a return to flying is possible, pending urology review.
- In the absence of a urological cause, a nephrology opinion is required for persistent haematuria or significant proteinuria.
    - If there is normal BP, renal function and imaging, unrestricted flying is possible pending nephrological assessment.

59.5 RENAL STONE DISEASE

- Lifetime risk is 15% in Europe, 25% in the Middle East (the hot and sunny climate predispose to dehydration and increased vitamin D synthesis).
- Male: female 2:1
- High recurrence rates, 50% in 10 years, 75% in 20 years.
- Peak recurrence at 2 years and 7–8 years after first stone (increased risk after second stone).
- Renal stone disease more common in aircrew:
  - Possibly caused by dehydration to reduce the need to urinate in-flight, hot conditions and wearing of bulky flying clothing.
  - Astronaut population also have an increased risk of stone formation, because of bone demineralization and the associated hypercalciuria.

AEROMEDICAL IMPLICATIONS

- Symptoms of renal stone disease in a pilot should lead to automatic grounding due to risk of renal colic, urinary frequency, dysuria or obstruction.
- Unrestricted flying may be possible once clinically and radiologically stone-free.
- Larger stones are treated with lithotripsy and ureteroscopy.
- Small, peripheral stones, proven by ureteroscopy to not be tubular, may be compatible with unrestricted flying.
- Ongoing restriction, such as unfit solo, may be necessary during observation.
- Regular imaging required to monitor residual stones and exclude new stone formation.
  - USS and AXR have similar sensitivities.
  - USS is better for radiolucent (urate) stones and utilises no radiation. AXR is ubiquitous and easy to compare to previous examinations (more so than USS images).
  - Frequency of surveillance imaging reflects the timings of recurrence – should occur at least at the 2- and 7-year point; in military single seat aircrew and recurrent stone formers, this may be as frequent as every 1–2 years.

59.6 DIALYSIS AND TRANSPLANTATION

- End-stage renal failure, peritoneal dialysis and haemodialysis are incompatible with flying and have high cardiovascular mortality rate.
- Renal transplantation may be acceptable:
  - Some civilian authorities allow restricted flying in those who are stable (e.g. after 1-year post-transplantation, on less than 10 mg of prednisolone, with stable renal function, normal BP, no surgical complications and immunosuppression within normal range).
  - High doses of steroids can cause psychosis.
  - The cardiovascular risk is lower than dialysis but still greater than that of the general population, and aircrew are required to undergo an annual exercise tolerance test.

59.7 SINGLE KIDNEY

- A functionally normal single kidney (secondary to nephrectomy, scarring or renal hypoplasia) in a pilot is compatible with flying if there is normal blood pressure, normal renal function, no proteinuria and no renal scarring (in that kidney).

- One-third of individuals with single kidney have extra-renal anomalies:
  - Some will not be compatible with flying (e.g. hearing impairment in bronchioto-renal syndrome, or visual disturbance in renal coloboma syndrome).

59.8 AUTOSOMAL DOMINANT POLYCYSTIC KIDNEY DISEASE (ADPKD)

- The most common form of inherited kidney disease.
- Fluid-filled cysts develop in the kidney (liver and pancreas) which increase in size and destroy normal renal tissue, leading to end stage renal failure.
- Before being considered for unrestricted flying duties, aircrew with ADPKD should undergo echocardiography, USS of the abdominal aorta and cerebral MRI due to risks of cardiac valvular abnormalities, abdominal aortic aneurysm and cerebral aneurysm (10%).

59.9 BENIGN PROSTATIC HYPERTROPHY

- Symptoms are related to bladder outflow obstruction.
- Management can be surgical (trans-urethral resection of prostate) or medical.

ALPHA-ADRENERGIC ANTAGONISTS

- Promote smooth muscle relaxation of the bladder neck, prostate capsule and prostatic urethra.
- Exert the same effect on vascular smooth muscle and can cause postural hypotension and syncope (exacerbated by +Gz).
- Tamsulosin and alfluzosin are more prostate-selective and may have a less pronounced effect on BP.
- Prior to return to flying, hypotension must be excluded by postural BP readings and ambulatory monitoring; high Gz flying generally excluded.

ALPHA REDUCTASE INHIBITORS

- Inhibit the conversion of testosterone to dihydrotestosterone and reduce prostatic size over several months.
- Side effects include reduction in libido and erectile dysfunction.
- Compatible with unrestricted flying when used alone; if used with alpha-blockers, then the above caveats for hypotension apply.

CHAPTER 60

Neurological disease

Contents

60.1 INTRODUCTION

- Neurological diseases can cause unpredictable, acute incapacitation.
- Neurological disease second only to cardiac disease in causing loss or restriction to aviation licences.
- Aeromedical assessment is challenging due to the unclear natural histories of many neurological conditions.
- Nonetheless, determining the likelihood of disease recurrence/progression, or the risk of incapacitation/distraction, are key.
- Neurological diseases may be viewed as static (e.g. nerve injury) or recurrent (e.g. epilepsy), and the medical examiner needs to understand the resultant disability of the former and risk of incapacitation of the latter:
  - Further subdivision is needed, as some static processes can promote subsequent episodic/progressive disease (e.g. head injury or strokes causing delayed seizures).
  - These conditions can have a low, moderate or high risk of progression (e.g. HIV), which can cause significant neurological disease.

60.2 STATIC WITH LOW RISK OF PROGRESSION

SPINAL CORD INJURY

- Recovery from spinal/nerve injury depends on the aetiology; acute spinal compression with rapid release may leave little residual deficit. However, predicting outcome is difficult.
- Static neurological deficits are usually incompatible with commercial flying but may still be compatible with recreational flying.
- Ejection can lead to spinal cord injury, and all aircrew must be assessed by a neurologist post-ejection.

PERIPHERAL NERVE INJURY

- Peripheral nerve injury resulting from trauma or Guillain-Barre syndrome is unlikely to progress, and the assessment should focus on disability/function.
- By contrast, peripheral neuropathy may cause progressive loss of function.
- Assessment of musculoskeletal function and flight simulation may be required.

CRANIAL NERVE INJURY

- Cranial nerve injury may affect the special senses.
- Injury to CNII (optic nerve), CNIII, IV and VI (ocular muscles), VII (facial nerve) and VIII (vestibular nerve) may result in loss of stereopsis, diplopia, reduction in blink reflex or hearing loss, all of which have potential flight safety ramifications and may lead to flying restriction or grounding.
- Neurological review is mandated.

60.3 STATIC WITH MODERATE/HIGH RISK OF PROGRESSION

CEREBROVASCULAR EVENTS (CVE)

- Cerebrovascular events (CVE) incorporate ischaemic stroke, transient ischaemic attacks (TIA) and haemorrhagic stroke.
- All are potentially disabling and usually associated with a high risk of recurrence (stroke risk at 5 years 10–40%).
- Ischaemic and haemorrhagic stroke, TIA, arteriovenous malformations and cavernous haemangiomas are nearly always incompatible with flying.

ARTERIOVENOUS MALFORMATIONS (AVM)

- AVM may cause headache, epilepsy and focal neurological deficits.
- Treatment with surgery, radio-frequency ablation or embolization (or a combination of these) can result in scar formation, and this may take up to 2 years to develop.
- The bleeding risk remains increased during this time.
- Risk of epilepsy in AVMs is the same whether or not a bleed occurs and, in most cases, precludes flying.
- Small numbers of individuals return to dual-crew flying after several years of observation.

CAVERNOUS HAEMANGIOMAS

- Cavernous haemangiomas are usually diagnosed following a seizure and the majority of these develop epilepsy.
- If associated with bleeding, epilepsy or focal neurological deficit, cavernoma are incompatible with flying privileges.
- If an incidental finding in aircrew, they require restriction to multi-crew flying duties.

HAEMORRHAGIC CVE/SUBARACHNOID HAEMORRHAGE

- Haemorrhagic CVE/subarachnoid haemorrhage (SAH) is associated with aneurysm or AVM rupture, and disqualification is usual.
- However, in the absence of seizure, and where treatment with clipping or coiling is successful *and* where short-term complications are avoided, a restricted return to aircrew duty may be possible.
- A prolonged period of observation (usually >2 years) is required.
- After successful intervention, recreational pilots may be able to return to unrestricted flying at 1 year.

PERIMESENCEPHALIC SAH

- Perimesencephalic SAH, in the absence of a vascular malformation, is associated with a lower risk of re-bleeding (<1% per annum).
- In normotensive aircrew, a return to flying duties at one year may be considered, depending on job role.
- Identification of unruptured aneurysms poses an occupational dilemma, with increased risk of events if left untreated weighed against the risks of intervention: both may cause bleeding and seizures.
- Aggressive management of risk factors (HTN, smoking and lipids) is essential, as is exclusion of associated conditions such as connective tissue disorders, cardiac malformations and polycystic disease.

OTHER CVEs

- Strokes associated with cervical arterial dissection are less concerning for disability or recurrence:
    - After a period of observation, younger aircrew may be permitted a return to restricted flying duties.
- The risk of recurrent stroke in patients with and without patent foramen ovale (PFO) is similar:
    - The risk may be reduced by PFO closure.
    - Decisions on aircrew undergoing PFO closure should be made case-by-case and jointly between a cardiologist and neurologist.
- Identification of white matter hyperintensities (WMH) on brain scanning is increasingly common, and the aetiological significance varies by individual:
    - WMH are associated with an increased risk of stroke (x3/x7.4 without/with stroke risk factors) and cognitive decline.
    - Neurology review, for stroke risk calculation, is recommended and risk factor management compulsory.

- The risk of WMH progression is greater still in high-altitude flight; aircrew found to have WMH warrant individual review and restriction from high altitude may ensue.

TRAUMATIC BRAIN INJURY

- Traumatic brain injury (TBI) encompasses a spectrum of severity from mild (e.g. concussion) to severe (new focal deficits).
- Determining the presence or absence of post-traumatic amnesia (PTA) is useful in determining severity:
  - PTA <30 min = mild.
  - PTA 1–7 days = severe.
- Severity predicts the risk of post-traumatic epilepsy (PTE), and this is used to determine if/when a return to flying duties is possible.
- PTE is especially common after penetrating trauma.
- The risk of PTE falls dramatically over time, with a risk reduction of 75% if free of epilepsy at 2 years post-event.
- Injury in childhood or adolescence may be associated with a higher rate of PTE.
- MRI evidence of brain injury is a useful marker of TBI severity and plays a role in risk assessment; however, electroencephalography (EEG) is not beneficial.
- Ongoing cognitive impairment following head injury is critical in aircrew, and even mild cognitive decline may be critical, depending on aircrew role.
  - Collaborative history from colleagues and family helps detect subtle changes.
- The severity of TBI determines the restriction in aircrew duties (see Table 60.1).

Table 60.1 Aircrew head injury observation periods

SEVERITY	SYMPTOMS	PERIOD OF GROUNDING
Mild	<30 minutes post-traumatic amnesia (PTA) No loss of consciousness No neurological deficit	1 week
	<30 minutes PTA Fleeting loss of consciousness No neurological deficit	2 months
Moderate	PTA >30 min <24 hr Neurological deficit Non-depressed fracture of skull base MRI evidence of haemosiderin	2 years
Severe	PTA >24 hr <7 days Neurological deficit Depressed skull fracture Traumatic dural penetration MRI evidence of haemosiderin and gliosis	5 years
Very severe	PTA >7 days Debilitating neurological deficit Penetration of brain parenchyma	Disqualifying

Table 60.2 Flight restrictions after neurological infection

TYPE	PERIOD OF GROUNDING	RESTRICTION ON FLYING
Viral or aseptic meningitis	6 months	Nil
Bacterial meningitis without early seizures	1 year	Nil
Bacterial meningitis with early seizures	2 years	Dual, 5 years
Viral encephalitis without early seizures	5 years	Dual, 5 years
Viral encephalitis with early seizures		Ground permanently
Cerebral abscess, cerebral malaria, neurocysticercosis		Ground permanently

60.4 EPISODIC AND INFECTIOUS DISEASE

- CNS infection may lead to epilepsy or behavioural/cognitive change.
- The risk of epilepsy does not increase with aseptic/viral meningitis but does with bacterial infection (2% if uncomplicated, 10–15% in complex disease).
- Encephalitis bestows a high risk, as does cerebral abscess, malaria and neurocysticercosis, all of which bar further flying.
- Suggested occupational disposition following CNS infection can be found in Table 60.2.

SEIZURES AND EPILEPSY

- Epilepsy is a major risk for incapacitation, and loss of consciousness is not the only concerning feature.
- Epilepsy can be subtle, and aircrew having seizures may demonstrate impaired judgement and performance.
- This may inadvertently interrupt the flight control panel with obvious consequences.
- Importantly, not all seizures are epilepsy:
  - If a fit occurs within a week of a neurological or systemic insult, it is termed an acute symptomatic seizure.
  - These may be caused by a variety of metabolic and other disorders.
  - Following a *symptomatic* seizure, the risk of developing epilepsy is approximately 20% over 10 years, with the main risk seen in the first 5.
  - Aircrew should be grounded for 4 years; if asymptomatic, off all medication, and with a normal MRI and EEG, they then may be considered for restricted flying duties.
- Unprovoked seizures are significantly more likely to herald the onset of epilepsy (>60%) unless occurring under the age of 5 years, when a more benign phenotype may be causative.
- Before being considered for flight duties, aircrew should be fit-free for 10 years and, if >5 years of age at time of seizure, should be restricted to multi-crew flying.
- EEG may be helpful to support the diagnosis of epilepsy (but there is a high false positive rate), and photic stimulation may be beneficial in rotary aircrew.

HEADACHE AND NEURALGIA

- Migraine is common:
  - It may present acutely, with/without visual or sensory aura, and is acutely debilitating in >50% sufferers.
  - Each of these features has clear implications for flight safety.
  - As such, migraine precludes military flying and many commercial aircrew roles.
  - Restricted flying duties may be possible in certain jobs when no aura or incapacitation is present.
  - Unfortunately, many migraine treatments are sedative and incompatible with flying.
- Trigeminal autonomic cephalgias and neuralgias (e.g. cluster headaches, trigeminal neuralgia) are erratic in their presentation, may be acutely incapacitating and are incompatible with flying duties.

PROGRESSIVE AND DEGENERATIVE DISORDERS

- To appropriately assess these conditions needs an understanding of rate of progression and type of disability conferred.
- Dementia is rare amongst aircrew, and cognitive decline warrants grounding and thorough investigation to exclude organic illness and reversible causes.
- Parkinson's disease, myasthenia gravis and most CNS tumours (usually metastatic) are incompatible with professional flying.
- A diagnosis of multiple sclerosis (MS) is a bar to initial licencing:
  - Depending on the subtype of MS, established aircrew who are free of epilepsy, trigeminal neuralgia, mood disorders or physical limitations may be able to continue to fly in a restricted capacity.
  - Optic neuritis and other isolated demyelinating syndromes, without dissemination in time and space, should be managed on a case-by-case basis but are usually incompatible with commercial flying.
  - Recreational flying may be possible with limitations.

CHAPTER

61

Ear, nose and throat

Contents

- Normal function of the ear (including hearing), nose and throat is important for communication and orientation in aircrew and controllers.
- Changes in atmospheric pressure, diseases and drugs may cause incapacitation.

61.1 CLINICAL EXAMINATION

- Clinical history should address:
    - Previous trouble with flying (e.g. barotrauma).
    - Ear: infections (otitis externa and media); tinnitus; vertigo; history of trauma (tympanic perforation or surgery); Eustachian tube dysfunction; hearing problems.
    - Nose: obstruction (polyps, hay fever, rhinitis medicamentosa); discharges (clear, purulent, blood); post-nasal drip; sinus blockage.
    - Oro-pharynx: dental; throat infections.
    - Social: smoking; alcohol; drug history.
- Physical examination should include:
    - Ears: auriscope examination of external auditory canals, tympanic membranes, middle ear; assessment of tympanic membrane whilst performing a Valsalva manoeuvre (but not always a good predictor of ability to clear ears in flight).

- Nasal airways: anterior rhinoscopy; nasal septum (perforation in cases of trauma or cocaine abuse); sinus drip.
- Oro-pharynx: teeth and gums; tongue; palate; salivary glands; uvula; tonsils; speech.
- CNS: nystagmus; cranial nerves; balance (gait, walking, standing, Romberg's test).
- Hearing tests:
  - Conversational voice test: standing 2 m behind, checking each side separately, in a normal voice the applicant is asked to repeat two-syllable words.
  - Tuning fork tests: Rinne and Weber; air and bone conduction helps distinguish different types of deafness.
  - Pure tone audiometry: for ATCOs, professional and instrument rated pilots.
  - Functional hearing assessment: the individual is tested in a background with noise representative of a cockpit, confirming the understanding of relevant radiotelephony phraseology and beacon identification.
  - Other tests are likely to require specialist intervention.

61.2 HEARING LOSS (HYPOACUSIS)

- Hearing loss may affect communications between crew and with ATC but may also reduce recognition of atypical noises during flight.
- Developing deafness should be picked up by regular checks.

NOISE-INDUCED HEARING LOSS (NIHL)

- Acquired sensorineural loss caused by noise exposure.
- Audiogram: Initial characteristic hearing loss at 4000–6000 Hz.

OTOSCLEROSIS

- Genetic neo-ossification in the capsule of the middle ear, especially between stapes and oval window, causing conductive deafness.
- In advanced cases, ossification will also involve the inner ear, thus adding sensorineural deafness.
- Surgery (stapedectomy or stapedotomy with fine fenestra technique and vein graft) may restore full hearing in some cases, but complications include dizziness and nystagmus in cases of poor sealing of the oval window.
- Recertification will require specialist reports confirming restoration of hearing and no complications.

PRESBYACUSIS

- Cumulative effect of aging on hearing.
- Insidious presentation of bilateral sensorineural loss.

AVIATION MANAGEMENT OF HEARING LOSS

- Certification will depend on the degree of hearing loss or post-treatment complications.
- Most pilots with moderate hearing loss prefer the amplification of sound in headsets to the use of hearing aids.

- Aviation-approved hearing aids (bone anchored or intra-aural) are not normally accepted for initial commercial or military certification but may be acceptable for already licenced civilian pilots and ATCOs.
- Functional hearing assessment may be required where hearing is outside required standards.

61.3 VESTIBULAR SCHWANNOMA (ACOUSTIC NEUROMA)

- Benign tumour, derived from the Schwann cells of the vestibulocochlear nerve.
- Typically presents with unilateral tinnitus and hearing loss, with or without vertigo.
- Diagnosis is by MRI scan.
- In cases of 'watchful waiting', some aircrew may temporarily be allowed to fly with restrictions.
- Surgical resection likely to result in damage to the nerve with subsequent irreversible ipsilateral hearing loss; other complications can include minimal facial weakness, tinnitus and/or late post-operative vertigo.
- Recertification will depend on remnant symptoms but at best will result in unfit military flying, restricted commercial flying, unlimited private flying.

61.4 VESTIBULAR FUNCTION DISTURBANCE

- Vertigo is the erroneous sensations of the world spinning or moving irregularly:
  - It is almost invariably secondary to inner ear disease or neurological disorders.
  - It is debilitating and will require grounding until diagnosis and full resolution is established.

MÉNIÈRE'S DISEASE

- Multifactorial origin.
- Typically, symptoms are acute attacks of vertigo, fluctuating tinnitus, increasing deafness and a feeling of pressure in the ear.
- Due to the unpredictable course of the disease (treated or not) and associated safety implications, the diagnosis of Ménière's disease is incompatible with military aircrew duties and civilian flying.

VIRAL VESTIBULAR NEURONITIS (LABYRINTHITIS)

- Viral inflammation of the inner ear.
- Symptoms can last from days to weeks; improves gradually with some slight unsteadiness for 2–3 months before symptoms clear completely.
- Recertification may be considered after weeks of being asymptomatic, usually with restrictions for a finite period for military and commercial pilots.

ALTERNOBARIC VERTIGO

- Abrupt onset of severe vertigo on aircraft climb or descent due to unequal pressures being exerted in the middle ear by Eustachian tube dysfunction.

- Tends to be self-limited; although it is distressing, the affected crew are usually able to maintain control of the aircraft.
- Depending on the cause (common cold vs. persistent perforated tympanic membrane), recertification may be possible after full investigation.

BENIGN PAROXYSMAL POSITIONAL VERTIGO (BPPV)

- Sudden short episodes (<30 seconds) of intense vertigo on moving the head in certain directions (e.g. looking behind).
- Caused by dislodged otoconia from the utricle to the semicircular canals, most commonly the posterior canal.
- Generally self-limited and will remit spontaneously (but may take months).
- Recurrence is not unusual (up to 20% in the first year; 50% within 5 years).
- Management includes several repositioning manoeuvres (e.g. Epley), medication or surgery.
- Due to the short presentations, unless it occurs during critical phases of flight, safety may not be compromised in multi-crew aircraft.
- Single pilot flying may not be acceptable.

61.5 OTHER ENT DISORDERS

BAROTRAUMA

- Middle ear cavity gas expansion on ascent will usually vent through Eustachian tube, but requires active process (e.g. yawning, swallowing) to open Eustachian tube on descent to equalise negative pressure.
- Venting of sinuses during descent may be obstructed by mucosal oedema, polyps or masses.
- Aviation-related barotrauma of the middle ear or sinus is rare; usually associated with an upper respiratory tract infection (i.e. self-limiting).
- Clinical grades of otitic barotrauma:
  - Grade 0 is symptoms of pressure within the ear with no signs.
  - Grade 1 is redness and retraction of the tympanic membrane.
  - Grade II is intratympanic membrane haemorrhage.
  - Grade III is gross tympanic membrane haemorrhage.
  - Grade IV is haemotympanum.
  - Grade V is perforation.
- Risk increases with chronic or recurrent disease, including sinusitis, hay fever (allergic rhinitis), nasal polyps, septal deviation or otitis media.
- Aircrew who cannot 'clear their ears' (e.g. with a Valsalva manoeuvre) remain grounded until the episode has ceased.
- Flying on aviation-approved medication for hay fever (e.g. non-sedating antihistamines) is allowed once it has been confirmed that no side effects have developed and symptoms have cleared.
- Following sinus surgery, a functional check of aircrew is sometimes conducted in a hypobaric chamber.
- Inner ear barotrauma (e.g. from excessive Valsalva manoeuvre) may cause perilymph fistula with sudden onset of vertigo with an accompanying hearing loss and tinnitus;

management may be conservative or surgical; flying not usually permitted until resolution.

TYMPANIC PERFORATION

- Requires a period of grounding until the membrane has healed; prophylactic use of antibiotics may reduce infection risk.
- In cases of permanent perforation, tympanoplasty may be required.
- Recertification will be permitted as long as there is obvious normal drum mobility.
- An audiogram may be required.

OTITIS MEDIA (ACUTE, WITH OR WITHOUT EFFUSION, AND CHRONIC SUPPURATIVE)

- Rare in adults.
- If ventilation tubes (grommets) are used, certification is only allowed in long stable dry cases for civilian flying.
- Not accepted for military flying duties.

CHOLESTEATOMA

- Usually associated with chronic otitis media.
- Following surgery, mastoid cavities are at risk of infection with water ingress.
- Return to flying is sometimes possible in long-term quiescent cases (no recurrences or need for frequent microsuction) with good Eustachian function and hearing.

CHAPTER 62

Orthopaedics

Contents

62.1 INTRODUCTION

- Aircrew suffer from similar orthopaedic disorders to the age-matched general population.
- Pilots may be more likely to engage in adventurous sports both on and off duty; therefore, more likely to suffer some form of sport-related trauma during their career.
- Flying may make aircrew more vulnerable to certain types of back and neck injury.
- The majority of patients suffering musculoskeletal symptoms will be managed successfully with analgesics and time, potentially with assistance from physiotherapists, osteopaths or chiropractors.

62.2 TRAUMA

- Advances in point of injury trauma care and rehabilitation may lead to challenging decisions in initial aircrew selection and fitness to fly following injury.
- The general categories used to help assess fitness to fly are:
    - Mobility.
    - Strength.
    - Dexterity.
    - Tendency for sudden change of function.
    - Pain.
- The overriding consideration should be to determine the ability of aircrew to perform all duties safely.
- Soft tissue injuries are a potent cause of morbidity and litigation:
    - For example, an ankle sprain could have potential flight safety implications with restriction of use of foot brakes or rudder bars.
    - The longer-term reduced range of movement (ROM) and loss of proprioception may be less obvious and should be anticipated and mitigated.

- Early referral to a multidisciplinary team is likely to give the patient the best chance of a swift recovery.
- Aircrew must be reminded that a safe return to flying duties will only be possible after a full functional assessment.

FRACTURES

- Plasters or splints: The aim of any treatment after a fracture is a return to maximum level of function as soon as possible; plaster or splints may be sufficient to allow fractures and damaged soft tissues to heal.
  - An undisplaced fracture may be discharged from a fracture clinic once it has united, but the residual pain and stiffness related to the soft tissue injury may pose a flight safety risk long after the splint or cast is removed.
- Plates, screws and intramedullary nails: may be needed to hold a fracture reduced whilst the bone heals:
  - An implant will have been chosen to allow stability at the fracture site whilst allowing early movement of soft tissues and joints.
  - Patients or therapists will often request the removal of metalwork once a fracture has healed.
  - There is significant morbidity associated with removal and unless significant local irritation of soft tissues is evident, it is to be discouraged.
  - There is no longer any place for routine removal of metalwork.
- Before a return to flying or controlling:
  - The treating team must be satisfied that the fracture has healed both radiologically and clinically; usually manifested by a lack of pain at the fracture site.
  - There should also be adequate function in the injured limb and no distracting pain.
  - Ideally a functional assessment should be carried out in an aircraft, but an equivalent assessment may be possible for the aeromedical examiner.
- Medical professionals are often asked to comment on fitness to fly of passengers subsequent to both trauma and increasingly elective surgery:
  - It is well known that patients with acute injuries should not fly with complete casts, but the possibility of medical complications after trauma and elective surgery such as deep venous thrombosis (DVT) and subsequent pulmonary embolus should be discussed, risk assessed and if needs be, mitigated before allowing patients to fly (see Chapter 43).

POST-TRAUMATIC ARTHRITIS

- Arthritis may occur if a fracture line extends into a joint; the injury to the cartilage of the joint surface is often much more significant.
- Any subsequent post-traumatic arthritis may cause long-term pain, reduced range of movement and stiffness, all of which can have flight safety implications.
- It is the cartilage damage that leads to any eventual degenerative change.
- Some fractures are 'high risk' for complications (e.g. intracapsular hip, scaphoid or talar neck fractures secondary to high-energy trauma); may lead to osteonecrosis of the area of devitalized bone.

- Aircrew sustaining such an injury should be followed very carefully to ensure that either the fracture unites or suitable assessment is in place to identify and quantify any long-term disability.

EJECTION SEAT INJURIES

- Aircrew are vulnerable to orthopaedic injuries during the ejection sequence; some of these may be subtle (see Chapter 18).
- Seat acceleration, wind flail and landing can all be potent sources of injury.
- The index of suspicion must be high for occult spinal injuries.
- Surviving aircrew should be managed by a trauma team, preferably in a level 1 trauma centre.
- Clinical evaluation and standard trauma imaging modalities must be supplemented by a whole spine MRI to identify occult spinal bony and soft tissue injuries.

62.3 ELECTIVE CARE

SOFT TISSUE JOINT SURGERY

- Knee and shoulder injuries and degenerative pathology are common.
- Many will be treated with arthroscopic surgery often as day-case episodes.
- DVT is a recognized complication of lower-limb surgery; should be considered before return to flying duties or flying as a passenger.
- Patients should demonstrate a full, functional, pain-free range of movement of the treated limb before returning to flying duties.
- Muscle tone is lost with as little as 2 weeks inactivity, and this must be addressed before a return to flying.

JOINT REPLACEMENT SURGERY

- Knee and hip replacement surgery are common, reliable and associated with high patient satisfaction; arthroplasty is associated with excellent relief of the pain and an improvement in the reduced movement associated with arthritis.
- Dislocation following total hip replacement is a recognised complication but usually occurs early. If the hip has proven stable at 3 months, it would be reasonable to attempt a cockpit functional assessment.
- Commercial aircrew may return to flying if they have:
  - Completed the prescribed rehabilitation process, following a standard arthroplasty procedure using a recognised technique, and
  - A functional assessment has been completed successfully.
- For military and private pilots, emergency egress, use of ejection seats and parachutes will need careful deliberation between the operating surgeon and qualified aviation medicine practitioner.

CHRONIC DISEASE

- Many aircrew with stable or slowly progressive chronic orthopaedic disease can enjoy safe and successful flying careers.

- This is dependent on their medical professional support network and an active system of regular review, functional assessment and acceptable medication.
- Low back pain:
  - Back pain is common in the population.
  - Factors that are thought to provoke back pain include vibration, posture and sudden maximal effort.
  - A higher incidence of back pain has been reported in certain groups of workers, such as truck drivers, heavy manual workers and nurses; higher incidence of back pain also reported in aviators.
  - Rotary-wing aircrew are at particular risk (see Chapter 2), but crews of all aircraft types report low back pain.
- Cervical pain:
  - As with the lumbar spine, degenerative change and symptoms of neck pain are common in the population.
  - An uninhibited and adequate range of movement to perform flight tasks such as lookout is required.
  - It is important to assess adequately aircrew with a history of neck pain before flight duties.
  - Risk of neck pain in aircrew is related to high +Gz exposure (see Chapter 16) and night vision goggle use (see Chapters 2 and 26).

CHAPTER 63

Haematology

Contents

63.1 ANAEMIA

- Haemoglobin (Hb) is needed for uptake of oxygen in the lungs and for transport and transfer of oxygen to peripheral tissues.
- Anaemia is not a diagnosis, but a consequence, and an underlying cause must be sought; normal values of Hb are 13.5–17.5 g/dL in males and 11.5–15.5 g/dL in females.
- Cardiovascular reserve can be impaired by anaemia and problematic in a pressurized cabin at 8000 ft (worse at higher altitudes).
- Passengers with Hb >7.5 g/dL are unlikely to experience problems with commercial travel unless there is associated cardiorespiratory disease.

- Acute anaemia may pose more problems than chronic anaemia (even when the latter has a lower Hb).
- Chronic anaemia may precipitate angina; Canadian Cardiac Society Guidelines recommend an Hb of >9 g/L prior to air travel in patients with a history of CABG.
- Features of haemodynamic instability such as chest pain, hypotension, dyspnoea and arrhythmia may be worse in flight.
- When assessing potential passengers for fitness to fly, do not rely on examination at rest but review exercise tolerance.
  - As a rough guide, those able to climb 10–12 stairs or walk 50 m should be able to tolerate commercial flight.

HAEMOLYTIC ANAEMIA

- An increase in the rate of destruction of erythrocytes (normal life span 120 days).
- Hereditary or acquired.
- Splenectomy may be indicated in those with significant anaemia.
- Autoimmune haemolytic anaemia can develop at any age:
  - Antibodies are targeted to red cell antigens and result in anaemia and splenomegaly.
  - Chronic course with relapses and remissions.
  - Permanent remission is not common and requirement for continuous therapy may preclude licencing.

SICKLE CELL DISEASE

- An inherited disorder of haemoglobin synthesis, resulting in abnormal haemoglobin molecules which are unstable and form precipitates.
- Sickle cell trait:
  - In heterozygous carriers is a benign condition as only 20–40% of the circulating haemoglobin is HbS; the rest is normal, HbA.
  - They have no clinical problems (as sickling only occurs when the pO_2 falls to 10 mmHg, in extreme hypoxia) and typically have normal haemoglobin levels.
  - Occasional reports of passengers with sickle cell trait experiencing problems during commercial air travel, possibly due to variable genotype penetrance.
  - Sickle cell trait is not a barrier to a career in commercial or civil aviation, or the licencing of military aircrew in the United Kingdom or United States.
- Sickle cell disease:
  - Homozygotes with sickle cell disease have a chronic anaemia (Hb <7–10 g/dL) and are prone to recurrent episodes of painful 'crises' due to intramedullary necrosis following occlusion of small vessels.
  - Sickle cell disease is not compatible with a career as an aviator.
  - Sickling crises and related problems in patients with homozygous sickle cell disease flying in pressurized commercial aircraft are extremely rare; passengers are encouraged to drink plenty of water.

THALASSAEMIA

- Autosomal recessive conditions characterised by decreased or absent synthesis of one of the two polypeptide chains (α or β) that form the normal adult human haemoglobin molecule (HbA, α2/β2).
- Alpha thalassaemia major is not compatible with life.

- Beta thalassaemia major is not compatible with medical certification as aircrew, as it produces a very severe anaemia, apparent within a few months after birth.
- Beta thalassaemia minor is the most common form in European countries and has no clinical problems:
  - There may be a mild anaemia (Hb 10–12 g/dL).
  - Beta thalassaemia minor is compatible with medical certification for flight duties.

63.2 MYELOPROLIFERATIVE DISORDERS

POLYCYTHAEMIA

- An increase in red cell mass, resulting Hb >17.5 g/dL in males, >15.5 g/dL in females.
- Symptoms are of hyperviscosity (headache, pruritus, night sweats, dyspnoea, blurred vision).
- Usually disqualifying from flight duties due to thromboembolic complications and unpredictable progression.

63.3 HAEMATOLOGICAL MALIGNANCIES

- Advances in recent years offer the prospect of a cure for many haematological malignancies, including acute leukaemias and lymphomas.
- Prolonged courses of chemotherapy or radiotherapy, and immunosuppression following bone marrow transplantation, may be required, with side effects potentially incompatible with flying.
- Consider effects of long-term treatment in pilots who have had successful treatment for childhood malignancy.

CHRONIC LYMPHOCYTIC LEUKAEMIA

- A disease of the elderly; often indolent and may be an incidental finding.
- Malignant proliferation of B lymphocytes.
- Increased susceptibility to infections and autoimmune haemolytic anaemia.
- Fitness may depend on age, WCC and complications, and would need to be discussed with the relevant medical authority and specialists.
- Requirement for active treatment, increasing WCC, infections or bone marrow suppression will likely be disqualifying.

CHRONIC MYELOID LEUKAEMIA

- Most frequently in those 40–60 years.
- Anaemia, thrombocytopaenia due to bone marrow infiltration.
- Imatinib has improved treatment and prognosis.
- Usually incompatible with flying duties.

MULTIPLE MYELOMA

- May affect older patients and run an indolent course.
- Insidious progression leads to late presentation during advanced disease.
- Multiple causes for incapacitation preclude certification and will require disqualification upon diagnosis.

63.4 DISORDERS OF HAEMOSTASIS

THROMBOCYTOPAENIA

- Caused by many conditions, and underlying cause will need to be considered when reviewing licencing, not just platelet count in isolation.
- Normal platelet range is 150–400 × 109/L.
- Platelet count <75 × 109/L is not compatible with certification as a pilot.
- Passenger threshold for safe flight is 40 × 109/L.
- Aspirin and non-steroidals are usually avoided.

AUTOIMMUNE THROMBOCYTOPAENIA

- Relatively common disorder in childhood; complete remission, without relapse, is usual.
  - Isolated ITP in childhood does not preclude licencing.
- However, ITP in adults has a chronic course:
  - With stable platelet count >75 × 109/L, certification to fly may be possible.

HAEMOPHILIA

- Haemophilia A – Hereditary deficiency of factor VIII.
- Haemophilia B (Christmas disease) – Deficiency of factor IX.
- Severe haemophilia is not compatible with licencing.
- However, those with mild forms are not at increased risk of sudden incapacitation and may be certified for civilian flying.
- No specific restrictions for passengers, but carriage of sufficient coagulation factor concentrate is advised.

VON WILLEBRAND DISEASE

- Congenital abnormality of platelet activation and adhesion.
- Diagnosis of vWD does not preclude licencing if disease is mild with no significant bleeding and no treatment requirements.

DEEP VENOUS THROMBOEMBOLISM

- A common indication for anticoagulation.
- 1% develop PE.
- 3–6 months of anticoagulation in first clot with no ongoing risk of VTE.
- 20% will have a recurrence in the next 5 years.
- DVT secondary to another condition (such as malignancy) may require disqualification for the underlying cause.

ANTICOAGULATION

- Heparin, warfarin, novel oral anticoagulants (NOACs).
- Consider indication for use as well as anticoagulant when reviewing licencing.
- Anticoagulation has a small but definite risk of bleeding complications, including intracranial haemorrhage.
- Risk is increased in older patients and INR >4.
- No specific restriction for passengers, but medication supply and access to monitoring is recommended.

- Sensitivity to warfarin is affected by changes in medication, diet, alcohol consumption and gastrointestinal illnesses.
- Some regulatory authorities will allow flying conditional on INR within range in the preceding 12 hr, and with the use of portable monitoring.
- NOACs such as apixaban, dabigatran and rivaroxaban are now routinely used in clinical practice.
- Aspirin has very little antithrombotic effect in the venous circulation; should not be used as an alternative to warfarin simply in order to avoid suspension of a medical certificate.

THROMBOPHILIA

- Congenital deficiency of natural anticoagulant (anti-thrombin, protein C or protein S).
- The most common is factor V Leiden genotype, resistance to activated protein C.
- 8 × increased risk of VTE (even more so with concurrent OCP use).
- Certification is acceptable in individuals with no history of previous thromboembolism and may be considered in those with a history of single thrombus, full recovery and no further anticoagulation.

63.5 AIR TRAVEL AND THROMBOSIS

- There is an association between long-distance travel and VTE, but absolute risk is low; incidence may be 0.5% for flights of 8 hr or more.

ASSESSING RISK OF TRAVEL-RELATED DEEP VEIN THROMBOSIS

Risk is low if:
- No history of DVT or PE, and
- No surgery in last 4 weeks, and
- No risk factors of moderate or high risk.

Risk is moderate if:
- Previous history of DVT or PE (but note that risk is considered low on anticoagulant treatment for recent DVT or PE).
- Surgery under general anaesthesia lasting more than 30 minutes in the previous 2 months but not in the last 4 weeks.
- Is pregnant or postpartum.
- Has a lower-limb fracture in plaster.
- Has congestive cardiac failure, recent myocardial infarction or other major acute illness (e.g. pneumonia).
- Is taking oestrogen therapy.
- Is obese (body mass index greater than 30 kg/m^2).
- Has varicose veins with phlebitis.
- Has a family history of venous thromboembolism in a 1st-degree relative.
- Has polycythaemia or thrombocythaemia.
- (Multiple risk factors will further increase the risk.)

Risk is high if:
- Surgery under general anaesthesia lasting more than 30 minutes in the previous 4 weeks.
- Has thrombophilia.
- Has cancer – Untreated or on treatment.

ADVICE FOR AIR TRAVEL LASTING MORE THAN 6 HOURS

- If low risk: General advice only.
- If moderate risk: Use graduated compression stockings (GCS) providing 15–30 mmHg pressure at the ankle.
- If high risk: Use GCS providing 15–30 mmHg pressure at the ankle and given a single prophylactic dose of low-molecular-weight heparin (LMWH) injected prior to departure; aspirin thrombo-prophylaxis lacks evidence, particularly in view of side effects.

OTHER FACTORS

- VTE is rare in flights <5 hr; more typically, flights >12 hr.
- Risk increases with age (>40, and especially >65).
- Symptoms often occur within 72 hr but not during flight and may occur up to 2 weeks later.
- Stasis is a contributing factor.
- Prolonged recent immobility (after a stroke) and significant dehydration (diarrhoea) also increase risk.
- Potentially, hypobaric hypoxia may activate the coagulation cascade.
- Mitigation may be achieved by avoidance of flight in higher-risk patients (i.e. post-surgery, fracture, etc.).
- Encouraging movement and adequate hydration, as well as avoiding restriction posed by under-seat luggage, may be beneficial.
- Sedative and excessive alcohol may discourage mobility.

63.6 BLOOD AND MARROW DONATION

- Pilots must wait 24 hr between donation of blood and commencing flying duties.
- Air traffic controllers must wait 12 hr between donation of blood and commencing flying duties.
- Pilots and controllers must wait 48 hr minimum between bone marrow donation and duties.

63.7 SPLENECTOMY

- Used to treat haematological disorders such as autoimmune thrombocytopaenia.
- Most commonly performed after traumatic rupture.
- Increased susceptibility to infection, particularly encapsulated organisms such as *Streptococcus pneumoniae*, *Haemophilus influenzae* and *Neisseria meningitidis*.
- Vaccination is given pre-splenectomy (where possible), and febrile illnesses require prompt antibiotic therapy.
- Antibiotic prophylaxis with penicillin V.
- Malarial prophylaxis is essential, as infection may be fatal.
- In stable individuals with no ongoing haematological contraindication, aircrew licencing is permissible.

Aviation psychiatry

Contents

64.1 BACKGROUND

- Psychiatric causes are amongst the most common reasons for in-flight medical incapacitation.
- These may be subtle via factors such as impaired concentration and sleep disturbance affecting neurocognitive functioning, or anxiety affecting decision making.
- There have also been several well-publicised pilot murder-suicides; however, such events are extremely rare, have many contributing factors other than psychiatric disorder and there is little or no evidence that they can be predicted or entirely prevented.

64.2 MEDICAL REGULATIONS

- Many severe disorders will be disqualifying indefinitely due to the severity and consequences upon recurrence (e.g. psychotic illnesses, bipolar disorder).
- Others may be acceptable after full recovery and subject to an assessment of risk of recurrence and acceptable maintenance medication, where indicated (e.g. depression, anxiety disorders, eating disorders).

64.3 GENERAL PSYCHIATRIC ASSESSMENT

- Psychiatric history and mental state examination form a key part of the initial medical examination and periodic medicals.
- Should be undertaken routinely by all aeromedical examiners.
- Important factors during a general medical examination include:
  - Obtain a full history of any past psychiatric episodes (most episodes will be seen and treated by general practitioners rather than specialists).
  - Observe mental state to determine features of common mental disorders (depression, anxiety, self-harm, alcohol use).
  - Always ask about thoughts of self-harm or suicide.
  - Assess presence of sleep disturbance, appetite or weight change, fatigue and concentration.
  - Determine presence of common risk factors for psychiatric disorder: childhood trauma, past self-harm, recent life events or stressors, ongoing stressors, alcohol use, multiple physical symptoms.
- Simple self-report screening tools such as the Patient Health Questionnaire (PHQ-9) could be useful in cases where symptoms are identified.

64.4 SPECIALIST PSYCHIATRIC ASSESSMENT

- Indicated for cases where there is:
  - Significant past psychiatric history.
  - Diagnostic uncertainty.
  - Assessment of resolution of episode, or potential effects on airmanship or controlling.
  - Concern regarding risk of future recurrence.
  - Need to monitor ongoing treatment.
- A specialist will undertake a full psychiatric assessment with a focus on:
  - Diagnosis.
  - History, including number of recurrences, triggering factors, previous treatments, duration of each episode of illness.
  - Treatment responsiveness.
  - Presence of psychosis.
  - Previous self-harm or suicide attempts, and any ongoing suicidal ideation.
  - Factors that might impair flying/controlling such as sleep disruption, impaired concentration, fatigue.
  - Any specific anxiety or flight phobic symptoms.
  - Factors that may indicate higher risk of relapse such as: severity, number of recurrences, chronicity, treatment resistance, high genetic loading (e.g. family psychiatric history in two 1st-degree relatives), significant childhood trauma, psychiatric co-morbidity (e.g. two or more diagnoses co-existing), ongoing residual/subclinical symptoms.
  - Alcohol/substance use (see Section 64.7).
  - Insight: did pilot present early with symptoms, accept diagnosis, adhere to treatment? Do they accept there is a risk of future recurrence, can they recognise early symptoms of relapse, will they disclose symptoms? Is there any history of

non-disclosure in the past, and/or do they inappropriately challenge previous clinical opinions?
- Use of standardised clinical ratings recommended (e.g. Hamilton Depression Rating Scale [HAM-D] if depression is presenting problem).

64.5 TREATMENT

- In order to regain fitness, any episode must have been fully treated and in stable remission:
  - The full course of any psychological treatments for the relevant condition should have been completed.
  - Some booster sessions (e.g. for ongoing relapse prevention) may be acceptable.
- Acceptability of pharmacological treatment needs to be checked against regulatory requirements:
  - Antipsychotic and mood-stabilising medication are not likely to be acceptable, in part because the conditions for which the drugs will be prescribed are disqualifying.

DEPRESSION

- Risk of relapse is highest in first month after entering remission, so symptoms must be stably absent for at least 1 month.
- Risk remains elevated for 6 months and continuation of antidepressant treatment is recommended for at least 6 months in all cases of depression:
  - Continuation and maintenance antidepressants reduce risk of depression recurrence by 2–3 fold for as long as they are taken.
- A full course of evidence-based psychological treatment for depression (e.g. cognitive behavioural therapy) also reduces risk of recurrence.
- Most antidepressants are incompatible with flying duties due to the potential for impairment from side effects (e.g. neurocognitive effects from sedative antidepressants, potential discontinuation effects due to short half-lives or novelty where safety data may not be sufficient).
  - Several selective serotonin reuptake inhibitors (SSRIs) are permitted by a number of regulatory authorities worldwide, as they have been judged to be sufficiently safe for use under controlled supervision with multi-crew limitation; usually supported by evidence that medication is having no impairing effects on an appropriately designed medical flight test.

TREATMENT DISCONTINUATION

- Antidepressant discontinuation symptoms are common, especially with serotonergic antidepressants like SSRIs but are usually short-lived and mild.
- A few percent may have more severe and potentially impairing symptoms:
  - Symptoms can include agitation, dizziness and electric shock-like bodily and head sensations ('brain zaps').
  - Any SSRI dose reduction or drug cessation requires a period of 'grounding' or away from controlling to ensure no ongoing discontinuation symptoms and no recurrence of symptoms.

64.6 FOLLOW-UP

- Once in remission, most cases can be followed up by aeromedical examiners for regulatory purposes.
- Periodic specialist review is needed for cases where antidepressant treatment is ongoing, to monitor:
  - Any side effects.
  - Adherence and any discontinuation.
  - Any re-emergence of illness, monitored using a structured assessment like HAM-D.
- Some regulatory authorities may permit return to duty at an earlier stage with restrictions until all therapy has ceased and a period allowed to ensure no recurrence.

64.7 ALCOHOL AND DRUG USE DISORDERS

GENERAL ASSESSMENT OF ALCOHOL AND DRUG DISORDERS

- Initial screening for alcohol and drug use usually carried out by the AME as part of the medical examination.
- This should complement the general psychiatric assessment and should include the following information:
  - Daily and weekly levels of alcohol consumption in units.
  - Use of questionnaires (e.g. AUDIT) to determine whether criteria for at-risk drinking are met.
  - Drug use history.
  - History of sleep disturbance (past, current).
  - History of alcohol-related medical conditions (e.g., hypertension; gastrointestinal disturbance).
  - Family history of alcohol and drug-related problems.
- Concerns may indicate the need for reports from family physician.

SPECIALIST ASSESSMENT OF ALCOHOL AND DRUG DISORDERS

- Indicated in the following situations:
  - Convictions related to drugs or driving (e.g. for possession or driving whilst under the influence).
  - Failed workplace testing, either random or for cause.
  - Third-party allegations of inappropriate alcohol/drug use.
  - Medical referral via AME/other medical doctor or health professional.
  - Self-referral to airline/AME.
  - History of alcohol and/or drug use disorders.
- Specialist assessment will involve taking a detailed history of the index event and whether this was a one-off 'out of character' event or an event reflecting recent 'concerns'.
- Key points of history include:
  - Family history of alcohol and/or drug use disorders.
  - Alcohol and drug use history, including:
    - Beverage/substance used.
    - Age at starting.

   – Context of use.
   – Quantity, frequency and pattern of use.
   – Medical, psychiatric and social complications.
   – History of treatment.
   – Insight.
 • Past psychiatric history.
 • Forensic history.
 • Risk indicators for alcohol and drug use disorders:
   – Male.
   – Parental alcohol/drug/psychiatric history.
   – Childhood trauma.
   – Anxiety/depression.
 • Resilience factors.
 • Social history.
 • Use of standardised questionnaires (e.g. AUDIT, Alcohol Problems
   Questionnaire [APQ], Severity of Alcohol Dependence Questionnaire
   [SADQ]).
• The aim is to establish whether the individual meets criteria for DSM-5 Alcohol/Drug
  Use Disorder and/or ICD10 Harmful Use of Alcohol or Another Substance/Substance
  Dependence.

TREATMENT AND FOLLOW-UP

• In the case of a moderate or severe Alcohol/Substance Use Disorder (DSM-5) or
  Alcohol/Substance Dependence (ICD-10), any return to flying duties is contingent
  upon total abstinence from alcohol, illicit and over-the-counter drugs, and a clean bill
  of health in relation to co-morbid psychiatric and physical disorders.
• Before a return to flying or controlling can be considered, individuals are required to
  have completed treatment for their alcohol and/or drug use disorder and have stopped
  taking any associated medication.
• Treatment may be either residential or outpatient.
• Aftercare may involve regular ongoing attendance at Alcoholics Anonymous or other
  similar meetings is the preferred option, though some will prefer to attend virtual
  meetings via videoconference or use AA online:
  • Some will opt not to attend 12-step meetings, and full discussion is needed to
    ascertain whether they can indeed maintain abstinence; individuals falling into
    this group will typically need to have good prognostic factors.
• Individuals may be followed up and monitored with testing (e.g. blood or hair sam-
  pling) for as long as they continue to fly:
  • Follow-up/monitoring is likely to be more frequent during the first 12 months
    and then gradually reduced if all goes well.
  • Reports may be obtained periodically from a nominated buddy.

64.8 FEAR OF FLYING

• Fear of flying is common in the general population (5–10% of adult population
  unable to fly).
• Military prevalence unknown but can impose severe career limitations.

- 'Break-off' phenomenon is a risk factor for anxiety problems and fear of flying in aircrew (see Chapter 27).
- Development of flying-related anxiety in experienced aircrew should lead to exploration of differential diagnosis (e.g. depressive illness, adjustment disorder, specific phobia, PTSD, panic disorder).
- Therapeutic approach usually includes cognitive behavioural group treatment, but in aircrew may also include virtual reality exposure therapy and other practical-based strategies.

Index